Small Animal Infectious Disease

Editor

ANNETTE L. LITSTER

VETERINARY CLINICS OF NORTH AMERICA: SMALL ANIMAL PRACTICE

www.vetsmall.theclinics.com

July 2019 • Volume 49 • Number 4

ELSEVIER

1600 John F. Kennedy Boulevard • Suite 1800 • Philadelphia, Pennsylvania, 19103-2899
http://www.vetsmall.theclinics.com

**VETERINARY CLINICS OF NORTH AMERICA: SMALL ANIMAL PRACTICE Volume 49, Number 4
July 2019 ISSN 0195-5616, ISBN-13: 978-0-323-67866-7**

Editor: Colleen Dietzler
Developmental Editor: Meredith Madeira

Veterinary Clinics of North America: Small Animal Practice (ISSN 0195-5616) is published bimonthly by Elsevier Inc., 360 Park Avenue South, New York, NY 10010-1710. Months of issue are January, March, May, July, September, and November. Business and Editorial Offices: 1600 John F. Kennedy Blvd., Ste. 1800, Philadelphia, PA 19103-2899. Customer Service Office: 3251 Riverport Lane, Maryland Heights, MO 63043. Periodicals postage paid at New York, NY and additional mailing offices. Subscription prices are $338.00 per year (domestic individuals), $662.00 per year (domestic institutions), $100.00 per year (domestic students/residents), $451.00 per year (Canadian individuals), $823.00 per year (Canadian institutions), $474.00 per year (international individuals), $823.00 per year (international institutions), and $220.00 per year (international and Canadian students/residents). To receive student/resident rate, orders must be accompanied by name of affiliated institution, date of term, and the *signature* of program/residency coordinator on institution letterhead. Orders will be billed at individual rate until proof of status is received. Foreign air speed delivery is included in all *Clinics* subscription prices. All prices are subject to change without notice. **POSTMASTER:** Send address changes to *Veterinary Clinics of North America: Small Animal Practice*, Elsevier Health Sciences Division, Subscription Customer Service, 3251 Riverport Lane, Maryland Heights, MO 63043. Customer Service (orders, claims, online, change of address): Elsevier Periodicals Customer Service, Elsevier Health Sciences Division Subscription **Customer Service 3251 Riverport Lane Maryland Heights, MO 63043. Tel: 1-800-654-2452 (U.S. and Canada); 314-447-8871 (outside U.S. and Canada). Fax: 314-447-8029. E-mail: journalscustomerservice-usa@elsevier.com (for print support); journalsonlinesupport-usa@elsevier.com (for online support).**

Reprints. For copies of 100 or more of articles in this publication, please contact the Commercial Reprints Department, Elsevier Inc., 360 Park Avenue South, New York, NY 10010-1710. Tel.: 212-633-3874; Fax: 212-633-3820; E-mail: reprints@elsevier.com.

Veterinary Clinics of North America: Small Animal Practice is also published in Japanese by Inter Zoo Publishing Co., Ltd., Aoyama Crystal-Bldg 5F, 3-5-12 Kitaaoyama, Minato-ku, Tokyo 107-0061, Japan.

Veterinary Clinics of North America: Small Animal Practice is covered in *Current Contents/Agriculture, Biology and Environmental Sciences, Science Citation Index, ASCA, MEDLINE/PubMed (Index Medicus), Excerpta Medica,* and *BIOSIS.*

Contributors

EDITOR

ANNETTE L. LITSTER, BVSc, PhD, FANZCVS (Feline Medicine), MMedSci (Clinical Epidemiology)
Senior Veterinary Specialist, Zoetis Petcare, Parsippany, New Jersey, USA

AUTHORS

MAUREEN E.C. ANDERSON, DVM, DVSc, PhD
Animal Health and Welfare Branch, Ontario Ministry of Agriculture, Food and Rural Affairs, Guelph, Ontario, Canada

EMI N. BARKER, BSc, BVSc, PhD, MRCVS
Diplomate, European College of Veterinary Internal Medicine–Companion Animals; Langford Vets, University of Bristol, Bristol, United Kingdom

VANESSA R. BARRS, BVSc(hons), PhD, MVetClinStud, FANZCVS
Professor of Feline Medicine and Infectious Diseases, Sydney School of Veterinary Science, Faculty of Science, Marie Bashir Institute of Infectious Diseases and Biosecurity, University of Sydney, New South Wales, Australia

JACQUELINE M. CARDWELL, MA, VetMB, MScVetEd, PhD, FHEA, MRCVS
Senior Lecturer in Epidemiology, Department of Pathobiology and Population Sciences, Royal Veterinary College, London, United Kingdom

STEFANO CORTELLINI, DMV, MVetMed, FHEA, MRCVS
Diplomate, American College of Veterinary Emergency and Critical Care; Diplomate, European College of Veterinary Emergency and Critical Care; Lecturer in Emergency and Critical Care, Department of Clinical Science and Services, Royal Veterinary College, Queen Mother Hospital for Animals, London, United Kingdom

LAURA HOLM, BVM&S, CertSAM, MRCVS
Staff Clinician in Small Animal Oncology and Internal Medicine, Anderson Moores Veterinary Specialists, Winchester, United Kingdom

JERILYN R. IZAC, BS
Student, Department of Microbiology and Immunology, School of Medicine, Virginia Commonwealth University Medical Center, Richmond, Virginia, USA

ROSANNE E. JEPSON, BVSc, MVetMed, PhD, FHEA, MRCVS
Diplomate, American College of Veterinary Internal Medicine–Small Animal Internal Medicine; Diplomate, European College of Veterinary Internal Medicine–Companion Animal; Senior Lecturer in Small Animal Internal Medicine, Department of Clinical Science and Services, Royal Veterinary College, Queen Mother Hospital for Animals, London, United Kingdom

LIN K. KAUFFMAN, DVM
Prairie View Animal Hospital, Grimes, Iowa, USA

LINDA KIDD, DVM, PhD
Diplomate, American College of Veterinary Internal Medicine–Small Animal Internal
Medicine; Associate Professor, Small Animal Internal Medicine, Western University of
Health Sciences College of Veterinary Medicine, Pomona, California, USA

RICHARD T. MARCONI, PhD
Professor, Department of Microbiology and Immunology, School of Medicine, Virginia
Commonwealth University Medical Center, Richmond, Virginia, USA

SUSAN M. MOORE, PhD, MS, BS, HCLD(ABB), MT(ASCP)SBB
Veterinary Diagnostic Laboratory, Kansas State University, Manhattan, Kansas, USA

COLIN ROSS PARRISH, BSc (Hons), PhD
Professor, Department of Microbiology and Immunology, Baker Institute for Animal
Health, College of Veterinary Medicine, Cornell University, Ithaca, New York, USA

CHRISTINE A. PETERSEN, DVM, PhD
Associate Professor, Department of Epidemiology, College of Public Health, University of
Iowa, Iowa City, Iowa, USA; Director, Center for Emerging Infectious Diseases, University
of Iowa Research Park, Coralville, Iowa, USA

KATHERINE POLAK, DVM, MPH, MS
Diplomate, American College of Veterinary Preventive Medicine; Diplomate,
American Board of Veterinary Practitioners–Shelter Medicine Practice; Head of Stray
Animal Care - Southeast Asia, FOUR PAWS International, Bangkok, Thailand

BARBARA QUROLLO, MS, DVM
Research Assistant Professor, Department of Clinical Sciences, College of Veterinary
Medicine, North Carolina State University, Raleigh, North Carolina, USA

KRYSTLE L. REAGAN, DVM, PhD
Infectious Disease Fellow, Veterinary Medical Teaching Hospital, University of California,
Davis, Davis, California, USA

KIM STEVENS, PhD, MScAgric, PGCAP
Lecturer in Veterinary Epidemiology, Department of Pathobiology and Population
Sciences, Royal Veterinary College, London, United Kingdom

JASON W. STULL, VMD, MPVM, PhD
Assistant Professor, Department of Veterinary Preventive Medicine, College of Veterinary
Medicine, The Ohio State University, Columbus, Ohio, USA; Assistant Professor,
Department of Health Management, Atlantic Veterinary College, University of Prince
Edward Island, Charlottetown, Prince Edward Island, Canada

JANE E. SYKES, BVSc(Hons), PhD
Professor of Small Animal Internal Medicine, Chief Veterinary Medical Officer, Associate
Dean for Veterinary Medical Center Operations, Department of Medicine and
Epidemiology, University of California, Davis, Davis, California, USA

IAN EUGENE HUBER VOORHEES, BA
Graduate Research Assistant, Department of Microbiology and Immunology, Baker
Institute for Animal Health, College of Veterinary Medicine, Cornell University, Ithaca,
New York, USA

DAVID WALKER, BVetMed (Hons), MRCVS
Diplomate, American College of Veterinary Internal Medicine–Small Animal Internal
Medicine, Diplomate, European College of Veterinary Internal Medicine–Companion
Animal; Head of Small Animal Internal Medicine, Anderson Moores Veterinary Specialists,
Winchester, United Kingdom

J. SCOTT WEESE, DVM, DVSc
Professor, Department of Pathobiology, Ontario Veterinary College, University of Guelph,
Guelph, Ontario, Canada

Contents

> Desensitization to rabies is a result of successfully eliminating canine rabies in the United States, which occurred in 2007; however, the need for mandatory rabies vaccination in pets remains. Rabies cases are rare in comparison with other vaccine-preventable diseases in companion animals; however, because it is a zoonotic disease with the highest case fatality rate of any infectious disease demands the establishment of strict laws for disease prevention. Preventive strategies include addressing current concerns in consideration of disease surveillance, appropriate vaccination recommendations, and local regulations protecting public health.

> Two different influenza A viruses have infected and spread among dogs since 2000, and both have been widespread in dogs in North America. The H3N8 canine influenza virus arose in the United States as a variant of equine influenza virus. The H3N2 canine influenza virus arose in Asia by transfer of an avian influenza virus to dogs. Both viruses cause mild respiratory disease and are associated with outbreaks in densely housed dogs or those with frequent connections to other dogs. The 2 canine influenza viruses each caused widespread epidemics over at least several years that were associated with localized outbreaks.

> Feline panleukopenia (FPL) is caused by a Carnivore protoparvovirus infection. Feline parvovirus (FPV) causes most cases. When Canine parvovirus 2 (CPV-2) first emerged, it could not replicate in cats. All current CPV variants (CPV-2a-c) can infect cats to cause subclinical disease or FPL. Feline panleukopenia has re-emerged in Australia in shelter cats associated with failure to vaccinate. Parvoviruses can remain latent in mononuclear cells post-infection. Molecular methods such as polymerase chain reaction are used to determine the infecting strain. Current perspectives on causes, epidemiology, diagnosis, treatment, prognostic indicators, and management of outbreaks in shelters are reviewed.

> The Lyme disease spirochetes are a highly diverse group of bacteria with unique biological properties. Their ability to cycle between ticks and mammals requires that they adapt to variable and constantly changing environmental conditions. Outer surface protein C is an essential virulence determinant that has received considerable attention in vaccine and diagnostic assay development. Knowledge of OspC diversity, its antigenic determinants, and its production patterns throughout the enzootic cycle, as

well as in the laboratory setting, is essential for understanding immune responses induced by infection or vaccination.

In North America, with the exceptions of Bartonella henselae and Cytauxzoon felis, feline vector-borne diseases (FVBDs) have been minimally studied in domestic cats. Cats can be infected with many of the same vector-borne pathogens that infect dogs. Nonspecific clinical signs linked to FVBDs and low prevalence of certain vector-borne pathogens contribute to a limited awareness of FVBDs in sick cats. As clinicians become informed about FVBDs and as vector-borne disease diagnostics are routinely applied to evaluate sick cats, we will gain a stronger understanding of vector-borne pathogens in cats. This article focuses on recent findings related to FVBDs.

Vector-borne disease and idiopathic immune-mediated disease present similarly. Diagnostic panels that include multiple organisms help detect infection and identify coinfections. Comprehensive diagnostic panels that combine polymerase chain reaction (PCR) and serology should be used in initial screening to maximize sensitivity and identify infection. Repeat testing using PCR is warranted in dogs at high risk of infection with organisms that circulate in blood in low numbers or intermittently. Convalescent serologic testing can help diagnose acute infection. This article discusses the pathophysiology and epidemiology of the organisms, panel selection, and how to recognize when more aggressive testing for an organism is warranted.

Several diagnostic tests are available to aid veterinarians in diagnosis of leptospirosis. Understanding the course of infection is imperative to determining which diagnostic test to order and sample to submit. Diagnostic tests for dogs suspected of having leptospirosis include antibody-based tests and polymerase chain reaction (PCR). Paired acute and convalescent microscopic agglutination test (MAT) are diagnostic for leptospirosis. PCR performed on blood and/or urine can be a valuable tool to aid in diagnosis of leptospirosis. Commercially available rapid point-of-care diagnostics have been validated in dogs and have value early in the course of illness before MAT and PCR results are available.

The wall-less, hemotropic, mycoplasma species *Mycoplasma haemofelis,* "*Candidatus* Mycoplasma turicensis" and, to a lesser extent, "*Candidatus*

Mycoplasma haemominutum" have the potential to induce clinical hemo-lytic anemia in infected cats. Prevalence varies markedly between infect-ing species, complicated by a chronic carrier state. Accurate and prompt confirmation of infection and identification of the infecting hemo-plasma species enables appropriate antibiotics (eg, tetracycline; fluoro-quinolone) to be prescribed. Although cats with hemoplasmosis respond rapidly to antibiosis and supportive care, initial monotherapy treatment rarely results in clearance of infection. A protocol now exists for the clear-ance of the most pathogenic feline hemoplasma *M haemofelis*.

Cutaneous renal glomerular vasculopathy (CRGV), colloquially named "Alabama rot," is an emerging condition in the United Kingdom, previously reported from the United States and Germany. The cause of CRGV is not yet determined; no definitive link to an infectious agent has been made. Dogs diagnosed with CRGV initially develop cutaneous lesions, and a pro-portion of these dogs go on to manifest acute kidney injury, which may result in oligoanuric acute renal failure. Antemortem diagnosis is chal-lenging given the lack of a specific diagnostic test, and confirmation of CRGV is therefore currently dependent on identification of thrombotic mi-croangiopathy on renal histopathology.

The genus *Brucella* is a primary cause of reproductive diseases. Widely known as a problem in livestock, *Brucella* is gaining notoriety as a cause of canine reproductive disease and as a scourge to dog breeders. Only within the last few decades has the risk of severe brucellosis in dogs, and the people who own and work with them, been more fully appreciated. This review summarizes the epidemiology, clinical signs, and advances in diagnosis and management of *Brucella canis*. Canine brucellosis preven-tion, owner education, and possible therapies for the future are also discussed.

VETERINARY CLINICS OF NORTH AMERICA: SMALL ANIMAL PRACTICE

SERIES OF RELATED INTEREST

Veterinary Clinics of North America: Exotic Animal Practice
https://www.vetexotic.theclinics.com/

THE CLINICS ARE NOW AVAILABLE ONLINE!
Access your subscription at:
www.theclinics.com

VETERINARY CLINICS OF
NORTH AMERICA: SMALL
ANIMAL PRACTICE

Preface

Small Animal Infectious Diseases

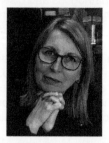

Annette L. Litster, BVSc, PhD, FANZCVS (Feline Medicine),
MMedSci (Clinical Epidemiology)
Editor

Changes to the environment, transportation, technology, and our attitudes toward the animals that we share our lives with have occurred at breakneck speed since the last Small Animal Infectious Diseases issue in *Veterinary Clinics of North America: Small Animal Practice* in 2011. The phenomenon of climate change has made natural disasters a regular occurrence, resulting in emergency transport of animals to localities that are sometimes unprepared for their arrival. Domestic and international pet transport is now an everyday reality, making a thorough travel history a mandatory component of any veterinary visit, and demanding much broader expertise in infectious diseases that were once considered irrelevant beyond our own neighborhoods. New diagnostic modalities have revised traditional notions of reference standard tests, challenging researchers to pit one test against another to determine where each one fits in optimal case management. The human-animal bond continues to strengthen as we depend on companion animals increasingly for companionship and emotional support. This bond not only means that our physical proximity to our pets is closer than ever before but also demands that we aim to provide the same standards of health care for our pets that we receive from medical providers. The One Health movement, which held its first international congress in 2011, links physicians and veterinarians to achieve better health outcomes for people and animals, by improving communication and knowledge exchange, especially concerning zoonotic diseases and combating antibiotic resistance. Information has never been as readily available or as boundless as it is today, but there is also a minefield of *mis*information for unwary consumers. Our ability to discriminate high-quality scientific evidence from opinion or ill-founded assertions is a skill that keeps yielding dividends for us and for our patients.

Does this make you feel like the world is spinning too fast for you to keep up? An important implication for practicing veterinarians is the need for at least a basic knowledge of an ever-growing list of infectious diseases. An understanding of practical, evidence-based infectious disease risk management for our patients and for us is also

Vet Clin Small Anim 49 (2019) xiii–xiv
https://doi.org/10.1016/j.cvsm.2019.04.001
0195-5616/19/© 2019 Published by Elsevier Inc.

vital in day-to-day practice. Critical and analytical skills are crucial to accessing reliable and accurate information from sources such as the Internet when more detailed information is required. This issue of *Veterinary Clinics of North America: Small Animal Practice* features an array of topical and practical science from our colleagues at the forefront of the world of small animal infectious disease research. Common themes throughout the issue are the emergence of new pathogens and diseases, the spread of known pathogens into new territories, new technologies to help prevent and control infectious disease, and troublingly, our growing awareness of the consequences of inadequate prevention and control programs.

We live in challenging and turbulent times in the infectious disease world, but I believe that excellent, innovative science is the best way forward. I would like to sincerely thank my friends and colleagues who so ably authored the articles in this issue. They lead our profession toward deeper understanding and control of the pathogens that torment us, so that we can continue to care for the animals that delight us.

Annette L. Litster, BVSc, PhD, FANZCVS (Feline Medicine), MMedSci (Clinical Epidemiology)
Zoetis Petcare
Parsippany, NJ 07054, USA

E-mail address:
Annette.Litster@zoetis.com

The Dynamic Nature of Canine and Feline Infectious Disease Risks in the Twenty-first Century

Jason W. Stull, VMD, MPVM, PhD[a,b],*,
Maureen E.C. Anderson, DVM, DVSc, PhD[c],
J. Scott Weese, DVM, DVSc[d]

KEYWORDS

- Driver • Infection • Climate • Surveillance • Emerging • Resistance • Virulence
- Travel

KEY POINTS

- Numerous factors influence the frequency, location, and emergence of canine and feline infectious diseases.
- Exploring each of these drivers assists in evaluating their impact on canine and feline health and potentially identifying modifiable components.
- Large data gaps exist (most importantly, reliable estimates of disease occurrence, by location and time) that currently prevent an in-depth evaluation and ranking of the relative importance of each driver.
- There is a need for a robust and dependable surveillance system for canine and feline infectious diseases to provide the data needed to model disease drivers and help anticipate the introduction of future pathogens and their emergence and spread and strengthen control measures.

Disclosure Statement: The authors have nothing to disclose.
[a] Department of Veterinary Preventive Medicine, College of Veterinary Medicine, The Ohio State University, 1920 Coffey Road, Columbus, OH 43210, USA; [b] Department of Health Management, Atlantic Veterinary College, University of Prince Edward Island, 550 University Avenue, Charlottetown, Prince Edward Island CIA 4P3, Canada; [c] Animal Health and Welfare Branch, Ontario Ministry of Agriculture, Food and Rural Affairs, 1 Stone Road West, 5th Floor Northwest (336), Guelph, Ontario N1G 4Y2, Canada; [d] Department of Pathobiology, Ontario Veterinary College, University of Guelph, 50 Stone Rd E, Guelph, ON N1G2W1, Canada
* Corresponding author. Department of Health Management, Atlantic Veterinary College, University of Prince Edward Island, 550 University Avenue, Charlottetown, Prince Edward Island CIA 4P3, Canada.
E-mail address: jstull@upei.ca

Vet Clin Small Anim 49 (2019) 587–598
https://doi.org/10.1016/j.cvsm.2019.02.002
vetsmall.theclinics.com

INTRODUCTION

Infectious diseases of dogs and cats seem to be in a state of rapid change, including changes in overall prevalence of established pathogens, geographic or spatial changes in disease incidence, inherent changes in the pathogenicity or virulence of known pathogens, and the emergence of newly identified pathogens. The proposed drivers for disease change in human populations are an area of great interest and research attention. Although many such drivers are likely similar for dog and cat populations, these groups differ from people to some extent.[1] Exploring the dynamic nature of canine and feline infectious diseases and the likely drivers of current and future shifts may help the veterinary community prepare for change and potentially modify those drivers determined to be most influential. From a public health standpoint, many pathogens affecting dogs and cats also are zoonotic; thus, changes in pathogen frequency in dog and cat populations can have important human health implications. Dogs and cats may be effective sentinels of exposure or disease for some human pathogens, based on factors, such as their susceptibility to disease, likelihood of exposure, and routine diagnostic testing (eg, tick-borne pathogen exposure as part of routine heartworm testing). Because it has been estimated that 60% to 80% of emerging diseases are zoonotic, the veterinary community plays a pivotal role in the identification, prevention, and control of emerging infectious diseases.[2]

An ecosystem approach to health, often referred to as the epidemiologic triad, considers disease occurrence to be at the intersection of the agent/pathogen, host (in this case, the dog or cat), and environment. Any shift in the interplay of the pathogen–host–environment characteristics can alter the risk of disease.[3] Thus, drivers of disease change come from an extensive list of factors involving 1 or more of these areas. The multitude of pathogen sources involved in feline and canine infections adds additional complexity. Wildlife, other companion animals, people, and vectors (eg, fleas and ticks) all serve as possible pathogen sources for dogs and cats, creating a web of infectious disease drivers (**Table 1**). In this article, these various theorized drivers of canine and feline infectious diseases are reviewed and explored to gain a better understanding of the challenges facing disease forecasting and to propose steps to provide improved disease monitoring in dog and cat populations. This will contribute to an improved understanding of, and means of modifying, disease drivers, to control and prevent infectious diseases in dogs and cats.

DRIVERS FOR CANINE AND FELINE INFECTIOUS DISEASE EMERGENCE AND CHANGE
Emergence of New Pathogens

In all biologic systems, existing members evolve and new pathogens emerge. Although less common than other mechanisms of disease change, novel feline and canine pathogens continue to be identified. This phenomenon has been most recently demonstrated with the emergence and rapid dissemination of novel influenza A viruses in dogs. In the early 2000s, a novel canine influenza virus (CIV) emerged from an established equine influenza virus (H3N8).[4] This canine-adapted variant, H3N8 CIV, first became established in racing greyhounds (presumably due to shared contact surfaces and close proximity to infected horses) and then rapidly spread into other dog groups (eg, shelters, kennels, and companion dogs), causing sporadic outbreaks with high canine morbidity throughout parts of the United States.[4–6] The more recent emergence of an avian-origin CIV (H3N2) has resulted in canine illness in parts of Asia, the United States, and Canada.[7,8]

Table 1
Theorized drivers and determinants of canine and feline infectious diseases: emergence and change in disease frequency and location

Driver	Description/Examples[a]	Pathogens Likely Influenced by Driver[a]
Pathogen emergence	New pathogen develops. Influenza viruses are notorious for genome changes (shift/drift) that allow for host switching.	CIV (H3N8 and H3N2) and canine parvovirus
Alteration in pathogen resistance or virulence	Change in the resistance or virulence of an existing pathogen. Such changes may occur due to natural permutations or be aided through a selective process (eg, antimicrobial use).	FCV-associated VSD; MDR organisms (eg, MRSP, MRSA, and ESBL producer)
Travel and trade	Movement of cats and dogs into geographically adjacent and distant locations. Can enable the importation of vectors and pathogens.	B canis; H3N2 CIV, Echinococcus multiloclularis; rabies virus; Leishmania infantum; and canine distemper virus
Climate	Changes in temperature, humidity, rainfall. Can have an impact on number and location of disease vectors and persistence of environmental and water-borne pathogens.	Vector-borne pathogens (eg, Borrelia burgdorferi and Dirofilaria immitis); L interrogans
Natural environment	Changes in vegetation, water resources, land use, habitats, and biodiversity. Can alter the range and abundance of vectors, hosts and reservoirs, and frequency and intensity of host interactions with vectors and wildlife reservoirs.	L interrogans; rabies virus; and canine distemper virus
High-risk groups	Extremes of age, immunocompromise, free-roaming, group settings (eg, shelter, daycare, and boarding), unique environments (eg, human health care facilities). Vulnerability can increase exposure and susceptibility to infectious diseases. Host contact with high-risk group animals increases infection risk.	B canis; H3N2 CIV; other CIRDC pathogens; papilloma virus; and MRSA
Prevention	Advances in vaccinations and preventative medications, adherence to treatment regimes, and appropriate prescription practices	CIV (H3N2 and H3N8); L infantum; tick-borne and flea-borne pathogens; D immitis; and MDR organisms
Surveillance and detection	Systematic, ongoing collection, collation, analysis, and dissemination of infectious disease data; advances in diagnostic methods	Feline morbillivirus; canine circovirus; and Sporothrix brasiliensis

Abbreviations: CIRDC, canine infectious respiratory disease complex; MRSA, methicillin-resistant Staphylococcus aureus.

[a] Examples purposely not exhaustive and should be considered illustrative. More than 1 driver may be involved in changes in a given pathogen.

(Adapted from Semenza JC, Lindgren E, Balkanyi L, et al. Determinants and drivers of infectious disease threat events in Europe. Emerg Infect Dis 2016;22(4):581–9; with permission. Available at: https://dx.doi.org/10.3201/eid2204.151073.)

Change in Existing Pathogens

Alterations in an existing pathogen can influence its pathogenicity, virulence, and resistance to treatment or prevention measures. Pathogens can develop novel traits while circulating in a host population, allowing the pathogen to unlock host resources that otherwise would remain unavailable, thereby improving the fitness of the pathogen.[3] An example of altered pathogen virulence is the hypervirulent feline calicivirus (FSV) associated with virulent systemic disease (VSD). Although a common cause of generally mild upper respiratory disease in cats, FCV mutants have been observed that result in a hypervirulent, systemic form of the disease, resulting in high mortality (22%–75%).[9] To date, several FCV-associated VSD outbreaks have been observed, identified in several geographically distinct locations.[9,10]

A prime example of pathogen resistance to treatment is highlighted by the antimicrobial resistance (AMR) epidemic currently affecting all species globally, including dogs and cats. The rapid emergence and spread of methicillin-resistant staphylococci and multidrug-resistant (MDR) *Escherichia coli*, including extended-spectrum β-lactamase (ESBL) producers, are at the forefront of concern for AMR in dogs and cats. Methicillin-resistant *Staphylococcus pseudintermedius* (MRSP) has rapidly spread in canine populations and to a lesser extent in feline populations.[11] This pathogen is a common cause of bacterial folliculitis, otitis, and surgical site infections, and treatment can be complicated because of high levels of resistance.[12,13] Although β-lactamase–producing bacterial isolates have been common for some time, there has been a recent emergence of ESBL producers, which are resultantly resistant to numerous β-lactam antimicrobials, including cephalosporins. Drivers for AMR are complex; however, recent antimicrobial administration seems important in the development of MRSP and MDR *E coli* colonization and infections.[13–15] Prudent antimicrobial use as a component of sound antimicrobial stewardship practices in all health care fields is desperately needed to reduce AMR and preserve the utility of existing and future antimicrobial drugs.[16]

Change in the Range of Existing Pathogens

Many pathogens have well-defined ranges that are restricted by factors, such as geography, weather, and the presence of pathogen reservoirs or vectors. Drivers that change these limiting factors can have profound impacts on local and global canine and feline disease incidence.

Land-use changes and changes in climate and weather that have an impact on host and vector habitats or pathogen survival may drive pathogen range expansion or contraction. Expanding ranges of various vector-borne diseases are particularly noteworthy. The influence of weather and climate on arthropod disease vectors and their transmission of disease-causing agents has been well-described. Examples include warming global temperatures that allow ticks and tick-borne diseases to move poleward, with range expansion into higher altitudes.[17] Additionally, such changes may increase the length of the transmission season, resulting in an increase in local vector-borne canine and feline disease. Similar trends are predicted to occur with canine and feline heartworm; the range of the parasite is likely to expand as warmer temperatures increase the heartworm development units (heat requirement for heartworms to complete incubation to the infective stage) past the minimum threshold in colder climates.[18] Conversely, elevated temperatures are expected to create environments not favorable for the development or survival of some tick species in locations, such as South Africa.[17]

Accompanying tick range expansion are a multitude of tick-borne pathogens that have demonstrated an ability to reproduce and be transmitted in novel areas. This is particularly well illustrated by the tick vector *Ixodes scapularis* and the pathogen *Borrelia burgdorferi*, the causative agent of canine borreliosis (Lyme disease), as noted by the steady movement of canine borreliosis within the United States and into Canada.[19] Between 1996 and 2016, the number of United States counties in which *I scapularis* or *I pacificus* was established doubled to 45% of all counties.[20] A similar range expansion has been documented with *I ricinus* in parts of Europe, including Sweden, the United Kingdom, and Russia.[21] A combination of changes in climate, agriculture, and land use is likely involved in these vector and pathogen extensions.[3]

Geographic jumps by pathogens often are facilitated by travel and trade, serving to connect distant landscapes and their respective host, vector, and pathogen communities. Such movements may be limited (ie, neighboring jurisdictions or within the same country) or extensive (ie, international or intercontinental). As an example, the pathogen *Brucella canis* is a troubling pathogen given its health impact on breeding dogs (eg, infertility, abortions, and other health manifestations), subclinical yet infectious period, and zoonotic potential. Among the factors linked to canine *B canis* outbreaks in the United States is intrastate and interstate movement of dogs. For instance, in Michigan over a 10-year period, most canine cases and human *B canis* exposures were associated with an influx of dogs from commercial dog production facilities where *B canis* was endemic (seropositivity 9%–83%). This included the movement of infected dogs from 22 Michigan counties and 11 states.[22] The concern for the spread of *B canis* is so great that some investigators have argued for mandatory testing of dogs before interjurisdictional or international movement.[23]

A similar situation has occurred with H3N2 CIV. This virus seemed to have been circulating in dogs in Asia for several years,[24] before first entering the United States in 2015, likely through international dog importation.[8] Additional introductions of infectious dogs from abroad, with resulting outbreaks, are suspected to have occurred into the United States and Canada, based on phylogenic analysis of virus isolates.[8] The consequences of this geographic movement are evident in the estimated tens of thousands of dogs that have been infected across the United States and Canada. Dog and cat importation has been involved or suspected to be involved in several other pathogen introductions[25] and is likely to increase in frequency, given the high mobility of these species through owner travel, rescue organizations, and distributors.

Geographic jumps also can occur with vectors. If imported vectors and their associated pathogens are introduced into a hospitable environment, or competent vectors are introduced into an environment where the pathogen already exists, novel pathogen transmission can occur. As an example, Public Health England established a tick surveillance program in part to track ticks entering the country on recently traveled or imported animals. Between 2005 and 2016, 10 tick species representing 6 genera were identified entering the United Kingdom from 15 countries. More than half of all identifications from animals with a history of travel were tick species non-native to England, illustrating the risks to dog, cat, and human health.[26]

Sometimes, unexpected changes in ranges occur. For example, West Nile virus emerged in North America in 1999, with tremendous long-lasting animal and human health consequences. This marked change in range could have occurred through intentional (legal or otherwise) movement of an infected reservoir host (eg, bird) or inadvertent movement of the infected mosquito vector. Although of minimal concern to canine and feline health, this highlights the potential severe consequences of pathogen movement.

Change in Frequency or Extent of Contact with Pathogen Reservoir Species

Anthropogenic changes to the environment are well-described contributors to changes in the presence and frequency of human infectious diseases, including zoonotic diseases.[27] Such changes may include or result in animal habitat fragmentation, habitat destruction, and urbanization. Each of these may alter wildlife population structures and increase emerging infectious diseases within wildlife.[1] For example, human density within a species' range is positively associated with zoonotic pathogen richness in mammals, which influences disease emergence.[28] Additionally, environmental changes often increase the frequency and magnitude of contact between wildlife species and domestic species, including dogs and cats, thereby increasing disease transmission risks.[3,29] Canine leptospirosis is an example of such canine-wildlife interface dynamics. Multiple wildlife species, including racoons, rodents, and opossums, carry distinct *Leptospira* serovars, which are shed in urine, and contact with infectious urine can result in canine disease. Over recent years, there has been an increase in the perceived incidence of canine leptospirosis, with reported outbreaks of unprecedented size and location. Studies suggest an important driver for this perceived increase in canine disease is increased direct and indirect contact between dogs and *Leptospira*-shedding wildlife, including the interactions of these species in urban locations.[30–32]

Dogs and cats themselves, along with other domestic animal species, also are involved in changes in canine and feline infectious disease spread, because changes in the frequency or intensity of contact with infectious animals drive disease dynamics. Shelter animals and free-roaming animals are important pathogen sources within their own populations but also drive pathogen spread into populations of owned dogs and cats that have direct or indirect contact with free-roaming animals or those recently adopted from a shelter. The impact of these populations on overall canine and feline infectious disease dynamics is difficult to quantify. Several examples are readily available, including the role free-roaming dogs likely serve as a reservoir for canine transmissible venereal tumor in many countries[33] and as a reservoir for rabies virus in Africa, Asia, and Central/South America.[33,34] In addition, shelter animals are considered a likely source for *B canis* transmission to the general canine population in certain areas; for instance, in Mississippi shelters where *B canis* was present, the mean modeled seroprevalence was high (18%).[35] Additionally, evaluation of H3N8 CIV transmission in the United States revealed that animal shelters likely served as important persistent sources for the virus. CIV had a high reproductive potential in these facilities (mean R_0 of 3.9), and these locations served as refugia from the sparsely connected majority of the dog population (for which R_0 was estimated to be close to 1, a level at which infection ceases to transmit in a population), allowing the virus to continue circulating.[36]

Close contact between pet dogs or cats also can drive infectious disease occurrence. Group settings, where many dogs or cats have direct or indirect contact, are becoming increasing popular. Such activities or environments include daycare facilities, boarding facilities, training classes, dog parks, shows, and sporting events. Veterinary clinics also can contribute to infectious disease spread if there is poor implementation of and compliance with infection control practices.[37] This is perhaps of greatest concern when group settings take place within veterinary clinics or during other opportunities for spread between clinics and group settings (eg, shared staff, kennels, and buildings). Disease transmission in these scenarios may result in an outbreak within a facility and/or spread into the general dog/cat populations once infected animals return home.[38,39] In many situations, animals may come from distant locations (nationally or internationally) and thus spread pathogens to distant locations on returning home. It is likely that canine group settings played a critical role in intensifying and spreading H3N2 CIV through the United States dog population.[8]

As highlighted previously, several of the pathogens infecting dogs and cats are zoonotic. Some of these organisms predominantly circulate between people, with spillover infections in dogs and cats. Once these pathogens have colonized or infected an individual dog or cat, further transmission often is possible to other dogs or cats or back to people. This phenomenon is particularly well described with *Staphylococcus aureus*.[40] Therefore, alterations in the frequency and intimacy of contact between infectious people and dogs/cats can further drive canine and feline infectious diseases. Although every person is likely infectious with some organism at any given time, this risk is greatly magnified in human health care settings. Dogs and cats frequently visit or even reside in many human health care facilities as part of animal-assisted therapy (or similar) programs often allowing for close interactions between these animals and patients. Anecdotally, this practice seems to be increasing in frequency. Despite guidelines aimed at reducing pathogen transmission to and from animals in these settings, many gaps are reported,[41,42] with pathogen transmission documented between the groups.[43,44] Although the frequency of transmission of pathogens to dogs/cats in these environments has been described, the risk and incidence of subsequent transmission to humans and other animal populations are unknown but certainly likely to occur.

Change in Host Susceptibility

Immune function is a key determinant of pathogen infectivity, pathogenicity, and virulence. Animals that are immunosuppressed often are at an increased risk for infection and generally experience more severe disease, disease of longer duration, or more severe or unexpected complications than others that are immunocompetent. Immunosuppression arises from many sources or reasons, including genetic/primary causes, infection with immunosuppressive pathogens, chemotherapy or immunosuppressive medical therapies, pregnancy, asplenia, and extremes of age. For example, immunosuppression can increase risk for clinical (especially severe) canine papilloma virus infection,[45] and feline leukemia virus (FeLV)-induced immunosuppression can be associated with several secondary infections (eg, coccidiosis and upper respiratory infections).[46] Some causes of immunosuppression seem stable or decreasing in frequency, such as FeLV infection in some regions,[47] whereas some advances in veterinary medical care (eg, cancer treatment) that result in immunosuppression, and thus increase infection risk, are increasing.

Change in Prevention Measures

Medical advances constantly are being made to prevent infectious disease transmission. Canine and feline vaccines against emerging and endemic pathogens continue to be developed and improved (eg, canine leishmaniasis, canine leptospirosis, and canine influenza). Advances in tick and flea prevention technologies have resulted in products with increased effectiveness and longer duration of effect, theoretically reducing vector-borne disease risks. Safe and effective environmental disinfectants are increasingly available. All these factors likely have contributed to reducing canine and feline infectious disease risk. Uptake of products resulting from such advances, however, may be hampered by factors, such as financial constraints, availability, or perceived need. Due to few data, the magnitude of such impacts are unknown.

Change in Ability to Detect

The perceived emergence of a disease sometimes may simply reflect advances in diagnostic testing, in particular the identification of viruses previously difficult to identify or classify. Differentiating new pathogens from new recognition of existing commensals can be a challenge. For example, feline morbillivirus is a novel paramyxovirus that has been identified in domestic cats in several countries.[48,49] Infection with the virus is suspected to be chronic and associated with feline renal diseases.[48,49] New diagnostic methods[50] undoubtably have assisted in the recent identification of this apparently common, persistent, globally distributed pathogen that has likely been present in cats for some time.

Surveillance programs, whereby specific infectious diseases or conditions are tracked, allow for early recognition of changes in disease occurrence and outbreaks. Such surveillance efforts can have important impacts on the perceived prevalence of canine and feline pathogens. For instance, efforts to systematically diagnose and record clinical cases of feline sporotrichosis were dramatically increased during a cat-associated human sporotrichosis outbreak.[51] A large, unprecedented epidemic of feline sporotrichosis was identified in Brazil, with more than 4000 cats diagnosed with sporotrichosis in Rio de Janeiro between 1998 and 2015, with an accompanying 4188 cat-associated human cases over a similar timeframe.[51] Without such human disease impacts, efforts and resources directed toward characterizing feline cases likely would have been limited and the extent of this outbreak underappreciated.

Currently, most countries have limited surveillance systems dedicated to canine and feline diseases. The paucity of canine and feline disease data is illustrated in the examples (discussed previously) for each driver. Disease outbreaks or unusual disease occurrences (eg, changes in pathogen virulence, emergence, and introduction through transport/travel) constitute the overwhelming majority of reports of disease occurrence in companion animals. There is limited information on changes in frequency or location of established, common pathogens. In comparison with human and livestock diseases, none of the international health agencies is mandated to coordinate surveillance of diseases in companion animals (with the possible exception of rabies).[52]

To address the gap in canine and feline surveillance data, several groups have independently initiated surveillance programs, through partnerships with wide-scale corporate laboratory testing (eg, Companion Animal Parasite Council in the United States and Canada) or private practice sentinel clinics (eg, Computer-based Investigation of Companion Animal Disease Awareness in the United Kingdom). Mining direct-feed, real-time data from private practices also recently has been used to investigate specific canine and feline health outcomes, although to date minimally used to investigate infectious diseases.[53] Although they are useful initiatives, these programs generally are inadequate for tracking disease trends, because they are fragmented and findings generally cannot be compared across programs/jurisdictions due to a lack of standardization of nomenclature, disease definitions, and means of diagnosis.[52]

NEXT STEPS

Dedicating additional resources to better tracking of canine and feline infectious diseases is needed to help inform prevention and control measures. Some of the drivers of disease, such as climate change, are likely to be critically important, but solutions to address/reduce its progression are complex and long term. Other drivers, such as pathogen introduction through travel and trade, probably are comparatively simple to address (eg, through control measures, such as quarantine and veterinarian pre/post-travel evaluation) and could have rapid, critical, and measurable impacts on the occurrence of canine and feline disease. Despite having identified several likely drivers of current and future canine and feline infectious diseases, however, the specific impacts of these drivers are poorly understood. This limited understanding challenges the ability to best direct resources to controlling canine and feline infectious disease spread and emergence.

In comparison, significant progress has been made in untangling these drivers in human infectious diseases. Between 2008 and 2013, 116 human infectious disease threat events were detected by the European Centre for Disease Prevention and Control.[27] In analyzing these events, researchers identified 17 unique drivers, with 2 or more drivers likely responsible for most of the events.[27] The top 5 contributing drivers were (in descending order based on overall frequency ranking of all events) (1) travel and tourism, (2) food and water quality, (3) natural environment, (4) global trade, and (5) climate. A hierarchical cluster analysis revealed travel and tourism to be separate from all the other drivers, suggesting that this driver should be considered distinct and that specific measures should be dedicated to addressing it.

Improving monitoring for canine and feline infectious diseases is a critically important step to facilitate the evaluation of changes in frequency, location, and impact of disease. Furthermore, such data would lend itself to modeling disease drivers to help prioritize risk-based surveillance actions; anticipate future pathogen introductions, emergence, and spread; and strengthen control measures. The most cost-effective strategy to address changes in infectious diseases in dogs and cats, as in other species, is to directly tackle the underlying infectious disease drivers rather than individual pathogens, diseases, and transmission events, whenever possible.

SUMMARY

Canine and feline infectious diseases are constantly changing in nature, frequency, and location. Due to limited surveillance efforts, the extent of these changes for the most part is unknown. Based on assumptions from human health data and documented outbreaks or other high-profile events, several drivers of these changes are suspected. There is a strong and immediate need for improved surveillance systems to reliably track feline and canine infectious diseases, both within and across political boundaries. Such data will allow for disease drivers to be further explored and ranked. Modifiable drivers should be prioritized and targeted to assist in preventing disease spread.

REFERENCES

1. Daszak P, Cunningham AA, Hyatt AD. Anthropogenic environmental change and the emergence of infectious diseases in wildlife. Acta Trop 2001;78(2):103–16.

2. Morens DM, Fauci AS. Emerging infectious diseases: threats to human health and global stability. PLoS Pathog 2013;9(7):e1003467.

3. Engering A, Hogerwerf L, Slingenbergh J. Pathogen-host-environment interplay and disease emergence. Emerg Microbes Infect 2013;2(2):e5.

4. Crawford PC, Dubovi EJ, Castleman WL, et al. Transmission of equine influenza virus to dogs. Science 2005;310(5747):482–5.

5. Anderson TC, Crawford PC, Dubovi EJ, et al. Prevalence of and exposure factors for seropositivity to H3N8 canine influenza virus in dogs with influenza-like illness in the United States. J Am Vet Med Assoc 2013;242(2):209–16.

6. Payungporn S, Crawford PC, Kouo TS, et al. Influenza A virus (H3N8) in dogs with respiratory disease, Florida. Emerg Infect Dis 2008;14(6):902–8.
7. Song D, Kang B, Lee C, et al. Transmission of avian influenza virus (H3N2) to dogs. Emerg Infect Dis 2008;14(5):741–6.
8. Voorhees IEH, Glaser AL, Toohey-Kurth K, et al. Spread of canine influenza A(H3N2) virus, United States. Emerg Infect Dis 2017;23(12):1950–7.
9. Deschamps JY, Topie E, Roux F. Nosocomial feline calicivirus-associated virulent systemic disease in a veterinary emergency and critical care unit in France. JFMS Open Rep 2015;1(2). 2055116915621581.
10. Hurley KE, Pesavento PA, Pedersen NC, et al. An outbreak of virulent systemic feline calicivirus disease. J Am Vet Med Assoc 2004;224(2):241–9.
11. Perreten V, Kadlec K, Schwarz S, et al. Clonal spread of methicillin-resistant *Staphylococcus pseudintermedius* in Europe and North America: an international multicentre study. J Antimicrob Chemother 2010;65(6):1145–54.
12. Videla R, Solyman SM, Brahmbhatt A, et al. Clonal complexes and antimicrobial susceptibility profiles of *Staphylococcus pseudintermedius* isolates from dogs in the United States. Microb Drug Resist 2018;24(1):83–8.
13. Saputra S, Jordan D, Worthing KA, et al. Antimicrobial resistance in coagulase-positive staphylococci isolated from companion animals in Australia: a one year study. PLoS One 2017;12(4):e0176379.
14. Weese JS, Faires MC, Frank LA, et al. Factors associated with methicillin-resistant versus methicillin-susceptible *Staphylococcus pseudintermedius* infection in dogs. J Am Vet Med Assoc 2012;240(12):1450–5.
15. Gibson JS, Morton JM, Cobbold RN, et al. Risk factors for dogs becoming rectal carriers of multidrug-resistant *Escherichia coli* during hospitalization. Epidemiol Infect 2011;139(10):1511–21.
16. Weese J, Giguère S, Guardabassi L, et al. ACVIM consensus statement on therapeutic antimicrobial use in animals and antimicrobial resistance. J Am Vet Med Assoc 2015;29(2):487–98.
17. Wikel SK. Ticks and tick-borne infections: complex ecology, agents, and host interactions. Vet Sci 2018;5(2). https://doi.org/10.3390/vetsci5020060.
18. Brown HE, Harrington LC, Kaufman PE, et al. Key factors influencing canine heartworm, *Dirofilaria immitis*, in the United States. Parasit Vectors 2012;5:245.
19. Bouchard C, Leonard E, Koffi JK, et al. The increasing risk of Lyme disease in Canada. Can Vet J 2015;56(7):693–9.
20. Eisen RJ, Eisen L, Beard CB. County-scale distribution of *Ixodes scapularis* and *Ixodes pacificus* (Acari: Ixodidae) in the continental United States. J Med Entomol 2016;53(2):349–86.
21. Korotkov Y, Kozlova T, Kozlovskaya L. Observations on changes in abundance of questing *Ixodes ricinus*, castor bean tick, over a 35-year period in the eastern part of its range (Russia, Tula region). Med Vet Entomol 2015;29(2):129–36.
22. Johnson CA, Carter TD, Dunn JR, et al. Investigation and characterization of *Brucella canis* infections in pet-quality dogs and associated human exposures during a 2007-2016 outbreak in Michigan. J Am Vet Med Assoc 2018;253(3):322–36.
23. Hensel ME, Negron M, Arenas-Gamboa AM. Brucellosis in dogs and public health risk. Emerg Infect Dis 2018;24(8):1401–6.
24. Zhu H, Hughes J, Murcia PR. Origins and evolutionary dynamics of H3N2 canine influenza virus. J Virol 2015;89(10):5406–18.
25. Verocai GG, Conboy G, Lejeune M, et al. *Onchocerca lupi* nematodes in dogs exported from the United States into Canada. Emerg Infect Dis 2016;22(8):1477–9.

26. Hansford KM, Pietzsch ME, Cull B, et al. Potential risk posed by the importation of ticks into the UK on animals: records from the tick surveillance scheme. Vet Rec 2018;182(4):107.

27. Semenza JC, Lindgren E, Balkanyi L, et al. Determinants and drivers of infectious disease threat events in Europe. Emerg Infect Dis 2016;22(4):581–9.

28. Olival KJ, Hosseini PR, Zambrana-Torrelio C, et al. Host and viral traits predict zoonotic spillover from mammals. Nature 2017;546(7660):646–50.

29. Smout FA, Skerratt LF, Johnson CN, et al. Zoonotic helminth diseases in dogs and dingoes utilising shared resources in an Australian aboriginal community. Trop Med Infect Dis 2018;3(4) [pii:E110].

30. Hennebelle JH, Sykes JE, Foley J. Risk factors associated with leptospirosis in dogs from Northern California: 2001-2010. Vector Borne Zoonotic Dis 2014; 14(10):733–9.

31. Richardson DJ, Gauthier JL. A serosurvey of leptospirosis in Connecticut peridomestic wildlife. Vector Borne Zoonotic Dis 2003;3(4):187–93.

32. Azócar-Aedo L, Monti G. Meta-analyses of factors associated with leptospirosis in domestic dogs. Zoonoses Public Health 2016;63(4):328–36.

33. Strakova A, Murchison EP. The changing global distribution and prevalence of canine transmissible venereal tumour. BMC Vet Res 2014;10:168.

34. Taylor LH, Wallace RM, Balaram D, et al. The role of dog population management in rabies elimination: a review of current approaches and future opportunities. Front Vet Sci 2017;4:109.

35. Hubbard K, Wang M, Smith DR. Seroprevalence of brucellosis in Mississippi shelter dogs. Prev Vet Med 2018;159:82–6.

36. Dalziel BD, Huang K, Geoghegan JL, et al. Contact heterogeneity, rather than transmission efficiency, limits the emergence and spread of canine influenza virus. PLoS Pathog 2014;23:10.

37. Weese JS, Stull J. Respiratory disease outbreak in a veterinary hospital associated with canine parainfluenza virus infection. Can Vet J 2013;54(1):79–82.

38. Stull JW, Kasten JI, Evason MD, et al. Risk reduction and management strategies to prevent transmission of infectious disease among dogs at dog shows, sporting events, and other canine group settings. J Am Vet Med Assoc 2016;249(6): 612–27.

39. Lane HE, Weese JS, Stull JW. Canine oral papillomavirus outbreak at a dog daycare facility. Can Vet J 2017;58(7):747–9.

40. Gomez-Sanz E, Torres C, Ceballos S, et al. Clonal dynamics of nasal Staphylococcus aureus and Staphylococcus pseudintermedius in dog-owning household members. Detection of MSSA ST(398.). PLoS one 2013;8(7):e69337.

41. Stull JW, Hoffman CC, Landers T. Health benefits and risks of pets in nursing homes: a survey of facilities in Ohio. J Gerontol Nurs 2018;44(5):39–45.

42. Murthy R, Bearman G, Brown S, et al. Animals in healthcare facilities: recommendations to minimize potential risks. Infect Control Hosp Epidemiol 2015;36(5): 495–516.

43. Lefebvre SL, Arroyo LG, Weese JS. Epidemic Clostridium difficile strain in hospital visitation dog. Emerg Infect Dis 2006;12(6):1036–7.

44. Lefebvre SL, Weese JS. Contamination of pet therapy dogs with MRSA and Clostridium difficile. J Hosp Infect 2009;72(3):268–9.

45. Goldschmidt MH, Kennedy JS, Kennedy DR, et al. Severe papillomavirus infection progressing to metastatic squamous cell carcinoma in bone marrow-transplanted X-linked SCID dogs. J Virol 2006;80(13):6621–8.

46. Reinacher M. Diseases associated with spontaneous feline leukemia virus (FeLV) infection in cats. Vet Immunol Immunopathol 1989;21(1):85–95.
47. Burling AN, Levy JK, Scott HM, et al. Seroprevalences of feline leukemia virus and feline immunodeficiency virus infection in cats in the United States and Canada and risk factors for seropositivity. J Am Vet Med Assoc 2017;251(2):187–94.
48. Park ES, Suzuki M, Kimura M, et al. Epidemiological and pathological study of feline morbillivirus infection in domestic cats in Japan. BMC Vet Res 2016;12(1): 228.
49. Sharp CR, Nambulli S, Acciardo AS, et al. Chronic infection of domestic cats with feline morbillivirus, United States. Emerg Infect Dis 2016;22(4):760–2.
50. De Luca E, Crisi PE, Di Domenico M, et al. A real-time RT-PCR assay for molecular identification and quantitation of feline morbillivirus RNA from biological specimens. J Virol Methods 2018;258:24–8.
51. Gremião ID, Miranda LH, Reis EG, et al. Zoonotic epidemic of sporotrichosis: cat to human transmission. PLoS Pathog 2017;13(1):e1006077.
52. Day MJ, Breitschwerdt E, Cleaveland S, et al. Surveillance of zoonotic infectious disease transmitted by small companion animals. Emerg Infect Dis 2012;18(12):e1.
53. Buckland EL, O'Neill D, Summers J, et al. Characterisation of antimicrobial usage in cats and dogs attending UK primary care companion animal veterinary practices. Vet Rec 2016;179(19):489.

Dog Transport and Infectious Disease Risk

An International Perspective

Katherine Polak, DVM, MPH, MS

KEYWORDS

- Animal relocation • Transport • Adoption • Dog • Animal shelter • Rabies
- Animal welfare • Rescue

KEY POINTS

- As animal shelters across North America make strides in lifesaving, many are looking internationally to help more animals. Although lifesaving for individual animals, transport is not without inherent risk.
- Infectious disease risk can be minimized through careful planning, collaborative partnerships between source and destination shelters, prescreening of dogs, preventive health care programs at the export site, and quarantine practices.
- Practical guidelines and resources are needed for all stakeholders to achieve positive animal outcomes while also mitigating disease.
- The author recommends that organizations performing international adoptions also focus on local, sustainable approaches to improve animal welfare.

INTRODUCTION

Over the past decade, interest in companion animal transport programs has grown considerably in North America and Europe in an effort to improve outcomes for dogs and cats in animal shelters.[1,2] These programs vary in type and scale but typically involve the transportation of dogs and cats from a geographic region with limited resources to one that has a greater capacity to provide better animal outcomes. Although some programs focus on the rehoming of animals in-country, others are significantly more resource-intensive, transporting animals from one part of the world to another. Some programs are operated by small, volunteer-based rescue groups whereas others are conducted by well-resourced international animal welfare organizations using a network of overseas shelter partners and well-established transportation routes.[3] Although lifesaving for individual animals, such programs are not without

Disclosure Statement: The author has nothing to disclose.
FOUR PAWS International, 89 AIA Capital Center, 20th Floor, Room 2081/2083, Ratchadapisek Road, Kwaeng Dindaeng, Khet Dindaeng, Bangkok 10400 Thailand
E-mail address: Katherine.polak@four-paws.us

Vet Clin Small Anim 49 (2019) 599–613
https://doi.org/10.1016/j.cvsm.2019.02.003
vetsmall.theclinics.com

controversy.[1] Veterinary professionals argue that transported animals pose a significant risk of the infectious disease introduction or transmission[4,5] and further saturate communities where healthy dogs are euthanized due to a lack of homes.[6]

Individual cases of disease introduction and transmission resulting from dog transport are well documented[7–9]; however, there is no formalized system to quantitatively track the number of dogs transported internationally for rescue or adoption purposes. This lack of a systematic approach to monitoring compromises the ability to quantify and properly address disease risk. Further information on common transportation routes, infectious diseases in transported dogs, and their frequency could help guide recommendations and the creation of resources to mitigate unintentional disease introduction. This article describes the motivating factors for international companion animal transportation, current regulatory mechanisms, infectious disease risks, and suggested measures to mitigate these risks.

TRENDS IN INTERNATIONAL DOG TRANSPORT

Animal welfare charities in the United States have been addressing geographic disparities of homeless shelter animals for years, relocating those from areas of overcrowding to places where certain types of dogs and cats are in short supply, thereby improving their chances of rehoming.[3] The United States saw a dramatic increase in relocation programs after Hurricane Katrina in 2005, when thousands of animals were abandoned, displaced, and later rehomed in shelters across the country.[10] Since then, international adoption programs began increasing in popularity, most likely due to dramatic strides in lifesaving in the United States and increasing awareness of international stray dog suffering.[2] According to a report published by the Canadian National Canine Importation Working Group, from 2013 to 2014, approximately 20% of all canine rescue organizations in Canada imported dogs from overseas.[11] This report speculated that the increasing interest in international dog rescue is due to the high veterinary costs associated with the adoption of local dogs from within Canada. Commercial airlines are also reporting sharp increases in requests for canine air transport.[12]

Social media has undoubtedly fueled the rapid increase in international adoptions, which has transformed the landscape of animal welfare, allowing charities from around the world to develop relationships with each other, engage with various stakeholders, and share their stories with the general public.[13] The creation of virtual networks and communities has facilitated a growing public awareness of international animal welfare issues, such as the dog and cat meat trade in Asia and mass dog culls before international sporting events, motivating many to take action through adoption.[14] International pet adoption and relocation programs generated significant media attention after the 2014 Olympics games in Sochi, Russia[15], and from Puerto Rico after Hurricane Maria in 2017.[16]

MOTIVATING FACTORS FOR INTERNATIONAL DOG TRANSPORT

In much of the developing world, rapid human population growth coupled with poor waste management and lapses in responsible pet ownership have led to increasing stray dog populations; some investigators estimate the population might exceed 500 million worldwide.[17] In countries with an overpopulation of stray dogs, animal welfare legislation is often weak, unenforced, or absent, affording companion animals little protecting from abuse, cruelty, or death.[18] As a result, there is high mortality of stray dogs due to starvation, infectious disease, and road traffic accidents (**Fig. 1**). Human-dog conflict often motivates government agencies to remove dogs through inhumane culling methods.[19] There also is a disparity in veterinary training worldwide, which ultimately affects stray animal care, spay/neuter capacity, and responsible pet ownership.

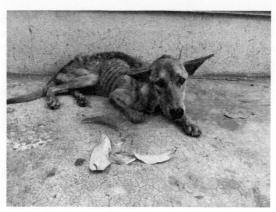

Fig. 1. Malnourished stray dog in Cambodia.

Approaches to managing free-roaming dogs are slowly changing.[20] During the past decade, numerous animal welfare organizations have started working internationally in limited-resource areas to address animal suffering through education, rescue, sheltering, and the provision of spay/neuter services. These activities promote long-term sustainable change; however, they may not address immediate animal suffering.

Exporting Organizations

Animal shelters in the developing world face incredible challenges. They operate in places with weak or absent animal welfare legislation and high levels of animal suffering, and few shelters are able to employ veterinarians to oversee and conduct medical practices on a full-time basis. Shelters are frequently under pressure to accept large numbers of suffering and abandoned dogs, yet the local capacity for adoptions usually is limited.[21] As a result, organizations have begun seeking partnerships with shelters outside their country, often in Europe or North America, that can provide dogs with better outcomes.[22] Besides being lifesaving for individual animals, transport also frees up resources to provide improved care for animals remaining at the shelter and fund programs that impact sustainable, long-term change.

Importing Organizations

Long-distance dog transport programs can benefit receiving agencies through positive publicity and increased adoptions.[23] Media coverage of imported rescued dogs often motivates the public to adopt and donate, increasing both public awareness and resources. Researchers from 1 study found that in 13% of sheltering organizations, their decision to accept transferred dogs was impacted by stories that evoked media attention.[1] This media attention also may be used to facilitate awareness of international animal welfare issues and mobilize support for associated campaigns. Transportation programs also can increase the diversity of dogs at sheltering facilities, which appeals to adopters.[22] Increased adoptions benefit not only the animals but also the shelter staff, who face the daily emotional burden of rehoming animals.[24]

METHODS OF TRANSPORTATION

Most international dog transport programs are collaborative, involving an exporting organization and a receiving animal shelter. Canada and the United States are preferred destinations for exported dogs due to their limited regulatory restrictions, lower flight costs, and presence of potential adopters.[11] Dogs typically are transported by either commercial airline or charter plane (**Fig. 2**). The cost of air travel varies, ranging from between $300 to $1200 per dog, depending on an animal's weight, size, and route.[25] In an effort to reduce the cost, rescue organizations may solicit volunteers already traveling on particular routes to accompany animals checked as excess baggage. (**Fig. 3**).

RISK OF DISEASE TRANSMISSION

Although well intentioned, international dog transport is not without inherent risk. The medical practices of exporting agencies vary depending on resources, location, and access to a veterinarian. Shelters located in developing countries often lack sufficient resources to diagnose, treat, and prevent infectious disease and operate in rabies-endemic areas.[18] International shelters are often prone to overcrowding, utilize group housing for dogs, and may lack suitable isolation facilities. Housing practices such as random co-mingling and group housing prior to or during transport may magnify the disease risk.[26]

Furthermore, in the developing world, shelter personnel frequently lack training in infectious disease control. For agencies fortunate enough to work with a local veterinarian, he or she may lack training in shelter medicine. Although shelter medicine is an emerging specialty in veterinary medicine in North America and Europe, it is relatively new or nonexistent in many other places around the world. Even with appropriate disease screening performed by trained personnel, subclinical infections can still pose a significant risk for introduction and transmission of numerous infectious agents.

Critics of transport programs argue that international animal transport facilitates an unpredictable spread of infectious disease globally.[5,27] Dog movement can introduce novel or re-emerging viral strains in places where animals are naïve and diseases were previously eradicated, and novel pathogens also can become endemic in the canine population and/or within wildlife.[4,9] Hotly debated topics involving disease and international dog transport include the following:

- In Central and Northern Europe, epidemiologic studies have documented the spread of *Dirofilaria immitis* after the movement of infected animals largely from Southern European countries considered endemic/hyperendemic.[28]
- The spread of vector-borne pathogens, including leishmaniasis and babesiosis, throughout Europe.[29,30]

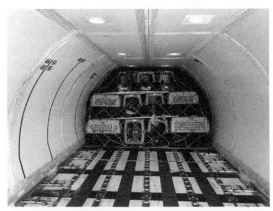

Fig. 2. Rescued dogs loaded in a chartered plane in Puerto Rico bound for adoptive homes in the United States.

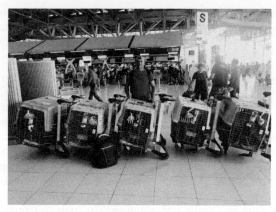

Fig. 3. A flight volunteer prepares to escort 5 rescued dogs from Thailand to the United States.

- Cases of canine rabies reported in imported rescue dogs in the United States and the United Kingdom from Egypt, India, and Sri Lanka.[31–33]
- The introduction of canine influenza H3N2 in the United States in 2015 highlighted the potential rapid spread of novel pathogens, although the exact source of this outbreak remains unknown.[34]

Table 1 provides a summary of select infectious diseases of concern in regard to the importation of dogs into the United States and Canada.

The transportation process itself also may compromise animal welfare given the prolonged confinement and limited monitoring during international routes. The stress

Table 1
Select infectious diseases of concern with regard to canine importation into the United States and Canada

	Rabies	Canine Influenza (H3N2)	Heartworm	Tick-borne Disease	*Brucella canis*
Federally reportable/ notifiable?	Yes	No	No	No	In livestock
Level of public health risk	High	Low	Low	Medium	Low for the general public, higher for those that are immunocompromised
Level of concern[a]	High	Medium	Low	Low	Medium
High-risk export countries/ regions	India and China, Africa, and Southeast Asia	China, Korea, Thailand	Worldwide distribution (temperate, tropical, and subtropical areas)	Worldwide distribution	Worldwide distribution

[a] Based on zoonotic potential, transmissibility, and virulence.

of transport can predispose dogs to longer-term issues, such as behavior problems, including phobias,[35] and increase viral shedding and susceptibility to infection.[36]

REGULATIONS

Transportation regulations vary depending on the country, territory, and state of importation and exportation (**Table 2**). Most attempt to strike a balance between an acceptable level of risk of disease introduction with freedom of animal movement, particularly for owned pets, but they do not specify how to ensure animal welfare and disease prevention for transport programs.[37] Federal transport requirements vary greatly depending on whether the importation is classified as personal or commercial. Personal importation typically has fewer requirements (primarily rabies vaccination), whereas commercial importation has more stringent requirements including vaccinations, health checks, permanent identification, and import permits.[38] Rescue groups may send dogs as "owner accompanied" animals to circumvent the stricter rules pertaining to commercial imports.[39] In many countries, an examination of the animal to be transported must be performed by a veterinarian with the exporting country's Ministry of Agriculture, or equivalent, before the animal is allowed to leave the country.

The United States and Canada are targeted by exporting organizations, in particular those in rabies-endemic countries, due to the relatively few importation requirements (see **Table 2**). Unlike New Zealand or the United Kingdom, dogs originating from countries with high-risk for rabies do not require quarantine or testing for rabies antibodies before entrance into the United States and Canada. Some rabies-free countries, such

Table 2
Comparison of various import requirements for cats and dogs in select countries

	United States	Canada	United Kingdom	New Zealand
Regulatory agency	US Department of Agriculture	Canadian Food Inspection Agency	Department for Environment, Food and Rural Affairs	Ministry for Primary Industries
Microchip or tattoo required	No	Yes	Yes	Yes
Infectious disease testing and/or treatment	None	None	*Echinococcus multilocularis*	• *Babesia gibsoni*[a] • *Brucella canis*[a] • Leptospirosis[a]
Quarantine requirement	None	None	None; however, titer testing is required 3 mo prior to entry	Minimum 10-d quarantine on arrival[a]
Rabies antibody test required	No	No	Yes[b]	Yes
Vaccination against rabies	Yes	Yes	Yes	Yes
Tapeworm treatment	No	No	Yes	Yes
Heartworm testing	No	No	No	Yes

[a] Dogs from all countries except Australia.
[b] If importing dogs from a country with high rabies prevalence.

as Australia and New Zealand, prohibit the entry of dogs directly from countries with high rabies prevalence.

Several prominent animal and public health organizations including the World Organisation for Animal[40] Health and the World Health Organization[41] have issued recommendations and guidelines pertaining to international companion animal transport and disease control. These standards typically vary depending on the rabies status of the exporting country and animal species involved. Regarding the transportation process itself, the International Air Transport Association (IATA) publishes an extensive set of guidelines annually for transporting live animals by air; these are considered to be the worldwide standard.[42] In 2018, the IATA launched a new standardized global certification program to improve the safety and welfare of animals traveling by air.

The World Trade Organization issues rules for international trade.[43] Its primary purpose is to ensure a system of rules-based trade to ensure universal access to free trade internationally. The World Trade Organization mandates that importing countries cannot impose conditions for import that are more restrictive than those of the importing country itself. This includes requiring proof of disease-free status or recent treatment of a particular disease, unless the importing country is also considered free of the disease and/or has a formal control program in place. For example, this means that a country lacking a formal brucellosis control program cannot require an exporting country to ensure exported animals are brucellosis free.

DISCUSSION

International adoptions are driven by the severity of animal welfare issues internationally, advances in global transportation networks, and societal interests. As the demand for imported dogs increases, so too will international dog transport despite the disease risk. Although international adoption fails to solve animal welfare issues in exporting communities, it can be lifesaving for individual animals and must be done in a way that mitigates disease risk. At the root of the issue, the animal welfare organizations looking to export dogs for adoption are often those that are the most limited resourced. Mitigating disease risk starts with addressing the practices of the exporting organization.

PARTNERSHIPS

International dog transport should involve a collaboration between well-established source and destination organizations rather than private individuals lacking expertise in disease control. Such organizational relationships facilitate clear and direct communication, an understanding of each organizations' capacity for medical care, and the ability to ensure transportation practices comply with federal and state guidelines. Partnerships also allow for information sharing, which can help exporting groups improve their medical practices and reduce the infectious disease risk. Ideally, staff from each organization should make an on-site visit to the partner facility to better understand their challenges and opportunities.

The decision to internationally rehome animals must begin with a thorough resource analysis by all agencies involved; the transport process can be long, tedious, and expensive.[36] Those involved in transport must be familiar with the import and export requirements for all countries involved, as well as airline requirements to ensure safe and responsible transport. All reasonable steps must be taken to ensure that the benefits of sending the animal outweigh the risks, and that all reasonable steps are taken to minimize disease risk.

Responsibilities of Exporting Agencies

Exporting agencies are responsible for ensuring transported animals are free from disease and eligible for import into the desired country. At a minimum, organizations exporting dogs must have the ability to screen dogs for infectious disease, isolate and quarantine dogs appropriately, and work with a local veterinarian familiar with the exportation process. The risk of disease transmission can be mitigated while dogs are still under the care of the exporting agency with a preventive health care program, well before the actual transportation date. Dogs should be housed individually or in stable groups, to minimize disease exposure prior to transport.

Animal selection should be performed carefully, based on the lowest risk of disease. Although there is frequent interest in puppies due to their high adoptability, they are immunologically naïve and the most susceptible to disease.[36] It is imperative that exporting agencies disclose any disease risks particular to their geographic region and any activities that might enhance the animal's risk for exposure to importing organizations.[44] Aside from physical health, behavioral health is equally important to ensure positive animal outcomes. Because adoption returns are costly and often impractical given the logistics of long-distance transport, it is imperative that behavioral assessments are performed on dogs prior to transport. It is common for former stray dogs to be transported for adoption purposes; however, these dogs may have never walked on a leash, lived indoors, or walked up stairs. A thorough and accurate behavioral assessment must be communicated to the importing agency to ensure placement success.

All dogs must be appropriately vaccinated for rabies. When stored at appropriate temperatures and administered according to manufacturer instructions, the 30 days required by most countries between the time of vaccination and travel should be sufficient to ensure sufficient protective antibodies.[45,46] A concern, however, is that 30 days may be inadequate to detect dogs incubating rabies at the time of vaccination.[47] For this reason, clear and timely communication with importing agencies, adopters, and private veterinarians for surveillance after transportation is crucial.

In an effort to reduce infectious disease risk, at a minimum exporting agencies should:

- Implant all dogs with an International Organization for Standards –compliant (15-digit, 134.2-kHz) microchip.
- Vaccinate all dogs for rabies and distemper/parvovirus using a modified live vaccine. Vaccination should not occur the day of transport; ideally dogs should be vaccinated at least 3 days to 5 days prior to transport to allow for the full onset of protection.[36]
- Fit dogs with appropriate visual identification, such as a collar or tag.
- Administer an endoparasiticide effective against hookworms and roundworms.
- Conduct a physical examination within 24 hours of transport.
- Apply an effective ectoparasiticide.

Spay/neuter procedures should ideally be performed prior to travel, which can facilitate the identification of underlying conditions, such as pyometra and pregnancy. Adequate time must be allowed between surgery and transport to allow for proper incisional healing. In an effort to minimize the stress of transport, some organizations may attempt to acclimatize dogs to their crates prior to transport. The administration of sedatives or tranquilizers, such as acepromazine prior to or during air transport is not recommended and may be prohibited.[44] If dogs are traveling via commercial air-lines, IATA requirements can be used to guide appropriate crate sizing.[42]

Specific recommendations exist for the management of heartworm infection in transported dogs.[48] The Association of Shelter Veterinarians and the American Heart-worm Society recommend the following:

- Dogs should be tested for microfilariae and heartworm antigen prior to transport if older than 6 months of age. If exporting organizations lack the resources to test, all dogs should be started on a macrocyclic lactone regardless prior to transport.
- Heartworm-infected dogs should be started on doxycycline therapy prior to transport.
- If treating infected dogs prior to transport is not possible, heartworm-positive dogs should be treated with topical moxidectin or a macrocyclic lactone in addi-tion to a topical canine insecticide.
- Dogs should not be transported within 30 days of receiving heartworm adulticidal therapy with melarsomine dihydrochloride.

Additional vaccination and diagnostic testing should be considered based on the disease risk of the exporting country.[49] These may include vaccination against *Borde-tella bronchiseptica*, parainfluenza virus, canine influenza, leptospirosis, and *Borrelia burgdorferi*. For example, dogs originating from South Korea or China should be vaccinated and appropriately screened for canine influenza; those from the Mediter-ranean basin should be screened for *Leishmania* antibodies.[50] In places where trans-missible venereal tumor is endemic, a full genital examination should be part of the routine physical examination. Tick-borne disease testing using point-of-care antibody tests requires special mention because positive results in asymptomatic dogs have the potential to create management dilemmas for both importing and exporting agencies, particularly if confirmatory testing is unavailable.[51] These tests should be interpreted with caution and in conjunction with clinical signs.

Every reasonable effort must be made to ensure that transported animals are free from disease. Aside from reducing disease transmission, early identification and treat-ment of sick dogs reduces the burden on importing organizations, because treatment typically is much less expensive in the exporting country. Medical records are critical to document preventive health practices and diagnostic testing results and should accompany all transported dogs.

Responsibilities of Importing Agencies

Importing agencies should have pretransfer medical requirements that exporting agencies are required to follow. On arrival in the destination country, dogs ideally should be quarantined based on age, source, and infectious disease risk to facilitate the identification of incubating infections. The quarantine period should be based on the disease risk of the exporting country.

The National Association of State Public Health Veterinarians suggests that all im-ported dogs undergo a minimum of 30 days in quarantine at an approved facility where veterinary supervision is present and records are maintained.[52] A compromised approach is to quarantine dogs for a minimum of 1 week on arrival, which should allow for clinical expression of common incubating infections including parvovirus, influ-enza, and kennel cough[53]; 1 week may be inadequate, however, to detect canine dis-temper virus and rabies infections. All dogs should receive a physical examination on arrival, and facilities should allow for the isolation of those with clinical signs of illness to prevent disease spread. Importing agencies have a duty to the local community and adopters to disclose the origin of the animal and all medical records.

ROLE OF VETERINARIANS IN THE IMPORTING COUNTRY

Veterinarians are often responsible for educating adopters, working with local shelters, and protecting both animal and human health. They play a key role in establishing effective surveillance systems to minimize disease transmission. Veterinarians may choose to engage with organizations importing dogs and private adopters to advise of the potential disease risks, ensure transported dogs are healthy, and facilitate the treatment of dogs that become ill after transport. Without this relationship, transported dogs that fall ill may go unreported and disease transmission unchecked.

RECOMMENDATIONS
Education and Resources

International dog transport is rapidly evolving and practical resources are desperately needed for all stakeholders to mitigate potential disease transmission. In the United States, the Association of Shelter Veterinarians,[26] American Veterinary Medical Association,[36] and Society of Animal Welfare Administrators[54] have issued guidelines for dog transport, but these may not address specific concerns pertaining to international transport. Additional research is required to better understand the needs of both source and destination agencies to create resources that are readily assessible, easy to understand, and in the local language of the target audience.

Exporting organizations

Most organizations exporting dogs strive to achieve minimum practices because it is in their best interest to ensure dogs arrive healthy. If receiving organizations believe that a partner organization has transported dogs without fully disclosing the dogs' medical conditions, they are inclined to terminate the cooperation.[1] Additional resources are needed to ensure exporting organizations and their veterinarians are familiar with general disease screening techniques, canine preventive health protocols, and general shelter management and infectious disease control practices.

Adopters

Veterinarians may consider developing and distributing educational materials that can be provided to clients that have adopted or are considering adopting an animal internationally. This is particularly important for adopters of dogs from countries with high-risk status for rabies. Resources should describe in detail any potential disease risks and what to do if an animal develops behavior change/neurologic signs in the 6 months after import.

Veterinarians

Veterinarians in importing countries must be made aware of increasing trends in international dog transport and should exercise increased vigilance for foreign diseases. Veterinarians in North America and Europe would benefit from resources to guide their diagnostic and treatment decisions for imported dogs, including a list of endemic diseases from the various source countries and recommended screening techniques. Diseases in imported dogs may pose a diagnostic conundrum for veterinarians who are unfamiliar with diseases in the exporting country, leading to a failure of diagnosis and treatment.[2] A low index of suspicion in regions with low or no prevalence may lead to under-diagnosis or misdiagnosis. In exporting countries, which are typically located in the developing world, veterinarians desperately need additional resources and training opportunities in shelter and small animal medicine to ensure the health of transported animals.

Voluntary Registry of Importers

A voluntary registry of canine rescue organizations that routinely import dogs could provide a vital communication link with at least a proportion of these groups. To ensure both interest and compliance, there needs to be a mechanism whereby compliance is incentivized; this could include discounted import permit fees.[11] Establishing this communication link would be particularly helpful in the event of emerging disease concerns. Crowd-sourced surveillance also could be a mechanism to bolster reporting.[55] Whatever the system used, it needs to be flexible enough to adjust to changing disease patterns and risks.

Regulatory Mechanisms

Although some veterinarians argue for stricter regulations on dog transport or a ban for rescue purposes, there is a danger of driving the transport underground, making risk mitigation far more difficult. Black market trading inevitably leads to deliberate smuggling across borders, document falsification, and ultimately a far larger risk for disease introduction. Although regulations may require modernizing to address increasing disease concerns, all stakeholders, including exporters, should be constructively engaged to strike a balance between disease control and freedom of animal movement, particularly for rescue purposes.

Sustainable Animal Welfare

Although international transport provides lifesaving outcomes for individual dogs, it fails to address the root causes of animal welfare issues in exporting communities. Improving canine welfare in the developing world almost always require a change in human behavior because populations of domesticated species are unable to facilitate welfare improvements for themselves.[56] Transport activities, therefore, should be coupled with programs that achieve in-country human behavior change and improved capacity for canine care and welfare. These might include public education campaigns to improve responsible pet ownership, veterinary training, and community engagement.

SUMMARY

The landscape of animal welfare is changing, and veterinary medicine must adapt. As interest in international dog transport continues to increase, veterinarians in countries where dogs are imported may need to modify their diagnostic practices to include screening for exotic canine diseases and advise importing agencies on best practices for dog transport. Until animal welfare improves on a global scale, international adoption may be one of the only options to address immediate animal suffering; however, it is not a sustainable or cost-effective solution. Although saving animals lives is a noble goal, it must be done responsibly to mitigate the risk of disease introduction and transmission. Guidelines, best practices, and operational procedures are needed for both importing and exporting agencies in addition to global cooperation and commitment to risk management and mitigation.

REFERENCES

1. Simmons K, Hoffman C. Dogs on the move: factors impacting animal shelter and rescue organizations' decisions to accept dogs from distant locations. Animals (Basel) 2016;6:11.

2. Allen G. With rescue dogs in demand, more shelters look far afield for Fido. 2015. Available at: http://www.npr.org/2015/01/01/374257591/with-rescue-dogs-in-dem and-more-shelters-look-far-afield-for-fido. Accessed March 25, 2018.

3. Zawistowski S. Introduction to animal sheltering. In: Miller L, Zawistowski S, editors. Shelter medicine for veterinarians and staff. Ames (IA): Blackwell Pub; 2004. p. 3–12.

4. O'Shea P. Shelter-animal relocation raises infectious disease concerns. 2018. Available at: http://www.veterinarynews.dvm360.com/shelter-animal-relocation-raises-infectious-disease-concerns. Accessed September 12, 2018.

5. Smith-Blackmore M, Kolb G. Animal rescue - transporting fido across state lines. 2011. Available at: https://www.avma.org/KB/Resources/Reference/AnimalWelfare/Pages/AVMA-Welfare-Focus-Featured-Article-Nov2011.aspx. Accessed September 12, 2018.

6. Avanzino R. Dog transport editorial. 2018. Available at: http://www.maddiesfund.org/dog-transport-editorial.htm. Accessed September 13, 2018.

7. Scarlett J. Population statistics. In: Miller L, Zawistowski S, editors. Shelter medicine for veterinarians and staff. Ames (IA): Wiley-Blackwell; 2013. p. 13–20.

8. Klevar S, Høgåsen H, Davidson R, et al. Cross-border transport of rescue dogs may spread rabies in Europe. Vet Rec 2015;176:672.

9. Trees A, Ridge A. Threat of imported diseases to UK dogs. Vet Rec 2016;178:347–8.

10. Levy J, Lappin M, Glaser A, et al. Prevalence of infectious diseases in cats and dogs rescued following Hurricane Katrina. J Am Vet Med Assoc 2011;238:311–7.

11. Anderson M, Douma D, Kostiuk D, et al. Report of the Canadian national canine importation working group. 2016. Available at: https://www.canadianveterinarians.net/documents/canadian-canine-importation-working-group-report. Accessed September 1, 2018.

12. Brulliard K. Fur and fury at 40,000 feet as more people bring animals on planes. The Washington Post 2018. Available at: https://www.washingtonpost.com/news/animalia/wp/2018/01/22/fur-and-fury-at-40000-feet-as-more-people-bring-animals-on-planes/?utm_term=.14be7ae7e91f. Accessed August 1, 2018.

13. Waters R, Burnett E, Lamm A, et al. Engaging stakeholders through social networking: How nonprofit organizations are using Facebook. Public Relat Rev 2009;35:102–6.

14. Aiello M. Olympian Gus Kenworthy plans to rescue more dogs from Pyeonchang. 2018. E! Online. Available at: https://www.eonline.com/news/912991/olympian-gus-kenworthy-plans-to-rescue-more-dogs-from-pyeonchang-after-2014-sochi-efforts. Accessed September 16, 2018.

15. Herszenhorn D. Racing to save the stray dogs of Sochi. The New York Times 2018. Available at: https://www.nytimes.com/2014/02/06/sports/olympics/racing-to-save-dogs-roaming-around-sochi.html. Accessed August 10, 2018.

16. Shrum J. Southwest Airlines helps save more than 60 animals stranded in Puerto Rico. CW33. 2018. Available at: https://cw33.com/2018/01/23/southwest-airlines-joins-rescue-group-to-save-more-than-60-stray-animals/. Accessed September 12, 2018.

17. Hsu Y, Liu Severinghaus L, Serpell J. Dog keeping in Taiwan: its contribution to the problem of free-roaming dogs. J Appl Anim Welf Sci 2003;6:1–23.

18. Kartal T, Rowan A. Stray dog population management. In: Polak K, Kommedal A, editors. Field manual for small animal medicine. Hoboken (NJ): Wiley; 2018. p. 15–28.

19. Dalla Villa P, Kahn S, Stuardo L, et al. Free-roaming dog control among OIE-member countries. Prev Vet Med 2010;97:58–63.
20. Jackman J, Rowan A. Free-roaming dogs in developing countries: the benefits of capture, neuter, and return programs. In: Salem DJ, Rowan AM, editors. The state of the animals. Washington, DC: Humane Society Press; 2007. p. 55–78.
21. Basic management guidelines for dog and cat shelters. 2010. Available at: https://www.animalsasia.org/. Accessed September 16, 2018.
22. Garrison L, Weiss E. What do people want? Factors people consider when acquiring dogs, the complexity of the choices they make, and implications for nonhuman animal relocation programs. J Appl Anim Welf Sci 2014;18:57–73.
23. Majchrowicz M. Spared from South Korean meat farm, dogs looking for new homes in Charleston. Post and Courier. 2018. Available at: https://www.postandcourier.com/news/spared-from-south-korean-meat-farm-dogs-looking-for-new/article_2bcf0898-aba6-11e8-9ff7-3f6a4184ecd5.html. Accessed September 16, 2018.
24. Rogelberg S, Reeve C, Spitzmüller C, et al. Impact of euthanasia rates, euthanasia practices, and human resource practices on employee turnover in animal shelters. J Am Vet Med Assoc 2007;230:713–9.
25. Pet shipping costs. Continental pet relocation; 2018. Available at: https://continentalpetrelocation.com/2017/02/pet-shipping-costs/. Accessed September 16, 2018.
26. Newbury S, Blinn M, Bushby P, et al. Animal transport. In: Guidelines for standards of care in animal shelters. Association of Shelter Veterinarians; 2010. p. 39–41.
27. Upham P, Thomas C, Gillingwater D, et al. Environmental capacity and airport operations: current issues and future prospects. J Air Transp Manag 2003;9:145–51.
28. Morchón R, Carretón E, González-Miguel J, et al. Heartworm disease (Dirofilaria immitis) and their vectors in Europe – New distribution trends. Front Physiol 2012;3:196.
29. Dujardin J-C, Campino L, Cañavate C, et al. Spread of vector-borne diseases and neglect of Leishmaniasis, Europe. Emerg Infect Dis 2008;14:1013–8.
30. Hamel D, Silaghi C, Lescai D, et al. Epidemiological aspects on vector-borne infections in stray and pet dogs from Romania and Hungary with focus on Babesia spp. Parasitol Res 2012;110:1537–45.
31. Sinclair J, Wallace R, Gruszynshi K, et al. Rabies in a dog imported from Egypt with a falsified rabies vaccination certificate—Virginia 2015. MMWR Morb Mortal Wkly Rep 2015;64:1359–62.
32. Castrodale L, Walker V, Baldwin J, et al. Rabies in a puppy imported from India to the USA. Zoonoses Public Health 2008;55:427–30.
33. Johnson N, Nunez A, Marston D, et al. Investigation of an imported case of rabies in a juvenile dog with atypical presentation. Animals (Basel) 2011;1:402–13.
34. Newbury S, Godhardt-Cooper J, Poulsen K, et al. Prolonged intermittent virus shedding during an outbreak of canine influenza A H3N2 virus infection in dogs in three Chicago area shelters: 16 cases (March to May 2015). J Am Vet Med Assoc 2016;248:1022–6.
35. Mariti C, Ricci E, Mengoli M. Survey of travel-related problems in dogs. Vet Rec 2012;170:542.
36. American Veterinary Medical Association best practices for the relocation of dogs and cats for adoption. 2014. Available at: https://www.avma.org/KB/Resources/Reference/AnimalWelfare/Documents/AVMA_BestPracticesAdoption_Brochure.pdf. Accessed on March 25, 2018.

37. Aziz M, Janeczko S, Gupta M. Infectious disease prevalence and factors associated with upper respiratory infection in cats following relocation. Animals (Basel) 2018;8:91.

38. Canadian Food Inspection Agency requirements for importing or travelling with domestic dogs. Available at: http://www.inspection.gc.ca/animals/terrestrial-animals/imports/policies/live-animals/pets/dogs/eng/1331876172009/1331876307796. Accessed January 28, 2015.

39. Canadian border control turns away dogs imported into Toronto. 2015. Available at: http://www.torontopetdaily.com/2015/07/canada-customs-turns-away-dogs-imported.html. Accessed May 5, 2016.

40. World Organisation for Animal Health (OIE). Terrestrial Animal Health Code, 15th edition. Paris (France); 2006.

41. World Health Organization. WHO expert consultation on rabies. Second report 2013. Available at: http://apps.who.int/. Accessed March 18, 2018.

42. International Air Transport Association. Live animals regulations. 2017. Available at: http://www.iata.org/publications/store/Pages/live-animals-regulations.aspx. Accessed December 2, 2018.

43. Thiermann A, Babcock S. Animal welfare and international trade. Rev Sci Tech 2005;24:747–55.

44. DiGangi B. Top 5 tips for animal transportation. In: Clinician's brief. 2018. Available at: https://www.cliniciansbrief.com/article/top-5-tips-animal-transportation. Accessed September 18, 2018.

45. Hanlon C, Niezgoda M, Rupprecht C. Postexposure prophylaxis for prevention of rabies in dogs. Am J Vet Res 2002;63:1096–100.

46. Manickam R, Basheer M, Jayakumar R. Post-exposure prophylaxis (PEP) of rabies-infected Indian street dogs. Vaccine 2008;26:6564–8.

47. Scientific Committee on Animal Health and Animal Welfare. Assessment of the risk of rabies introduction into the UK, Ireland, Sweden and Malta as a consequence of abandoning serological tests measuring protective antibodies to rabies. EFSA J 2006;426:1–54.

48. Minimizing heartworm transmission in relocated dogs. 2018. Available at: https://www.heartwormsociety.org/images/A-News/SKO_Transport_Guidelines2018.pdf. Accessed July 14, 2018.

49. American Animal Hospital Association. Vaccination recommendations for general practice. 2018. Available at: https://www.aaha.org/guidelines/canine_vaccination_guidelines/practice_vaccination.aspx. Accessed September 22, 2018.

50. Solano-Gallego L, Miró G, Koutinas A, et al. LeishVet guidelines for the practical management of canine leishmaniosis. Parasit Vectors 2011;4:86.

51. Bolser J. Point-of-care testing. In: Polak K, Kommedal A, editors. Field manual for small animal medicine. Hoboken (NJ): Wiley; 2018. p. 418–39.

52. Eidson M. Comments from the National Association of State Public Health Veterinarians (NASPHV) on "Proposed Revision of HHS/CDC Animal-Importation Regulations. National Association of State Public Health Veterinarians; 2007. Available at: http://www.nasphv.org/Documents/CorrespondenceANPRM-Dog-Cat-Ferret.pdf. Accessed March 3, 2018.

53. Levy J. Pro tips: relocation of animals displaced by Hurricanes Irma and Harvey. University of Florida Maddie's Shelter Medicine Program. 2018. Available at: https://sheltermedicine.vetmed.ufl.edu/files/2017/09/2017-UF-Hurricane-Shelter-Pet-Relocation-Guidelines.pdf. Accessed February 3, 2018.

54. Society of Animal Welfare Administrators companion animal transport programs best practices. Available at: http://c.ymcdn.com/sites/www.sawanetwork.org/resource/resmgr/files/SAWA_ Companion_Animal_Transp.pdf. Accessed March 25, 2018.
55. Chunara R, Smolinski M, Brownstein J. Why we need crowdsourced data in infectious disease surveillance. Curr Infect Dis Rep 2013;15:316–9.
56. Reed K, Upjohn M. Better lives for dogs: incorporating human behavior change into a theory of change to improve canine welfare worldwide. Front Vet Sci 2018; 5:93.

Impact of Dog Transport on High-Risk Infectious Diseases

Maureen E.C. Anderson, DVM, DVSc, PhD[a],*,
Jason W. Stull, VMD, MPVM, PhD[b,c], J. Scott Weese, DVM, DVSc[d]

KEYWORDS

- Importation • Translocation • Transportation • Companion animals
- Infectious disease risk

KEY POINTS

- Translocation of dogs inherently poses infectious disease risks when pathogen distributions vary between regions, even within the same country.
- Concerns include introduction of novel pathogens that can infect dogs, zoonotic pathogens, pathogens that can become established in existing reservoirs or vectors, and vectors that might carry pathogens and/or become established in a new region.
- Implementation of mandatory screening or testing programs before interregional movement or importation of dogs is not feasible in many cases because of a plethora of economic, practical, and political reasons.
- Education of all stakeholders involved to raise awareness of the potential disease consequences of translocation events via the movement of dogs needs to be a priority.

INTRODUCTION

Geographic boundaries and barriers that previously helped to keep infectious diseases regionally contained can now be bridged in a matter of hours, by plane, train, or automobile. Even many political boundaries pose minimal challenge to temporary visitors, and with them come their infectious pathogens, both foreign and familiar. Given the strength of the human-animal bond and frequent inclusion of dogs in the

Disclosure: The authors have nothing to disclose.
[a] Animal Health and Welfare Branch, Ontario Ministry of Agriculture, Food and Rural Affairs, Guelph, Ontario, Canada; [b] Department of Veterinary Preventive Medicine, The Ohio State University, College of Veterinary Medicine, Columbus, OH, USA; [c] Department of Health Management, University of Prince Edward Island, Atlantic Veterinary College, 550 University Avenue, Charlottetown, Prince Edward Island CIA 4P3, Canada; [d] Department of Pathobiology, Ontario Veterinary College, University of Guelph, Guelph, Ontario N1G 2W1, Canada
* Corresponding author. 1 Stone Road West, 5th Floor Northwest (336), Guelph, Ontario N1G 4Y2, Canada.
E-mail address: maureen.e.c.anderson@ontario.ca

Vet Clin Small Anim 49 (2019) 615–627
https://doi.org/10.1016/j.cvsm.2019.02.004
0195-5616/19/© 2019 Elsevier Inc. All rights reserved.

family unit, it is not surprising that where people go, dogs seem to eventually follow, and they bring all of their microbes along as well. Although both temporary and permanent translocation of dogs is clearly a common occurrence, it is extremely difficult to accurately quantify, largely because of a lack of importation regulations by which the data may be collected, and lack of sharing of these data by the agencies responsible. For example, in Canada, the Canadian Border Services Agency ostensibly collects data regarding dog entry and applies separate codes to dogs that are imported either personally or commercially. However, the number of animals imported under each category and any additional data on the origin or destination of these animals are not available.[1] Based on an independent estimate, at least 6189 dogs from 29 different countries were imported into Canada in 2013 to 2014 through 218 rescue organizations alone.[1] This number is likely a gross underestimation of the actual number of imported dogs, because there is no registration or licensing requirement for rescue organizations to ensure they were all identified, and these numbers do not include animals that were personally imported by individuals for a variety of reasons, such as vacation, seasonal residence, breeding, or competition, in addition to adoption. It was estimated that more than 287,000 dogs were imported into the United States in 2006 through land border crossings and airports.[2] There is even less information available on illegal movement of dogs that may occur, particularly by ground transportation over poorly protected borders such as that between the United States and Canada or those of some European countries.

Translocation of dogs, regulated or unregulated, legal or covert, small or large scale, inherently poses infectious disease risks when pathogen distributions vary between regions, even within the same country. There are many drivers of this kind of canine traffic, and the transportation process itself can exacerbate the risks. Concerns include introduction of novel pathogens that can infect dogs (eg, canine influenza virus), introduction of pathogens that can infect people (eg, rabies virus), introduction of pathogens that can become established in existing reservoirs or vectors (eg, tick-borne or mosquito-borne pathogens), and introduction of vectors that might carry pathogens and/or become established in a new region (eg, ticks).

DRIVERS OF CANINE MOVEMENT

The drivers of long-distance dog transport are many and varied, and the risks of pathogen movement vary by the reason for translocation. **Table 1** provides reasons/means and examples of canine importation into a country with minimal importation requirements, such as Canada.

Because of the scarcity of data available regarding canine importation, it is not possible to accurately quantify each of these drivers, but dogs transported by rescue organization and puppies imported for retail sale (which are not mutually exclusive groups) represent the largest number of high-risk animals.[2,4] The reasons for rescuing dogs are equally many and varied, including displacement of dogs by natural disasters (eg, hurricanes),[5–7] high-profile international events (eg, Olympic games),[8,9] the canine meat industry in Asia,[10] and puppy mills.[11] In addition, it has been reported that at least 1 commercial puppy mill in the United States has set up its own so-called rescue organization in order to circumvent regulations and bylaws designed to deter sales of dogs from such facilities, by essentially laundering the puppies through the rescue before sale to retailers.[12] The medical requirements stipulated by rescues, shelters, and other organizations that may receive rescue dogs, including quarantine periods, are highly variable and in many cases are nonexistent.[13]

Table 1
Reasons for, and means of, canine importation into Canada

Reason/Means	Examples	Risk Mitigating Factors	Risk Enhancing Factors
Personal pet reentering country with owner after short-term trip	Dog returning with resident vacationing seasonally in another country; show or breeding animal that was exported for a short term	Dog ownership is clear, strong owner attachment, dog likely receives some veterinary care in order to fulfill minimum requirements to cross the border (eg, rabies vaccination certificate)	Owners may not be aware of disease risks in other regions, and may not consult a local veterinarian. May increase likelihood of regionally dependent carriage/infection on entry
Personal pet entering country with owner for first time or reentering after long-term trip	Family moving to country for work bringing the family dog; refugees with pet dog	Dog ownership is clear, strong owner attachment, more likely to provide care if dog is/becomes ill	Long duration or wider variety of potential exposures to diseases in country/region of origin. May increase likelihood of regionally dependent pathogen carriage/infection on entry
Recently adopted pet entering country with owner who is either entering or reentering	Vacationer returning with an adopted street dog; military personnel returning from overseas deployment with an adopted dog	Dog ownership is clear, well-intentioned owner more likely to provide care if dog is/becomes ill	Animal history is typically unknown, dog may have only received cursory veterinary care before importation (eg, to obtain rabies vaccination certificate), dog may be too young for some vaccinations (eg, rabies), vaccination in some countries may be less reliable (eg, poor vaccine quality, cold chain not maintained, falsified certificates)
Animal being imported for a specific commercial purpose (eg, research, breeding, competition, prearranged individual sale)	Purpose-bred specific pathogen–free dogs being imported by a research facility; individual purebred puppy imported for sale to a specific individual (ie, not a retailer)	Dog ownership is clear, high sentimental and/or commercial value, more likely to provide care if dog is/becomes ill, typically increased requirements for entry compared with personal dogs	Importer may not be aware of disease risks in other regions, may be at increased risk of pathogen carriage/infection in competition and breeding dogs because of high exposure to other dogs, or antimicrobial use practices[3]

(continued on next page)

Table 1
(continued)

Reason/Means	Examples	Risk Mitigating Factors	Risk Enhancing Factors
Rescue animal being imported under commercial dog rules (including animals from puppy mills)	Group of dogs arriving with an individual working for a rescue organization	Typically increased requirements for entry compared with personal dogs (eg, import permit, microchip or tattoo, veterinary health certificate, rabies vaccination certificate)	Dog's final owner is unknown, adoptability may be unknown, animal history is typically unknown. Other risks as above, plus typically originating from high-risk facility or area (eg, crowded, suboptimal care/sanitation)
Rescue animal being imported under guise of personal pet (including animals from puppy mills)	Lead rescue individual travels to a foreign country and returns with several dogs at once, claiming them all as personal pets when in fact hoping to adopt them out once in the country	Few to none. High-risk rescue dog imported with the requirements for a low-risk personal dog. Sentimental or commercial value questionable/variable	Dog's final owner is unknown, adoptability may be unknown, animal history is typically unknown, minimal entry requirements (ie, rabies vaccination). Other risks as above
Rescue animal being imported on behalf of owner/adopter who has never seen the dog (including animals from puppy mills)	Dog adopted via an Internet campaign through a rescue organization, brought in by third party to be delivered to new owner in new country	Well-intentioned owner more likely to provide care if dog is/becomes ill, assuming adoption goes through	Unclear how to verify ownership, owner may ultimately decide not to adopt dog after importation. Other risks as above
Personal pet entering country for veterinary care	Dog requiring a highly specialized surgical procedure for which the nearest expertise and equipment is across the border at a referral hospital in an adjacent country (eg, Canada, United States)	Primarily occurs for referral/tertiary care of personal pets, not typically sought for rescue/unadopted animals, dog ownership is clear, being taken directly to a veterinary facility so likely to have limited contact with local dogs	Inherently animals are not healthy. Personnel at referral centers near the border or near major ports of entry need to be particularly aware of risks of imported diseases

Adapted from Report of the Canadian National Canine Importation Working Group. 2016. Available at: https://www.wormsandgermsblog.com/files/2016/06/CIWG-Report-2016-06-09-FINAL-w-Apx.pdf. Accessed October 1, 2018; with permission.

STRESS DURING TRANSPORT

The way in which dogs are transported can also have a significant impact on their susceptibility to disease, pathogen shedding, and overall likelihood of disease transmission before, during, and after transport. Individuals or organizations often import groups of dogs, from a few dogs to several dozen at a time. These animals may come from a single source or multiple sources in the country of origin but be brought together in the same holding area and loaded into the same cargo area of a plane or a truck. Health screening, vaccination, and other preventive medicine measures at this and other stages are highly variable and often unregulated. Even if they are individually caged, the mixing, crowding, potentially poor ventilation, and the inability to adequately control fecal and urinary contamination lead to ideal conditions for transmission of respiratory and gastrointestinal pathogens. On commercial carriers, there is potential for multiple shipments of dogs to be transported on the same vessel, along with individually owned personal animals, and in the event of a disease outbreak it can be extremely difficult to trace back these contacts to determine which animals may be at risk and to alert their owners. There may also be undocumented contact with various individuals throughout the transportation process, which can be dangerously problematic if the animals in question are subsequently diagnosed with a zoonotic disease (eg, rabies). The entire transportation process can also cause both physiologic and psychological stress, particularly on long trips during which dogs may receive marginally adequate to inadequate food, water, and exercise; thermal stress from fluctuating temperatures; and sudden exposure to entirely unfamiliar environments, such as airports, which are often loud and chaotic. In combination, these factors are likely to have an important effect on immune function,[14,15] which may lead to both increased shedding of pathogens already harbored by the dog (clinically and subclinically) and susceptibility to new pathogens. In some cases, these factors also constitute a significant welfare issue, particularly in the case of dogs that are already clinically ill or injured, because appropriate veterinary care typically cannot be provided en route. Furthermore, even after arrival at their final destination, these dogs continue to be stressed by further changes in environment and diet. In most countries there is no regulatory requirement or support for any form of postarrival quarantine, and only a minority of rescue organizations implement such quarantine on a voluntary basis.[13] New owners or caretakers therefore often introduce the animals to other resident dogs soon after arrival at their final destination, in an attempt to begin socializing the new dogs, which presents risks to both the new and resident dogs. Dispersal of groups of dogs to numerous locations further increases the risk of spread of pathogens transmitted within the group during transport.

EXAMPLES OF POTENTIAL IMPACT OF HIGH-RISK DISEASES

The following are examples of specific diseases that are considered high risk with regard to interregional movement and importation of dogs, particularly to North America and much of Europe. This list is not exhaustive, and the relative risk of each disease varies by region based on current disease prevalence, host, vector, and habitat availability. These diseases are used to show how different pathogen characteristics and transmission pathways affect the impact of movement of infected dogs.

Rabies

Because rabies is not transmitted via respiratory secretions or the fecal-oral route as many other common pathogens are, and because the disease is rapidly fatal within a short time from when a dog begins shedding the virus and subsequently develops clinical signs, movement of an infected dog is less likely to have a significant impact on the local epidemiology of rabies in developed or other rabies-endemic countries compared with other canine diseases. Instead, the most significant risk is the potential for human exposure either in transit or on arrival, depending on the time frame of infectivity. Trace-backs of contacts in such cases can often be extremely challenging, because dogs may move through multiple jurisdictions and large public transport hubs, such as airports.[16] From 2001 to 2013, 18 cases of rabies in dogs (and 1 in a kitten) imported from rabies-enzootic countries were reported in western Europe, of which only 2 animals were identified by customs officials and placed under quarantine.[17] For each case, an average of 34 (range, 0–187) persons and other animals required postexposure prophylaxis, and 1 case resulted in infection and the deaths of 2 resident dogs in France.[17]

Regulations requiring animals to be vaccinated for rabies before importation only serve to help protect the dog from infection if it is exposed after arrival. The incubation period for rabies in dogs can exceed 6 months, and a dog that is vaccinated before travel but after exposure may still harbor the virus and go on to develop clinical disease. Six of the 19 rabid animals imported into western Europe from 2001 to 2013 were reportedly vaccinated for rabies, but most of the vaccinated pets did not meet the recommendations for age of vaccination, revaccination interval, or serologic analysis before import.[17]

Importantly, rabies vaccines are only licensed for puppies older than a certain age (2–3 months), but infection can occur before this age and may affect multiple animals within a litter. Rabies infection in puppies is particularly problematic from a public health standpoint because of the potential for dispersal of the puppies to multiple owners and regions, high animal-human contact because of the way in which puppies are often closely and extensively handled by people, and the tendency for young untrained puppies to bite, causing minor wounds that may not be considered significant but can nonetheless potentially transmit rabies.

In 2011 to 2012, nearly 2800 dogs that were unvaccinated for rabies entered the United States and were placed under confinement agreements, which stipulated that contact with humans and other animals must be restricted until they were fully immunized.[4] Most of these were puppies imported for commercial sale or rescue purposes.[4] However, there is often poor compliance with such confinement agreements; more than 4000 confinement agreement violations were recorded in 2006 in the United States.[2] Falsified rabies vaccination certificates (and possibly other health documents required for importation) are also a growing concern.[18]

Canine Influenza

Canine influenza virus (CIV; H3N8 and H3N2) generally causes self-limiting mild to moderate clinical disease in dogs. However, like other influenza A viruses, it is highly transmissible, particularly within naive and high-density populations such as shelters, and can cause serious and even fatal infections in some animals. A single-point introduction of H3N2 CIV from a dog imported from South Korea is suspected to have initiated the 2015 outbreak in the Chicago, Illinois, area and, within a year, H3N2 CIV had spread to multiple eastern and southeastern US states, with smaller isolated outbreaks in other areas of the country.[19] Subsequent significant outbreaks have been identified in California, Nevada, and New York, as well as Ontario, Canada, through the movement of infected dogs from Asia or from other affected states.[20–22] Testing for CIV before movement of dogs is problematic in terms of timing requirements. Viral shedding precedes clinical signs and persists (possibly intermittently) for up to 24 days.[23] Commercially available vaccines can decrease the likelihood and severity of infection but are not 100% effective for preventing infection or active shedding, and products are strain specific. Based on its short incubation period, the most effective means of controlling the risk of CIV in translocated dogs would be quarantine for 48 to 96 hours along with polymerase chain reaction testing to detect shedding in sub-clinically infected dogs, but the potentially significant costs of implementing such precautions must be weighed against the currently limited risk to public and animal health. To date, there is no evidence of dog-to-human transmission of either circulating strain of CIV, but concern regarding the potential for a reassortment event should a dog (or a person) be concurrently infected with both CIV and a human seasonal influenza virus remains.[19]

Echinococcosis

Echinococcus multilocularis (EM) is a parasite of public health significance that can also be carried by domestic dogs. It is widely distributed in the northern hemisphere, including parts of central Europe, most of northern and central Eurasia, and parts of North America, specifically the northern tundra zone and the north central region.[24] In recent decades, the risk areas in Europe and North America seem to have expanded significantly.[24,25] Several European countries require treatment of dogs before importation in order to prevent the introduction of this particular tapeworm.[1] More recently, EM has been identified in southern Ontario, Canada,[26] and could potentially be present but as-yet undetected in adjacent northeastern US states. Its spread in this case was likely primarily through wildlife involved in the tapeworm's sylvatic life cycle (ie, wild canids, rodents), but it is possible that importation of dogs with patent intestinal infections from more endemic areas (eg, central Europe, China) may have also played a role. Strain typing of EM in emerging areas could potentially contribute significantly to the current understanding of the spread of this parasite in some areas.[25] Imported animals harboring intestinal infection with EM are capable of causing significant environmental contamination with parasite eggs, potentially resulting in serious infections in people in the form of alveolar echinococcosis (the intermediate stage of the parasite), and infection of rodents or other small mammals, leading to increased risk of spread to both wild canids and other domestic dogs. Although treatment and control of EM in dogs with intestinal infection is straightforward and effective, once the wildlife cycle is established it becomes essentially impossible to eradicate, resulting in ongoing risk to domestic dogs and a significant public health risk, particularly in densely populated regions.[24]

Leishmaniasis

Leishmania infantum is endemic to the Mediterranean basin, the Middle East, southern Asia, Iran, Armenia, Afghanistan, and central Asia; *Leishmania chagasi* is endemic in Central and South America, and *Leishmania mexicana* is endemic to parts of south-central Texas.[27] Although there is some potential for direct transmission of these protozoa between dogs and humans via direct contact with cutaneous lesions or other infected tissues, the parasite is normally transmitted by certain phlebotomine sandflies (*Lutzomyia* or *Phlebotomus* spp). In areas where no known competent vector is thought to exist, the risk of transmission to other animals and people should be limited, but there is always a risk that an infected dog may encounter an as-yet unknown competent vector. Subsequent spread to other susceptible hosts, including wildlife, can rapidly lead to establishment of a sylvatic cycle, after which eradication is essentially impossible. Furthermore, treatment of infected dogs, even with long-term antimicrobials, is generally ineffective at eliminating the infection; therefore, dogs are lifelong carriers and reservoirs of infection. Despite the lack of a known competent vector species in the eastern United States and Canada, in 1999 there was a large outbreak of visceral leishmaniasis in foxhounds in New York. A subsequent serosurvey showed that canine visceral leishmaniasis was enzootic in foxhounds specifically in 18 US states and 2 Canadian provinces (Ontario, Nova Scotia).[28] The range of *Lutzomyia shannoni* sandflies overlapped with many of the affected hunt clubs along the east coast,[28] and it was later discovered that *Lutzomyia vexator* were widespread in the New York area, but it is unknown whether they played a role in local transmission,[29] and no evidence of human infection was identified.[28] It is highly likely that the importation of infected dogs from other endemic regions was involved in the early stages of the outbreak,[27] and infection was then propagated through direct transmission between dogs within specific breed groups, via contact such as bites, breeding, needle reuse, and vertical transmission.[28]

Heartworm

When imported into nonendemic or low-endemic areas, dogs infected by heartworm (*Dirofilaria immitis*) pose a significant threat to local dogs. Unlike a pathogen such as *Leishmania* spp that requires a specific insect vector, or tick-borne pathogens of which dogs are end hosts and therefore cannot infect other tick vectors, competent mosquito vectors for *D immitis* are widespread and can easily acquire the parasite from a microfilaremic dog and transmit it to others. In 2005, thousands of dogs were dispersed from the Gulf coast to other areas of the United States and Canada following Hurricane Katrina, and one study showed 48.8% of these animals were heartworm antigen positive.[5] Many of the locations to which these dogs were transported throughout the United States and Canada had low prevalences of *D immitis* in the mosquito and dog populations. The ultimate effects of such movement on *D immitis* risk are unquantified. A similar exodus of dogs from high-risk southern US states occurred in 2017 following Hurricane Harvey and Hurricane Irma.[6,7] Wild canids such as coyotes can also be infected and thus establish a wildlife reservoir that is nearly impossible to eradicate; in endemic areas of North America, coyotes are considered likely to be the most important heartworm reservoirs.[30] Testing for heartworm is simple and noninvasive, but the long incubation period of the parasite poses an additional challenge, necessitating testing of dogs before transport and also at 6 to 12 months following relocation, depending on documentation of preventive treatment, in order to ensure they are free from infection.[31]

Screwworm

New-world and old-world screwworm (*Cochliomyia hominivorax* and *Chrysomyia bezziana*, respectively) can have significant trade implications for some countries, primarily because of their potential to affect livestock. The larvae can infect any warm-blooded or cold-blooded animal, but mammals are most commonly affected. Although the flies cannot complete their life cycle when the soil temperature is consistently less than 8°C,[32] climate change may increase their potential range. Eradication of screwworm from the southern United States, Mexico, and most of Central America required the development and release of sterile male flies, in addition to control of animal movements.[32] During a subsequent incursion in 2016 in the Florida Keys, which included 3 confirmed canine infections, checkpoints were established at which all people and animals (including dogs) had to be verified as free of suspicious lesions, in order to prevent further spread of the parasite to the mainland.[33] That particular outbreak severely threatened the survival of the endangered key deer, many of which became infected.[33] Although the source of the incursion was never definitively determined, the outbreak shows the potential effects of any infected animal, including a dog, traveling to an area with a suitable climate to complete the insect's life cycle. Fortunately, lesions associated with infection are typically readily visible, and diagnosis and treatment are usually straightforward once the larvae are found.

Ticks and Tick-Borne Diseases

The role of translocated dogs in the spread of ticks and tick-borne diseases is fairly small compared with the effect of climate change on the expansion of suitable tick habitats[34,35] and the natural migration of ticks into these areas via wildlife hosts such as migratory birds, which may disperse hundreds of millions of ticks across vast geographic areas annually.[36] However, recognition of tick-borne diseases in dogs that have been transported from high-endemic to low-endemic regions is a concern,[37] particularly because early clinical signs of infection can be nonspecific, and local veterinary practitioners may not be aware of the need to consider such pathogens in their differential diagnoses. Even when they are considered, testing can be problematic because most readily available serologic tests cannot differentiate active infection from previous exposure. There is also risk of zoonotic transmission of pathogens to owners or veterinary personnel who attempt to remove infected ticks from dogs, should the tick be accidently crushed in the process.[38]

Adventitial ticks on imported dogs are generally of limited concern in terms of their ability to establish new tick populations or to spread infection by subsequently attaching to a new host, but there are exceptions. *Rhipicephalus sanguineus* (brown dog tick) is already one of the most widely distributed ticks in the world but is also a vector of *Ehrlichia canis*, *Babesia canis*, *Anaplasma platys*, and several rickettsial species, including *Rickettsia rickettsii*.[37] Unlike most other ticks, it is capable of completing its entire life cycle indoors (and on 1 host), thus infected ticks on an imported dog can pose a risk to other dogs living on or visiting the premises (eg, kennel, shelter, veterinary clinic). *Haemaphysalis longicornis* (longhorned tick) was recently found in the northeastern United States.[39] Although primarily considered a livestock pest in east Asia, Australia, and New Zealand, the tick feeds on a variety of hosts, including humans and dogs.[37,39] Its ability to transmit pathogens of concern in North America remains unclear, but specimens infected with *Borrelia* spp, *Ehrlichia* spp, *Anaplasma* spp, and *Rickettsia* spp have been found in Asia.[39] This tick has also been implicated in the transmission of a bunyavirus, associated with severe fever with thrombocytopenia syndrome.[39] One of the risks associated with *H longicornis* is related to its unusual ability to reproduce by parthenogenesis; that is, females can reproduce without mating.[39] This ability facilitates the establishment of an invasive population even if only a small number of ticks, or even a single tick, is translocated on a dog or other animal or person. Prompt removal of ticks on such individuals, either immediately after or ideally before transport, therefore remains prudent.

Reproductive Diseases

Purebred animals with highly desirable genetics may be transported long distances, even transcontinentally, for breeding. There can also be substantial movement of breeding stock between large, high-volume breeding kennels,[40] which may be associated with far less medical scrutiny based on lower value of individual animals. Imported rescue dogs are also often sexually intact, particularly when they come from regions where the availability of veterinary services is limited, and then they may or may not be spayed or neutered on arrival at their final destinations. Breeding animals are at a higher risk for spreading specific reproductive diseases. Infected breeding sires in particular have the potential to be point sources of disease by breeding with multiple bitches. Canine brucellosis, caused by *Brucella canis*, can be transmitted during mating and is also a zoonotic concern. This bacterium is thought to be an under-recognized pathogen in dogs and humans worldwide, but few countries have *B canis*–specific regulations.[41] Outbreaks in breeding kennels in several countries have been linked to interregional movement and importation of dogs from these types of facilities and are a significant source of economic loss in breeding facilities in the United States.[40,41] Canine transmissible venereal tumor (CTVT) is spread by transfer of living cancer cells during copulation. It is endemic in at least 90 countries worldwide, and is associated with free-roaming intact dogs.[42] Although its prevalence has significantly decreased in northern Europe, in the United States and Australia, the disease remains endemic in remote indigenous communities.[42] Some of these populations of free-roaming dogs may be targeted by individuals or organizations hoping to relocate the animals, increasing the risk of spread of CTVT to other areas. Although CTVT is also a risk with the movement of intact dogs, unlike *B canis*, it can be easily and effectively diagnosed and treated in most cases if these measures are performed promptly.[43]

Vaccine-Preventable Diseases

Exposure to vaccine-preventable diseases from translocated dogs is a common risk that tends to attract far less attention than exposure to higher-profile exotic or zoonotic diseases. These diseases include, but are not limited to, canine distemper virus (CDV), canine parvovirus (CPV), and pathogens comprising the canine infectious respiratory disease complex. Rescued dogs that may have previously received little to no veterinary care, perhaps coming from or transported under high-density conditions, are at particularly high risk. Although few published reports are available, CDV is likely the single largest cause of import-associated illness and mortality in dogs, through both acute disease that develops after arrival and, perhaps more importantly, severe neurologic disease that may only develop later in dogs that were clinically normal on arrival. Transmission of CDV from imported dogs to housemates has (anecdotally) also occurred on numerous occasions. One study of a shipment of 15 rescue dogs imported from Hungary to Switzerland reported that 85% of the dogs had active CDV infection, despite all dogs having been vaccinated 7 to 30 days before import.[44] Shedding persisted for up to 4 months in at least 2 dogs, but none of the resident in-contact dogs (all of which had been vaccinated for CDV at least once in the past) developed clinical signs of infection.[44] The estimated vaccination rate for CDV in dogs in Switzerland is 60% to 70%, which is inadequate to provide population immunity, and leaves a substantial number of individual dogs unprotected in case of exposure.[44] Companion animal vaccination rates in other regions are largely unknown but are likely to be similar or lower.

SUMMARY

Many of the drivers of canine movement stem from a strong human-animal bond and a desire to alleviate animal suffering. However, the individuals and organizations involved often do not realize the variable risk of disease transmission associated with many of these scenarios, and thus the potential greater long-term impact of their actions beyond the individual dogs. For many of the diseases discussed here, the implementation of mandatory screening or testing programs before interregional movement or importation of dogs is not feasible because of a plethora of economic, practical, and political reasons.[1] Education of stakeholders, including the public, rescue organizations, shelters, transportation companies, and veterinarians, to raise awareness of these diseases, and the potential consequences of translocation events via the movement of dogs, needs to be a priority. Those motivated by a genuine desire to do the right thing are likely to be the most receptive to information and guidance about how to mitigate disease risks associated with the long-distance movement of dogs. Those involved in the industry purely for profit are more likely to only respond to requirements imposed on them by others, including recipients, transporters, and various levels of government. As the world becomes "smaller" and long-distance travel becomes faster and easier for both people and animals alike, it is critical that all stakeholders involved in the movement of dogs do their part to help mitigate these disease risks.

REFERENCES

1. Anderson MEC, Bourque T, Douma D, et al. Report of the Canadian National Canine Importation Working Group. 2016. Available at: https://www.wormsandgermsblog.com/files/2016/06/CIWG-Report-2016-06-09-FINAL-w-Apx.pdf. Accessed October 1, 2018.
2. McQuiston JH, Wilson T, Harris S, et al. Importation of dogs into the United States: Risks from rabies and other zoonotic diseases. Zoonoses Public Health 2008;55: 421–6.
3. Dendoncker PA, Moons C, Sarrazin S, et al. Biosecurity and management practices in different dog breeding systems have considerable margin for improvements. Vet Rec 2018;183:381.
4. Sinclair JR, Washburn F, Fox S, et al. Dogs entering the United States from rabies-endemic countries, 2011-2012. Zoonoses Public Health 2015;62:393–400.
5. Levy JK, Lappin MR, Glaser AL, et al. Prevalence of infectious diseases in cats and dogs rescued following Hurricane Katrina. J Am Vet Med Assoc 2011;238: 311–7.
6. Drake J, Wiseman S. Increasing incidence of Dirofilaria immitis in dogs in USA with focus on the southeast region 2013–2016. Parasit Vectors 2018;11:39.
7. American Heartworm Society. Heartworm Incidence Maps 2001-2016. Available at: https://www.heartwormsociety.org/veterinary-resources/incidence-maps. Accessed October 1, 2018.
8. Deluca AN. Rescued Sochi dogs adjusting to an American life. National Geographic. 2014. Available at: https://news.nationalgeographic.com/news/2014/10/141003-dogs-rescued-sochi-extermination-family/. Accessed October 1, 2018.
9. World Animal Protection. Olympic gold medalists support animals rescued at Rio 2016. 2016. Available at: https://www.worldanimalprotection.ca/news/olympic-gold-medallists-support-animals-rescued-rio-2016. Accessed October 1, 2018.
10. Fiest R. Canadians rescuing animals from South Korean dog meat farms. Global News 2018. Available at: https://globalnews.ca/news/4024624/dog-meat-farms-south-korea-rescue/. Accessed October 1, 2018.
11. CTV News Montreal. 70 dogs rescued, 4 dead in suspected Quebec puppy mill. 2017. Available at: https://www.ctvnews.ca/canada/70-dogs-rescued-4-dead-in-suspected-quebec-puppy-mill-1.3629308. Accessed October 1, 2018.
12. Chicago Tribune. Puppy laundering in Chicago. Editorial. 2018. Available at: http://www.chicagotribune.com/news/opinion/editorials/ct-edit-puppy-mills-chicago-rescue-20180529-story.html#. Accessed October 1, 2018.
13. Simmons KE, Hoffman CL. Dogs on the move: Factors impacting animal shelter and rescue Organizations' decisions to accept dogs from distant locations. Animals (Basel) 2016;6 [pii:E11].

14. Hekman JP, Karas AZ, Sharp CR. Psychogenic stress in hospitalized dogs: Cross species comparisons, implications for health care, and the challenges of evaluation. Animals (Basel) 2014;4(2):331–47.
15. Protopopova A. Effects of sheltering on physiology, immune function, behavior, and the welfare of dogs. Physiol Behav 2016;159:95–103.
16. Curry PS, Kostiuk D, Werker DH, et al. Translocated dogs from Nunavut and the spread of rabies. Can Commun Dis Rep 2016;42:121–4.
17. Ribadeau-Dumas F, Cliquet F, Gautret P, et al. Travel-associated rabies in pets and residual rabies risk, western Europe. Emerg Infect Dis 2016;22:1268–71.
18. Sinclair JR, Wallace RM, Gruszynski K, et al. Rabies in a dog imported from Egypt with a falsified rabies vaccination certificate: Virginia, 2015. MMWR Morb Mortal Wkly Rep 2015;64:1359–62.
19. Voorhees I, Glaser AL, Toohey-Kurth KL, et al. Spread of canine influenza A (H3N2) virus, United States. Emerg Infect Dis 2017;23:1950–7.
20. Canine Influenza Virus Surveillance Network. H3N2 test results from March 2015 to present. Available at: https://ahdc.vet.cornell.edu/news/civchicago.cfm. Accessed October 1, 2018.
21. Weese JS. Canine influenza: Ontario. In: Worms & Germs Blog. 2018. Available at: https://www.wormsandgermsblog.com/2018/01/articles/animals/dogs/canine-influenza-ontario/. Accessed October 1, 2018.
22. Weese JS. Update: canine influenza, US and Canada (May 2018). In: Worms & Germs Blog. 2018. Available at: https://www.wormsandgermsblog.com/2018/05/articles/animals/dogs/canine-influenza-update-us-and-canada-march-18-2018/. Accessed October 1, 2018.
23. Newbury S, Godhardt-Cooper J, Poulsen KP, et al. Prolonged intermittent virus shedding during an outbreak of canine influenza A H3N2 virus infection in dogs in three Chicago area shelters: 16 cases (March to May 2015). J Am Vet Med Assoc 2016;248:1022–6.
24. Eckert J, Deplazes P. Biological, epidemiological, and clinical aspects of echinococcosis, a zoonosis of increasing concern. Clin Microbiol Rev 2004;17:107–35.
25. Massolo A, Liccioli S, Budke C, et al. *Echinococcus multilocularis* in North America: the great unknown. Parasite 2014;21:73.
26. Kotwa J, Jardine C, Isaksson M, et al. Prevalence and geographic distribution of Echinococcus multilocularis in wild canids across southern Ontario, Canada. In: Proceedings of the 26th International Conference of the World Association for the Advancement of Veterinary Parasitology. Kuala Lumpur, Malaysia, September 4–8, 2017. abstract #4742. 2017.
27. Petersen CA. Leishmaniasis, an emerging disease found in companion animals in the United States. Top Companion Anim Med 2009;24:182–8.
28. Duprey ZH, Steurer FJ, Rooney JA, et al. Canine visceral leishmaniasis, United States and Canada, 2000–2003. Emerg Infect Dis 2006;12:440–6.
29. Ostfeld RS, Roy P, Haumaier W, et al. Sand fly (*Lutzomyia vexator*) (Diptera: Psychodidae) populations in upstate New York: abundance, microhabitat, and phenology. J Med Entomol 2004;41:774–8.
30. Brown HE, Harrington LC, Kaufman PE, et al. Key factors influencing canine heartworm, *Dirofilaria immitis*, in the United States. Parasit Vectors 2012;5:245.
31. American Heartworm Society. Current canine guidelines for the prevention, management, and diagnosis of heartworm infection in dogs. 2014. Available at: https://www.heartwormsociety.org/images/pdf/2014-AHS-Canine-Guidelines.pdf. Accessed October 1, 2018.

32. Screwworm. In: Spickler AR, Roth JA, Galyon J, et al, editors. Emerging and exotic diseases of animals. 4th edition. Ames (IA): Iowa State University, College of Veterinary Medicine; 2010. p. 271–3.
33. United States Department of Agriculture – Animal and Plant Health Inspection Service. New World Screwworm. 2018. Available at: https://www.aphis. usda.gov/aphis/ourfocus/animalhealth/animal-disease-information/cattle-disease-information/nws/new-world-screwworm. Accessed October 1, 2018.
34. Bouchard C, Leonard E, Koffi JK, et al. The increasing risk of Lyme disease in Canada. Can Vet J 2015;56:693–9.
35. Jaenson TG, Lindgren E. The range of *Ixodes ricinus* and the risk of contracting Lyme borreliosis will increase northwards when the vegetation period becomes longer. Ticks Tick Borne Dis 2011;2(1):44–9.
36. Ogden NH, Lindsay LR, Hanincová K, et al. Role of migratory birds in introduction and range expansion of *Ixodes scapularis* ticks and of *Borrelia burgdorferi* and *Anaplasma phagocytophilum* in Canada. Appl Environ Microbiol 2008;74: 1780–90.
37. Chomel B. Tick-borne infections in dogs-an emerging infectious threat. Vet Parasitol 2011;179:294–301.
38. Parola P, Raoult D. Ticks and tickborne bacterial diseases in humans: an emerging infectious threat. Clin Infect Dis 2001;32:897–928.
39. Rainey T, Occi JL, Robbins RG, et al. Discovery of *Haemaphysalis longicornis* (Ixodida: Ixodidae) parasitizing a sheep in New Jersey, United States. J Med Entomol 2018;55:757–9.
40. Brower A, Okwumabua O, Massengill C, et al. Investigation of the spread of *Brucella canis* via the U.S. interstate dog trade. Int J Infect Dis 2007;11:454–8.
41. Hensel ME, Negron M, Arenas-Gamboa AM. Brucellosis in dogs and public health risk. Emerg Infect Dis 2018;24:1401–6.
42. Strakova A, Murchison EP. The changing global distribution and prevalence of canine transmissible venereal tumour. BMC Vet Res 2014;10:168.
43. Ganguly B, Das U, Das AK. Canine transmissible venereal tumour: a review. Vet Comp Oncol 2016;14:1–12.
44. Willi B, Spiri AM, Meli ML, et al. Clinical and molecular investigation of a canine distemper outbreak and vector-borne infections in a group of rescue dogs imported from Hungary to Switzerland. BMC Vet Res 2015;11:154.

Rabies

Current Preventive Strategies

Susan M. Moore, PhD, MS, BS, HCLD(ABB), MT(ASCP)SBB

KEYWORDS

- Rabies • Serology • Diagnostics • Disease surveillance • Vaccination

KEY POINTS

- Rabies control regulations have provided effective protection to humans and pets; however, in some areas the lack of updates in response to evolving risk situations occurs.
- Pet owner concerns about vaccination have led to the consideration of alterative vaccine schedules.
- Use of rabies serology in lieu of current recommended booster vaccination, while supported by studies, remains problematic.

INTRODUCTION

As difficult as it is to imagine, the presence of rabid dogs in cities and the countryside was of great concern after World War II in the United States.[1] The urgency of the problem led to the creation of the National Rabies Program, which began operations in 1947. The program consisted of 3 main pillars: (1) education, (2) dog control, and (3) vaccination. Relatively quickly, control of urban rabies epizootics was achieved by the early 1950s.[2] This same program was endorsed by the World Health Organization (WHO)[3] and resulted in successful rabies control programs in places such as Taiwan, Malaya, and Hong Kong. As early as 1983, the idea of a world rabies program was discussed by the WHO, including the cost of such a large endeavor.[4] Thirty-two years later, in 2015, after years of separate efforts by veterinary health and human health organizations, a joint declaration to eliminate human deaths caused by dog-mediated rabies by the year 2030 was made by WHO, the World Organization for Animal Health (OIE), the Food and Agriculture Organization of the United Nations, and the Global Alliance for Rabies Control.[5] The time to invest in ending human rabies death had arrived: rabies is a model infectious disease for the One Health approach; several pilot efforts at dog rabies control have provided proof of concept; and the United Nation's sustainable development Goal Three targets ending epidemics of neglected tropical diseases (of which rabies is one) by 2030. Using a blueprint for each country that essentially

The author has nothing to disclose.
Veterinary Diagnostic Laboratory, Kansas State University, Manhattan, KS 66502, USA
E-mail address: smoore@vet.k-state.edu

mimics the early 3-pillar plan of education, dog control, and vaccination, the effort is in place.[6] In countries and regions that have achieved and sustained rabies control in dogs, epizootics of rabies involving other animals have become the focus. This does not mean the National Rabies Program is ended; it expands to include control of wildlife rabies, constant surveillance, and strict import regulations. Education, dog control, and vaccination is still needed to protect human from rabies exposure. The basic components of rabies control are as follows:

- Vaccinate pets: 70% vaccine coverage is the minimum required.
- Have policies and protocols for treatment of exposed pets and livestock.
- Have policies and procedures for animals that bite humans.
- Provide rabies diagnostic testing.
- Provide preexposure and postexposure vaccination for humans.
- Provide education and training for bite prevention, rabies exposure prevention, and rabies prophylaxis.
- Control stray dog and cat populations.
- Perform surveillance for rabies and maintain current epidemiology maps and information.
- Control rabies in wildlife.

LEGAL AND REGULATORY CONTROL

As a global model One Health infectious disease, rabies control and prevention is guided by the WHO and the OIE.[7,8] In the United States, the Compendium for Animal Rabies Control and Prevention, which contains recommendations of the National Association of State Public Health Veterinarians, is updated regularly by consideration of new/current data on rabies epidemiology, vaccines, and knowledge of the disease. For example, in 2016 the Compendium was updated to allow postexposure management of dogs, cats, and ferrets that were previously rabies-vaccinated but out of date, the same as currently vaccinated pets (**Table 1**).[9] This change was in response to a study that demonstrated there was no significant difference in the antibody response to booster vaccination in currently vaccinated and out-of-date pets.[10]

Unfortunately, state and local laws and regulations, for which the Compendium recommendations act as a guide, are not always reviewed and updated in a timely

Table 1		
Recommendations of the National Association of State Public Health Veterinarians for rabies postexposure management of dogs and cats based on their vaccination status from the 2016 of the Compendium for Animals Rabies Control and Prevention guidelines		
Vaccination Status	Type of Confinement	Vaccinate
Current	Observation/Owner's control for 45 d	Booster
Never vaccinated	A. None: euthanize	NA
	B. 4 mo strict quarantine: dogs and cats 6 mo strict quarantine: ferrets	Vaccinate (<96 h) Vaccinate (<96 h)
Out of date/ documented	Observation/Owner's control for 45 d	Booster
Out of date/ undocumented	A. None: euthanize	NA
	B. 4 mo strict quarantine: dogs and cats	Vaccinate (<96 h)
	C. Observation/Owner's control for 45 d[a]	Booster

[a] Provided serologic proof of prior rabies vaccination is obtained.

manner. This results in differing regulations between states as well as within states. Certainly, there can be valid reasons for differences based on epidemiology, populations, resources, and other variables. However, if rabies regulations and laws have not been reviewed and updated in years, it is likely there are regulations outside current best practices in place. As rabies surveillance data, data from exposure and quarantine practices, vaccination rates, and evaluation of the response to vaccination are analyzed, further updates to laws and regulations are expected.

ASSESSING THE RISK OF RABIES

Every year the rabies case data are analyzed and reported by the Rabies Section at the Centers for Disease Control and Prevention in the *Journal of the American Veterinary Medical Association*.[11] This information has been used to track and illustrate trends in the spread of rabies variants. Rabies variants are viral strains that circulate in reservoir species to which the virus has adapted. Vector species are mammals that are susceptible to rabies infection and are able to infect other susceptible individuals. Rabies is an RNA virus, making it susceptible to mutation and thus adaption into vector species; surveillance is meant to identify such events. An example of rabies virus cross-species transmission occurred when positive rabies cases in skunks were reported in an area of Arizona in which skunk strain of rabies had not previously been identified.[12] Viral sequencing of the positive cases determined the variant had passed from bats in the area and adapted to skunks. This demonstrates that just because an area is free of terrestrial rabies, it is not absolutely free of the risk of rabies exposure to pets and domestic animals, and hence humans. Another point to consider when assessing rabies risk in an area or region, is the "discovery" of rabies in the ferret badger population in Taiwan. Taiwan was believed to be rabies-free since 1961.[13] Further study determined that rabies had been circulating in this population for years.[14] Poor surveillance for rabies can create this peril by not being aware of or controlling rabies exposures from reservoir species. Both examples illustrate the key point that rabies control measures, including education and surveillance, must be sufficient and sustainable. In the Americas, all rabies variants are within the classic rabies lyssavirus species. However, companion animals travel with their owners, sometimes to areas of the world in which other lyssavirus species are present. Rabies vaccine covers many of the other lyssavirus species in phylogroup I, but those in phylogroups II and III are not.[15]

PREVENTING INTRODUCTION INTO RABIES-FREE AREAS

Pet owners have come to view their pets as family members, so much so that pet travel is a thriving industry. When pets travel from rabies-endemic areas into rabies-free areas, it is of primary importance that they are not incubating rabies, thereby risking the introduction of rabies into a susceptible population. The incubation period for rabies in dogs and cats is reported to be approximately 4 months.[9] In the past, pets traveling or moving to rabies-free areas were subjected to long quarantines periods, established (in consideration of the incubation period) to ensure the pet was not incubating rabies. Starting in the 1990s, rabies-free areas instituted the use of rabies serology as a surrogate for protection. A defined concentration (level) of rabies virus neutralizing antibodies (RVNA), typically 0.5 IU/mL, demonstrates proof of adequate response to rabies vaccination. Once adequate vaccine response is established, a defined waiting period to account for a prevaccination infection and incubation must be achieved before the pet can enter the rabies-free area. This procedure was initiated by Hawaii in 1997 and now many rabies-free areas use similar procedures.[16]

POSTVACCINATION SEROLOGY

Studies analyzing rabies antibody level data from pets have provided information about the immune response to rabies vaccination in dogs and cats, by age, size, and number of vaccines and timing of vaccination.[17–21] The major factors correlated with a robust rabies vaccine response are vaccination after maternal antibody has declined, small size, more than 1 vaccination, and time interval between vaccination and blood draw of 15 to 30 days. Evidence from previous studies has indicated that type of vaccine (multivalent vs monovalent, and manufacturer) can also play a role.[17,18] Rabies serology results from The Kansas State University (KSU) Rabies Laboratory from June 2015 to July 2017 were used to evaluate factors affecting RVNA levels in dogs. Evaluation of RVNA levels from 2 groups of pet dogs, that is, dogs being prepared to travel to rabies-free areas (export group) and dogs whose owners prefer to check rabies titer rather than revaccinate (core vaccine group), demonstrated that timing of blood sampling influences the probability that the pet was adequately vaccinated (**Fig. 1**). In the export group, pet owners and their veterinarians were highly motivated to test at the expected time interval to coincide with the peak response (15–30 days after vaccination). In this group, only 4.5% of the dogs had a result less than 0.5 IU/mL, compared with 16.1% of in the core vaccine group. The proportion of dogs with inadequate rabies antibody levels in the core vaccine group was similar to the proportion of dogs with nonprotective antibody levels to other core vaccines, at 18%, 13%, and 14% for canine distemper, canine adenovirus, and canine parvovirus, respectively.

A repeated observation in these studies is the higher probability of failure to mount or sustain a robust RVNA response in young animals. The presence of maternal antibodies has been identified as one reason for this finding, due to interference by maternally derived rabies with vaccine antigen presentation to the immune system.[22,23] However, the decline of the primary humoral immune response to below detectable levels before 6 months of age is also a factor. Both duration and magnitude of response is affected by the number of vaccinations administered.[20] The influence of age on the probability of inadequate response to rabies vaccination is consistent, even when data are stratified by dog size. Results of rabies serology testing of 20,447 dogs being prepared for travel to rabies-free areas, performed at KSU Rabies Laboratory from July 2016 to April 2017, demonstrated the influence of age by breed size (**Fig. 2**). Breed size was defined by American Kennel Club standards. The largest group that failed to respond to vaccination was younger than 2 years (48.5% <2 years of age; 29.0% 1–2 years of age; 19.5% <1 year of age). These findings, combined with a positive correlation between increase in antibody level and probability of survival in

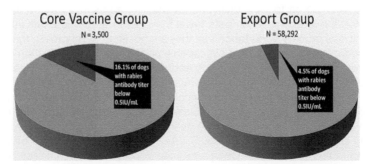

Fig. 1. Proportion of dogs having antibody titer check for core vaccine response compared with dogs being prepared for export to rabies-free areas. Rabies serology for RVNA performed at KSU from June 2015 to July 2017.

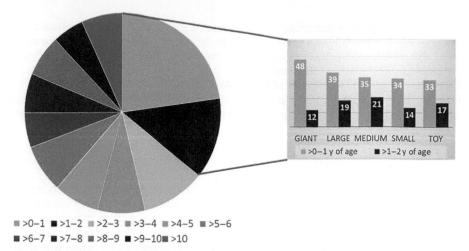

■ >0–1 ■ >1–2 ■ >2–3 ■ >3–4 ■ >4–5 ■ >5–6
■ >6–7 ■ >7–8 ■ >8–9 ■ >9–10■ >10

Fig. 2. Percentage of dogs with inadequate rabies vaccine response by age (in years) and breed size group, from a data set of 20,447 dogs tested for rabies antibody at KSU from July 2016 to April 2017.

challenge studies,[24] has brought into question the practice of waiting until 1 year of age to give the first booster vaccination. Because we know that pets younger than 1 year are at increased risk of an inadequate response to vaccination, providing a booster vaccination at 6 months of age could be considered for pets at increased risk of rabies exposure.

VACCINATION CONCERNS BY PET OWNERS AND VETERINARIANS

Rabies control in the United States has been so effective that the canine variant was eliminated from the United States in 2007.[25] This achievement is also a challenge for maintaining a sufficient level of awareness of the continued risk of rabies exposure, particularly lowering awareness of the importance of rabies vaccination by pet owners. In addition, an increasing focus on the human-animal bond has changed how pet vaccination is evaluated and consequently, is either valued or questioned. Concerns regarding adverse reactions and immune modulation caused by vaccination have increased among pet owners and some veterinarians, who have suggested the use of smaller doses of rabies vaccine to potentially reduce reaction rates, and using rabies serology to provide proof of immunity and thus waive routine booster vaccinations. The frequency of reactions to rabies vaccines has been evaluated by industry groups and organizations. The following are potential vaccine adverse reactions in dogs and cats according to the American Animal Hospital Association Canine Vaccine Guidelines, 2017[26] and the American Association of Feline Practitioners, Feline Vaccination Advisory Panel Report, 2013,[27] respectively:

- Injection-site reactions
- Allergic or immune-mediated reactions
- Tumorigenesis
- Vaccine-induced immunosuppression
- Anaphylaxis
- Injection-site sarcomas

A 2007 study of approximately 1.2 million dogs whose medical records were in a large veterinary database reported that the rate of vaccine-associated adverse events

(VAAE) within 3 days of vaccination in dogs was 38.2 of 10,000 dogs vaccinated.[28] A study of VAAE within 30 days of vaccination in almost 500,000 cats in the same database and performed by the same group reported a VAAE rate of 51.6 of 10,000 cats vaccinated; 92.0% were diagnosed within 3 days after vaccination. Anaphylaxis comprised 17 of 2560 total cases of feline VAAE (0.7%).[29] These organizations recognize that adverse reactions are likely to be underreported by both veterinarians and pet owners[27] and that in veterinary medicine there is no requirement to report VAAE, either known or suspected.[26]

RABIES VACCINE REGIMENS

Fear of vaccine adverse reaction/immune modulation or questioning the need for vaccination among pet owners parallels the similar concerns for human vaccination that has existed for many decades. It may be useful to compare rabies vaccines and vaccine regimens for humans and pets for perspective. For humans who are at increased risk of rabies exposure and thus rabies preexposure vaccinated with a series of 3 vaccinations,[30] 2 booster vaccines are given at day 0 and day 3 on exposure, regardless of titer. Titer does not affect the recommendations for people because it is absolutely necessary to stimulate an anamnestic response. This is to ensure (1) the highest level of RVNA is present to neutralize the virus; and (2) that other immune system components are stimulated (T memory cells), to help with B-cell antibody production and cytokine responses, which alert immune effectors to the threat. For animals that are preexposure vaccinated, after a known or suspected rabies exposure, regardless of titer, a single booster vaccine is given on day 0 (or as soon as seen by a veterinarian), for the same reasons as stated previously. One vaccine booster is administered rather than 2, because to ensure effective prevention in humans for a fatal disease such as rabies, no risk of understimulating the anamnestic response is tolerated. However, for animals, protection from rabies is intended to prevent rabies exposure to humans; thus, different standards, different regimens/policies are applied. Humans who have had preexposure vaccination and continue to be at risk of rabies exposure due to occupation or travel are recommended by the Advisory Committee on Immunization Practices (ACIP) and WHO to have routine titer checks to ensure an adequate level exists to ensure a fast, robust rise in immune defenses on postexposure vaccinations, and to protect from unrecognized exposures.[7,31] In addition, humans who have been preexposure vaccinated are informed to recognize rabies exposure and to seek postexposure treatment, including wound care, which alone can reduce the chance of infection by up to 60%,[32,33] whereas pets cannot. Although rare, vaccinated pets have succumbed to rabies after exposure to rabid animals.[34,35]

The dose of human rabies vaccine used is related to the antigenic content and the route. Human rabies vaccines must provide 2.5 IU antigen by intramuscular (IM) injection, whether in 1 mL or in 0.5 mL of diluent. An intradermal (ID) dose uses a tenth of the antigen in an IM dose and can be given for preexposure and postexposure rabies vaccination. Although ID rabies vaccination is not approved in the United States, it is recognized by the WHO. Some rabies ID regimens require multiple ID injections per day at different sites on the body.[7] Horses, cows, and pigs typically receive a 2-mL dose, and dogs and cats, 1 mL; the entire list of US-approved veterinary vaccines are listed in Compendium for Animals Rabies Control and Prevention.[9] As with human vaccines, all rabies vaccines must meet minimum standards for safety, efficacy, and immunogenicity. The Code of Federal Regulations (CFR) defines standard requirements for both human and animal vaccines.[36]

THE IMMUNE RESPONSE TO RABIES VACCINATION

Vaccines must contain sufficient antigen to induce an adequate immune response in the target species that affords protection from infection, disease, or in some cases, reduction in severity of disease. Vaccines induce immune responses based on amount of antigen and the corresponding immune cell receptor availability and degree of specificity (including avidity and affinity). Receptor specificity is controlled by the major histocompatibility complex (MHC), which is polygenic, meaning there is a great diversity of MHC genes and hence molecules within a species. MHC molecules on the surface of immune cells take up, process, and present antigen to immune cells for the induction immune response. Alongside the diversity of immunity induced by MHC molecules, there is variation between animals in a population in terms of protective response. A vaccine must show the ability to produce a robust and protective immune response among representative animals of the intended species. The notion that size of animal is the major factor in vaccine response, with larger animals mounting a lower response than smaller animals for a defined antigenic dose, or that smaller animals require a smaller dose is prevalent among those who fear the effects of vaccination. The role of immune genetics and mechanisms of the immune response, as described previously, argues against this. Moreover, further analysis of the KSU study of the canine RVNA response (see **Fig. 2**), by breed and by size, indicated that breed also influences the probability of mounting an adequate RVNA response to vaccination (**Fig. 3**). In both the 10 breeds with the highest percentage of dogs with inadequate RVNA (<0.5 IU/mL), and the 10 breeds with the lowest percentage of dogs with inadequate RVNA, small, medium, and large breeds were represented. However, in the group with the lowest percentage of inadequate RVNA, there were 3 large breeds

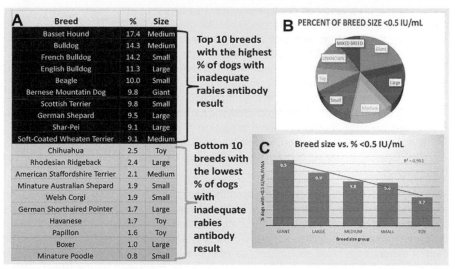

Fig. 3. (A) Ranking of dog breeds by percentage of dogs with inadequate rabies vaccine response into the 10 breeds with the highest and the 10 breeds with the lowest percentage. (B) Pie chart displaying the percentage distribution of breed size groups with inadequate rabies vaccine response within the entire data set of dogs. (C) Bar chart displaying the percentage of dogs in each breed size group with inadequate rabies vaccine response. All data are from a data set of 20,447 dogs tested for rabies antibody at KSU from July 2016 to April 2017.

and no giant breeds; in the group with the highest percentage of inadequate RVNA, there was no toy breed and 1 giant breed represented, indicating size is also a factor. These findings are supported by the study by Kennedy and colleagues,[20] who demonstrated that although for some breeds, RVNA level was associated with size, for other breeds this was not the case. There were also some MHC gene associations demonstrated in that study. Moreover, as has been shown with human rabies vaccine, diluted (reduced) doses result, on average, in reduced RVNA levels.[37] Human adults, children, and infants all receive the same size dose of rabies vaccine. It would be difficult, based on these findings, to recommend dosing vaccines for dogs and cats by size alone.

TITER TESTING TO INFORM VACCINATION DECISIONS

One way to address concerns over vaccine adverse reactions/immune modulation is allowance of RVNA titer checks in lieu of routine vaccination. Indeed, in general, revaccination of an animal already protected does not result in enhanced disease resistance. However, the main challenge for a particular disease or infection for which vaccination is available is to provide proof of "already protected." Peer-reviewed data regarding proof of rabies protection afforded by vaccination, as well as the predictive ability of rabies serology results, is primarily obtained from published rabies challenge studies. Per the CFR, studies for vaccine approval must demonstrate protection by survival of the challenged animals; included in the requirement is proof of immunogenicity by the measurement of rabies antibody levels.[36] The following list includes information from challenge studies publications,[24,38,39] the 9 CFR 113.209,[36] and the Compendium,[9] regarding rabies vaccines:

- Vaccines for dogs and cats: At least 86% to 87% of animals must survive challenge and at least 80% of unvaccinated controls must succumb to challenge.
- Current rabies vaccines are licensed for 1 to 3 years.
- Dogs and cats with rabies serology results greater than 0.5 IU/mL survive more frequently than dogs and cats with results less than 0.5 IU/mL; there are almost 100% survival rates in animals with RVNA greater than 0.5 IU/mL.
- There are a few reported animals with an RVNA result greater than 0.5 IU/mL that succumbed to challenge.
- Challenge studies require experimental challenge through the intracerebral route, which is considered an extreme challenge route of exposure for pets.
- Rabies serology methods have a precision (CV%) of 50% (or less), meaning an RVNA level of 0.5 IU/mL could actually be 0.25 to 1.0 IU/mL in any given assay run. Greater or lesser variability may occur between laboratories and assay types.

The 0.5 IU/mL "adequate level" was identified as robust based on this knowledge. In the conclusions made by Aubert[38] in a 1992 publication presenting a comprehensive review of challenge studies in dogs and cats, it was stated "The security of the protection constituted by this threshold [RVNA level] would be increased by the extent to which it exceeds the level recognized as effective against experimental challenge in cats and dogs 0.1 IU/mL and 0.2 IU/mL, respectively, measured by the RFFIT" (rapid fluorescent focus inhibition test). Even before this study was published, a study by Bunn and Ridpath[24] (1984) analyzed the probability of survival by RFFIT level using challenge study data and concluded that survival rate increased as RVNA level increased up to approximately 1.0 IU/mL, with a survival probability of approximately 99% at level of 0.5 IU/mL. Whether these findings can be extrapolated to pets without current vaccination status is the question at hand.

IMMUNOLOGIC PROTECTION IN THE FACE OF EXPOSURE

Currently, limited published studies provide rabies serology to correlate with survival data in dogs and cats. A study by Lawson and Crawley[40] provides some information. The investigators challenged vaccinated dogs and cats at 5 and 4 years, respectively, after vaccination and reported that 92% of dogs and 100% of cats survived; 54% of dogs and 87% of cats had detectable RVNA before challenge. Assuming that immune protection extends for an indeterminate period beyond the due date for a booster is reasonable, based on immunologic principles. An argument supporting this idea is that for human postexposure prophylaxis (PEP), a single dose (40 IU/kg bodyweight) of heterologous antirabies serum was protective in combination with vaccination.[41] In the case of an unrecognized rabies exposure in a pet, it is assumed that stimulation of memory immune cells to become effector cells would provide protection, rather than vaccination. There is evidence of this kind of response in a report of a human organ recipient of a rabies-infected liver, who survived even though their last rabies vaccination was many years previously,[42] due to a robust protective anamnestic response. However, this was a single case, and the outcome cannot be reliably generalized to larger groups, as exposures and the probability of infection can vary considerably.[32] PEPs and other protocols are based on the level of risk regulatory authorities and policy makers consider acceptable.

SEROLOGIC DATA TO DEMONSTRATE PROTECTION AGAINST RABIES

Based on the data from challenge studies, there is a valid argument for use of rabies serology to estimate rabies protection. However, several critical parameters need to be defined before confidently using rabies serology as a correlate of protection:

- Definition of an adequate antibody response (correlation of protection level)
- Significance of a rise or fall in antibody level
- Method (assay used) of measurement (correlate with protection, with ample data)
- Reported value: IU/mL or titer
- Timing of blood sampling and how often is the level assessed
  - 4 weeks after vaccination? Yearly? After exposure to rabies?
  - Will there be different acceptance levels based on timing of blood draws?
- Approval for laboratories providing testing; routine proficiency testing required for approval (as for rabies serology for pet travel and equine infectious anemia/Coggins for horses).

In an article that attempted to define rabies antibody level as proof of protection in different wildlife species using rabies serology results, few conclusions could be drawn from a systematic review of published studies, due to the highly variable study designs and results.[39] Also, in this article, sets of serum samples from challenge studies in dogs, foxes, skunks, raccoons, raccoon dogs, and mongooses were tested using 2 types of assay: serum neutralization (RFFIT) and a blocking enzyme-linked immunosorbent assay (ELISA). it was concluded that a level of 0.25 IU/mL and 40% inhibition by RFFIT and ELISA, respectively, were reasonably associated with survival; however, species differences were noted. Similarly, a study comparing RFFIT results with indirect ELISA results for a human rabies vaccine trial demonstrated that results from the assays were variously correlated by time since vaccination; results at day 14 were very poorly correlated, whereas results at day 90 had good correlation.[43] Although there are studies that have demonstrated good correlation between serum neutralization and ELISA techniques for rabies antibody measurement,[44–46] it is necessary to establish requirements by method validation, including diagnostic specificity and sensitivity, before approval of an assay for a specific use, such a proof of adequate vaccine response in lieu of booster vaccination.[47]

PRACTICAL USE OF TITER TESTING

The use of serology for verification of rabies immunity should be reserved for well-vaccinated pets (dogs and cats that have received a primary vaccination, followed by 1 or 2 boosters). Rabies titer checks in animals could also be used for prospective serologic monitoring to help determine whether an animal has been previously vaccinated.[9] In addition, they can be used if public health officials need to determine the risk of an exposed pet becoming infected after a nonstandard postexposure treatment or other unusual circumstances (eg, vaccinated animal for which no licensed vaccine is approved, such as an alpaca or monkey), or in pets for which routine vaccinations are contraindicated because of health concerns.[48] In a perfect world, defining pet risk would also be part of the decision to perform titer testing.

ADVANTAGES AND DISADVANTAGES OF USING SEROLOGY IN LIEU OF REVACCINATION

Advantages

- Reduces the number of vaccinations, hence reduces the risk of VAAEs.
- If required yearly for pet licensing, would identify pets that fail to respond to vaccination or have low titers, making them at higher risk of vaccine failure on rabies exposure.

Disadvantages

- The accuracy of the RVNA level to predict protection in pets for which vaccination is out of date is unknown because there have not been any studies to determine this.
- Routine vaccination stimulates/activates both humoral and cellular immune effectors.
- Enhanced assurance of human protection to humans is achieved by routine vaccination of pets, based on current knowledge.

SUMMARY

Current measures to prevent and control rabies in animals work very well, but there are challenges, such as decreased awareness of rabies risks, given the shift of rabies cases from primarily dogs before the establishment of the National Rabies Program in the 1940s, to wildlife. The threat of rabies virus variants adapting to new wildlife species is real, requiring continuous surveillance and prevention procedures. Viewpoints and opinions toward vaccination of pets and the compilation of robust data correlating rabies serology with adequate protection will drive changes in rabies control policies. An RVNA level of 0.5 IU/mL in a dog or cat demonstrates a continuing robust response to rabies vaccination and there is an expectation of sufficient immunologic memory to produce a protective response following exposure. Ideally, the animal would also receive postexposure treatment (wound care/cleaning and booster vaccination). Without postexposure treatment, complete protection is somewhere between expected and probable, but is unknown at this time, given lack of published data and variability in immune status at the time of exposure and exposure type. No vaccine can be 100% effective in every animal because of these variables. Given the importance of rabies protection in pets to human protection, an abundance of caution regarding defining the protective level and how it is measured in pets is warranted.

Rabies serology testing is not regulated, except for the recommendation of the ACIP to measure RVNA by the RFFIT. Experts in public health administration are responsible for weighing the risks of recognizing RVNA levels in animals solely as proof of rabies protection. Science is just one part of the equation; public health decisions in light of scientific data is another, and a multitude of factors, including the enforcement of laws both technically and politically, must be considered.

REFERENCES

1. Blanton JD, Palmer D, Christian KA, et al. Rabies surveillance in the United States during 2007. J Am Vet Med Assoc 2008;233(6):884–97.
2. Steele JH, Tierkel ES. Rabies problems and control. Public Health Rep 1949; 64(25):785–96.
3. World Health Organization. WHO Expert Committee on Rabies & World Health Organization. In: WHO expert committee on rabies: sixth report. 1973. Geneva (Switzerland). p. 1–54.
4. World Health Organization. Guideline for rabies control. 1983. Geneva (Switzerland). p. 1–92.
5. Zero by 30: the global strategic plan to prevent human deaths from dog-transmitted rabies by 2030. 2015. Available at: http://www.who.int/rabies/Executive_summary_draft_V3_wlogo.pdf?ua=1. Accessed October 14, 2018.
6. World Health Organization WOfAH. Global elimination of dog-mediated human rabies report of the Rabies Global Conference, Geneva, Switzerland, December 10–11, 2015. Geneva, Switzerland, June 2016. p. 1–33.
7. World Health Organization. WHO expert consultation on rabies third report. Geneva (Switzerland): WHO; 2018.
8. Fooks A. Rabies (infection with rabies virus and other lyssaviruses). In: (OIE) WOfAH, editor. Manual of diagnostic tests and vaccines for terrestrial animals 2018. 2018. p. 1–35. Available at: http://www.oie.int/fileadmin/Home/eng/Health_standards/tahm/3.01.17_RABIES.pdf. Accessed March 21, 2019.
9. Brown CM, Slavinski S, Ettestad P, et al. Compendium of Animal Rabies Prevention and Control, 2016. J Am Vet Med Assoc 2016;248(5):505–17.
10. Moore MC, Davis RD, Kang Q, et al. Comparison of anamnestic responses to rabies vaccination in dogs and cats with current and out-of-date vaccination status. J Am Vet Med Assoc 2015;246(2):205–11.
11. Birhane MG, Cleaton JM, Monroe BP, et al. Rabies surveillance in the United States during 2015. J Am Vet Med Assoc 2017;250(10):1117–30.
12. Leslie MJ, Messenger S, Rohde RE, et al. Bat-associated rabies virus in skunks. Emerg Infect Dis 2006;12(8):1274–7.
13. Wu H, Chang SS, Tsai HJ, et al. Notes from the field: wildlife rabies on an island free from canine rabies for 52 years—Taiwan, 2013. MMWR Morb Mortal Wkly Rep 2014;63(8):178.
14. Lin YC, Chu PY, Chang MY, et al. Spatial temporal dynamics and molecular evolution of re-emerging rabies virus in Taiwan. Int J Mol Sci 2016;17(3):392.
15. Evans JS, Wu G, Selden D, et al. Utilisation of chimeric lyssaviruses to assess vaccine protection against highly divergent lyssaviruses. Viruses 2018;10(3) [pii:E130].
16. Lopez T. Quarantine changes take effect in Hawaii. J Am Vet Med Assoc 1997; 211(7):817, 819.
17. Cliquet F, Verdier Y, Sagne L, et al. Neutralising antibody titration in 25,000 sera of dogs and cats vaccinated against rabies in France, in the framework of the new

regulations that offer an alternative to quarantine. Rev Sci Tech 2003;22(3): 857–66.

18. Mansfield KL, Burr PD, Snodgrass DR, et al. Factors affecting the serological response of dogs and cats to rabies vaccination. Vet Rec 2004;154(14):423–6.

19. Jakel V, Konig M, Cussler K, et al. Factors influencing the antibody response to vaccination against rabies. Dev Biol (Basel) 2008;131:431–7.

20. Kennedy LJ, Lunt M, Barnes A, et al. Factors influencing the antibody response of dogs vaccinated against rabies. Vaccine 2007;25(51):8500–7.

21. Wallace RM, Pees A, Blanton JB, et al. Risk factors for inadequate antibody response to primary rabies vaccination in dogs under one year of age. PLoS Negl Trop Dis 2017;11(7):e0005761.

22. Morters MK, McNabb S, Horton DL, et al. Effective vaccination against rabies in puppies in rabies endemic regions. Vet Rec 2015;177(6):150.

23. Muller TF, Schuster P, Vos AC, et al. Effect of maternal immunity on the immune response to oral vaccination against rabies in young foxes. Am J Vet Res 2001;62(7):1154–8.

24. Bunn TO, Ridpath HD. The relationship between rabies antibody titers in dogs and cats and protection from challenge, vol.11. Lawrenceville (GA): U S Department of Health, Education and Welfare, Public Health; 1984. p. 43–5.

25. Velasco-Villa A, Reeder SA, Orciari LA, et al. Enzootic rabies elimination from dogs and reemergence in wild terrestrial carnivores, United States. Emerg Infect Dis 2008;14(12):1849–54.

26. Ford RB, Larson LJ, McClure KD, et al. 2017 AAHA Canine Vaccination Guidelines. J Am Anim Hosp Assoc 2017;53(5):243–51.

27. Scherk MA, Ford RB, Gaskell RM, et al. 2013 AAFP Feline Vaccination Advisory Panel Report. J Feline Med Surg 2013;15(9):785–808.

28. Moore GE, Guptill LF, Ward MP, et al. Adverse events diagnosed within three days of vaccine administration in dogs. J Am Vet Med Assoc 2005;227(7):1102–8.

29. Moore GE, DeSantis-Kerr AC, Guptill LF, et al. Adverse events after vaccine administration in cats: 2,560 cases (2002-2005). J Am Vet Med Assoc 2007; 231(1):94–100.

30. Centers for Disease Control. Vaccine recommendations and guidelines of the ACIP. 2015. Available at: https://www.cdc.gov/vaccines/hcp/acip-recs/vacc-specific/rabies.html. Accessed October 23, 2018.

31. Manning SE, Rupprecht CE, Fishbein D, et al, Advisory Committee on Immunization Practices Centers for Disease Control and Prevention (CDC). Human rabies prevention - United States, 2008 recommendations of the Advisory Committee on Immunization Practices. MMWR Recomm Rep 2008;57(RR-3):1–28. Atlanta, GA.

32. Fishbein DB, Robinson LE. Rabies. N Engl J Med 1993;329(22):1632–8.

33. Dean DJ, Baer GM, Thompson WR. Studies on the local treatment of rabies-infected wounds. Bull World Health Organ 1963;28(4):477–86.

34. Murray KO, Holmes KC, Hanlon CA. Rabies in vaccinated dogs and cats in the United States, 1997-2001. J Am Vet Med Assoc 2009;235(6):691–5.

35. Eng TR, Hamaker TA, Dobbins JG, et al. Rabies surveillance, United States, 1988. MMWR CDC Surveill Summ 1989;38(1):1–21.

36. Rabies vaccine, killed. In: Regulations CoF, vol. 9. U.S. National Archives and records Administration; 2007. Available at: https://www.govregs.com/regulations/9/113.209. Accessed March 21, 2019.

37. Beran J, Honegr K, Banzhoff A, et al. How far can the antigen content of tissue culture rabies vaccine be reduced safely? Vaccine 2006;24(13):2223–4.

38. Aubert MF. Practical significance of rabies antibodies in cats and dogs. Rev Sci Tech 1992;11(3):735–60.
39. Moore SM, Gilbert A, Vos A, et al. Rabies virus antibodies from oral vaccination as a correlate of protection against lethal infection in wildlife. Trop Med Infect Dis 2017;2(3) [pii:E31].
40. Lawson KF, Crawley JF. The ERA strain of rabies vaccine. Can J Comp Med 1972; 36(4):339–44.
41. Bahmanyar M, Fayaz A, Nour-Salehi S, et al. Successful protection of humans exposed to rabies infection. Postexposure treatment with the new human diploid cell rabies vaccine and antirabies serum. JAMA 1976;236(24):2751–4.
42. Lu XX, Zhu WY, Wu GZ. Rabies virus transmission via solid organs or tissue allo-transplantation. Infect Dis Poverty 2018;7(1):82.
43. Moore SM, Pralle S, Engelman L, et al. Rabies vaccine response measurement is assay dependent. Biologicals 2016;44(6):481–6.
44. Feyssaguet M, Dacheux L, Audry L, et al. Multicenter comparative study of a new ELISA, PLATELIA RABIES II, for the detection and titration of anti-rabies glycoprotein antibodies and comparison with the rapid fluorescent focus inhibition test (RFFIT) on human samples from vaccinated and non-vaccinated people. Vaccine 2007;25(12):2244–51.
45. Servat A, Feyssaguet M, Blanchard I, et al. A quantitative indirect ELISA to monitor the effectiveness of rabies vaccination in domestic and wild carnivores. J Immunol Methods 2007;318(1–2):1–10.
46. Wasniewski M, Guiot AL, Schereffer JL, et al. Evaluation of an ELISA to detect rabies antibodies in orally vaccinated foxes and raccoon dogs sampled in the field. J Virol Methods 2013;187(2):264–70.
47. Moore SM, Hanlon CA. Rabies-specific antibodies: measuring surrogates of protection against a fatal disease. PLoS Negl Trop Dis 2010;4(3):e595.
48. Wallace RM, Niezgoda M, Waggoner EA, et al. Serologic response in eight alpacas vaccinated by extralabel use of a large animal rabies vaccine during a public health response to a rabid alpaca in South Carolina. J Am Vet Med Assoc 2016;249(6):678–81.

H3N8 and H3N2 Canine Influenza Viruses
Understanding These New Viruses in Dogs

Colin Ross Parrish, PhD*, Ian Eugene Huber Voorhees, BA

KEYWORDS

- Canine influenza virus • H3N8 • H3N2 • Emergence • Host range • Outbreak

KEY POINTS

- Influenza A viruses are able to emerge and spread among dogs, including specific canine influenza viruses (H3N8 and H3N2) and occasional infections by human or other influenza viruses.
- Virus infections seem to cause mostly mild disease, with respiratory signs developing.
- The H3N8 canine influenza virus emerged in 2000, was recognized in 2004, and spread widely in the United States for several years, but since 2016 has been rarely seen.
- The H3N2 canine influenza virus emerged around 2005 in Asia, was first introduced into the United States in 2015, and has caused widespread outbreaks.

INTRODUCTION

Canine influenza viruses (CIVs) are members of the genus that includes the influenza A viruses (IAVs), among the family Orthomyxoviridae. The IAVs have a complex natural history, with most viruses being found as common and endemic gastrointestinal tract infections of bird populations that live in flocks in marine or fresh water environments.[1] Occasionally, members of the avian IAVs spill over to infect terrestrial bird populations, such as domestic chickens or turkeys, or into certain mammalian populations.[2] Among mammals, the viruses have been commonly seen to cause outbreaks among humans, swine, horses, seals, mink, and, in recent years, dogs and cats have been involved in epidemics or outbreaks. Our detailed understanding of the IAVs only extends back to about 1918, when the H1N1 virus emerged to cause parallel pandemics in humans and swine. In the twentieth century, pandemic IAVs have emerged in humans in 1918 and 2009 after the transfer of entire viruses from other hosts, while

Disclosure statement: Dr. Parrish was supported by NIH grant GM080533 and Dr. Voorhees was supported by NSF Award DGE-1650441.
Department of Microbiology and Immunology, Baker Institute for Animal Health, College of Veterinary Medicine, Cornell University, Ithaca, NY 14853, USA
* Corresponding author.
E-mail address: crp3@cornell.edu

pandemic variants of these viruses emerged in humans in 1957 and 1968 after the replacement of 3 or 2 of the viral gene segments from avian virus sources.[3] In addition, there have been many other avian to human (or other animal) spill-over events or small outbreaks that have resulted in serious infections, but with little or no onward transmission.

INFLUENZA VIRUSES AND THE ORIGINS OF THE CANINE INFLUENZA VIRUSES

The IAVs have an enveloped virion, which packages an RNA genome that is made up of 8 different segments that are packaged as a set. The virions display 2 major glycoproteins on their surface—hemagglutinin and neuraminidase—and virus isolates are identified by the hemagglutinin and neuraminidase subtypes they contain. For example, H3N2 and H3N8 are the viruses found in dogs. The virus (**Fig. 1**) is not very stable in the environment and is inactivated within a few minutes to hours under most environmental conditions, although it may survive longer—perhaps for days—in cool, dark, damp conditions. The viruses are readily inactivated by hot water and detergent. When infecting mammals, the viruses are transmitted by respiratory routes. Whether particular viruses are spread by aerosol, direct contact, or on fomites, or through more than one of those routes, is not known. However, for both CIVs, it seems that direct contact is generally required to allow transmission to a susceptible recipient.

Epidemics of influenza viruses in dogs are relatively recent developments. Before 2004, there was little suggestion that dogs would be a natural host for influenza infection or epidemic spread. However, in that year the H3N8 variant of the equine influenza virus was isolated and identified as the cause of an epidemic in dogs.[4] The H3N8 CIV emerging around 1999 in Florida by transfer of an intact H3N8 equine influenza virus to dogs and then that virus circulated continuously among dogs in the United States for

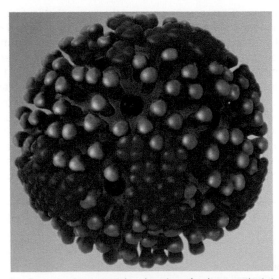

Fig. 1. Structure of influenza virus particle, showing the hemagglutinin (*blue*) and neuraminidase (*red*) glycoproteins on the surface. The viral RNA and internal proteins are inside the membrane. (*Courtesy of* Centers for Disease Control and Prevention, National Center for Immunization and Respiratory Diseases (NCIRD), Atlanta, GA.)

more than a decade, with most continuing spread occurring in Colorado and the Northeast states after about 2005.[5] It seems that the virus did not spread efficiently among household dogs, and after about 2012 the H3N8 CIV was restricted to only a few small geographic pockets where it was found primarily among animal shelter dogs. By 2016, it was reduced to very low levels.

A second CIV, the avian-origin H3N2 CIV, emerged in dogs in China or Korea in 2004 or 2005, and then spread widely within both China and Korea during 2005 and 2006.[6(p2)] That virus was also reported in Thailand, where it caused an outbreak but likely did not continue to spread.[7] The H3N2 CIV was first introduced into the United States in the area around Chicago in February 2015, and has since caused ongoing epidemics of disease,[8] with multiple introductions from Asia reseeding the disease on at least 2 occasions.[9]

It is clear that each of the CIV epidemics ultimately derived from a single cross-species transfer event, with the H3N8 subtype transferring from horses,[4,10] while the H3N2 subtype arose from a virus in an avian reservoir.[6] A recent study showed that, in Southern China, dogs may be frequently infected by various swine, canine, and other influenza viruses,[11] although such high levels of infection have not so far been reported elsewhere.

CANINE INFLUENZA VIRUS-ASSOCIATED DISEASES

Both H3N8 and H3N2 CIV infections in dogs are associated with mild upper respiratory tract disease, often including frequent coughing and fever.[12–14] Where it has been examined, infection of the lungs may occur, and that is rarely associated with more severe disease and sometimes death.[4,15] The more severe disease is likely associated with mixed infections by other viruses or bacteria, or with other health issues for the dogs. The natural risks to other animals, including humans, are largely unknown, but no human infections by either strain of CIV have been reported. The H3N8 CIV seems to be restricted to dogs, has not been reported to infect other animals, and does not infect horses when infected dogs are housed with susceptible horses.[16,17] Natural infection of cats by H3N2 CIV transferred from dogs has been documented in Korea and in the United States, but the cat outbreaks have been confined to the shelter populations where they emerged.[18,19] Despite high levels of viral replication and shedding by the canine H3N2 viruses, the relatively unsocial nature of and lack of contact between populations of household cats suggests that a cat-adapted influenza virus would not transmit for very long. In experimental studies, the H3N2 CIV has been shown to infect ferrets and guinea pigs, as well as cats.[20] The experimental inoculation of Korean or US strains of H3N2 CIV into swine resulted in poor replication, suggesting that sustained transmission of the virus after transfer from dogs to swine is unlikely, despite swine being a common host of other H3N2 IAV strains.[21]

OTHER INFLUENZA VIRUSES IN DOGS, HUMAN INFECTIONS, AND MIXED INFECTIONS

No infections by either CIV subtype have been reported in humans. However, human seasonal IAV subtypes may infect dogs occasionally, including both H1N1 strains (the original seasonal and the 2009 pandemic variants) and H3N2 seasonal viruses,[11,22,23] and some avian viruses.[24] None of these infections seem to result in much onward transmission among dogs, but they may provide opportunities for human IAVs to reassort with CIVs during natural coinfections in dogs. One H3N1 virus in a Korean dog seems to have arisen from the reassortment of an H3N2 CIV (hemagglutinin segment) and pandemic H1N1/09 virus (the other 7 genomic segments).[25] A novel reassortant H3N2 CIV containing the PA genomic segment from an H9N2 pandemic avian IAV was isolated from a Korean dog in 2015.[26(p2)] In addition, dogs and humans express a similar diversity of sialic acid variants and linkages, which may be associated with variation in IAV infection and host range.

INFLUENZA VIRUS EPIDEMICS IN DOGS
H3N8 Canine Influenza Virus

As mentioned, the H3N8 CIV emerged around 1999 by transfer of an equine influenza virus into dogs. The virus was recognized in 2004, when it was isolated from greyhounds in Florida. The virus then spread widely between 2004 and 2006, although after that time it was maintained in only a few areas, including Colorado and some of the Northeastern states.[10,27] Areas of continuous transmission included Denver and Colorado Springs, as well as New York City. More limited outbreaks of disease occurred in smaller cities and regions, likely seeded from the major centers of transmission, but those secondary outbreaks generally died out in a few weeks or months. The virus outbreak in Colorado died out around 2012, and it was at very low levels in New York by mid-2016, with very little disease being reported after that time.[4,5,13(p8)]

H3N2 Canine Influenza Virus

The H3N2 CIV was first recognized in South Korea and China around 2006, and it seems to have arisen by transfer of a single avian virus into dogs around 2005. The virus circulated widely in dogs in both countries after it was recognized and was also found in both Northern and Southern China, with some genetic differences developing between the viruses in the different regions suggesting that they were circulating locally for a number of years with less long-range movement. In early 2015, an outbreak of respiratory disease in the area of Chicago, Illinois, was identified as being caused by the H3N2 virus strain, and that soon after caused an outbreak of disease in Georgia and nearby states.[8] Although the outbreak in the Southeastern states died out relatively quickly, there were continuing infections in Chicago and nearby areas, which seemed not to cause any other major secondary outbreaks. A second wave of virus emerged in 2017, and that virus spread widely for the next year, being first recognized in Florida and also causing outbreaks in many areas of the country over the next several months. The virus involved in that outbreak was a new introduction from Asia, most likely from South Korea.[9] A third wave of infections occurred in 2018, with an initial outbreak in California near San Francisco, followed by a second outbreak in the New York City area (**Fig. 2**).

Vaccination Against Canine Influenza Viruses

Vaccines to both strains of influenza virus in dogs are available. Those are inactivated virus vaccines that are given as 2 doses, 3 or more weeks apart. Combined (bivalent) vaccines that contain both the H3N2 and H3N8 strains are also available. The most important virus is currently the H3N2 strain because it is still circulating widely in the United States. Vaccination is most recommended for use in dogs that attend canine day care centers, travel widely including to dog shows, spend time in kennels, or frequently go to dog parks.

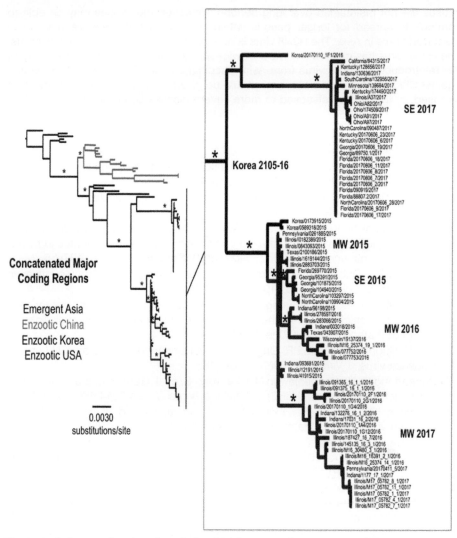

Fig. 2. A phylogeny showing the relationships between the sequences of the H3N2 CIVs in the United States compared with those in Asia. MW, Midwest; SE, Southeast. Asterisk: High statistical support for clades of interest.

SUMMARY

The influenza viruses that infect dogs are a threat to canine health, and it now seems that dogs are a susceptible host, so that we should consider influenza viruses in cases of contagious respiratory disease in dogs. The 2 CIVs both cause relatively uncomplicated upper respiratory tract diseases in dogs, with relatively short periods (3–4 days) of high level viral shedding, but with clinical signs continuing for several days or more. In some cases, persistent viral shedding of the H3N2 CIV has been reported.[28] More severe disease is occasionally reported, which may be associated with higher growth of the virus and infection of the lungs.[28,29] The viruses seem to require relatively close contact to give transmission, so that in most populations of household dogs the viruses are not maintained over long periods. However, the viruses may be able to continue to spread for longer periods within large animal shelters, kennels, or in meat dog farms in Asia. The H3N8 virus is now present in US dogs at very low levels. The H3N2 virus has caused a number of widespread outbreaks, apparently owing to the reintroduction of the virus from Asia. Vaccinations provide a level of protection against CIV infection or disease, and should be given to animals that are likely to be exposed, or that are predisposed to more severe disease by comorbidities or other factors.

REFERENCES

1. Yoon S-W, Webby RJ, Webster RG. Evolution and ecology of influenza A viruses. Curr Top Microbiol Immunol 2014;385:359–75.
2. Webster RG, Govorkova EA. Continuing challenges in influenza. Ann N Y Acad Sci 2014;1323:115–39.
3. Herfst S, Imai M, Kawaoka Y, et al. Avian influenza virus transmission to mammals. In: influenza pathogenesis and control - volume I. Current topics in microbiology and immunology. Cham (Switzerland): Springer; 2014. p. 137–55.
4. Crawford PC, Dubovi EJ, Castleman WL, et al. Transmission of equine influenza virus to dogs. Science 2005;310(5747):482–5.
5. Dalziel BD, Huang K, Geoghegan JL, et al. Contact heterogeneity, rather than transmission efficiency, limits the emergence and spread of canine influenza virus. PLoS Pathog 2014;10(10):e1004455.
6. Zhu H, Hughes J, Murcia PR. Origins and evolutionary dynamics of H3N2 canine influenza virus. J Virol 2015;89(10):5406–18.
7. Bunpapong N, Nonthabenjawan N, Chaiwong S, et al. Genetic characterization of canine influenza A virus (H3N2) in Thailand. Virus Genes 2014;48(1):56–63.
8. Voorhees IEH, Glaser AL, Toohey-Kurth K, et al. Spread of canine influenza A(H3N2) virus, United States. Emerg Infect Dis 2017;23(12):1950–7.
9. Voorhees IEH, Dalziel BD, Glaser A, et al. Multiple incursions and recurrent epidemic fade-out of H3N2 canine influenza A virus in the United States. J Virol 2018. https://doi.org/10.1128/JVI.00323-18.
10. Hayward JJ, Dubovi EJ, Scarlett JM, et al. Microevolution of canine influenza virus in shelters and its molecular epidemiology in the United States. J Virol 2010; 84(24):12636–45.
11. Chen Y, Trovão NS, Wang G, et al. Emergence and evolution of novel reassortant influenza A viruses in canines in Southern China. MBio 2018;9(3). https://doi.org/10.1128/mBio.00909-18.
12. Song D, Moon H, Jung K, et al. Association between nasal shedding and fever that influenza A (H3N2) induces in dogs. Virol J 2011;8:1.
13. Castleman WL, Powe JR, Crawford PC, et al. Canine H3N8 influenza virus infection in dogs and mice. Vet Pathol 2010;47(3):507–17.
14. Pulit-Penaloza JA, Simpson N, Yang H, et al. Assessment of molecular, antigenic, and pathological features of canine influenza A(H3N2) viruses that emerged in the United States. J Infect Dis 2017;216(suppl_4):S499–507.
15. Lee Y-N, Lee H-J, Lee D-H, et al. Severe canine influenza in dogs correlates with hyperchemokinemia and high viral load. Virology 2011;417(1):57–63.
16. Yamanaka T, Nemoto M, Bannai H, et al. No evidence of horizontal infection in horses kept in close contact with dogs experimentally infected with canine influenza A virus (H3N8). Acta Vet Scand 2012;54:25.

17. Quintana AM, Hussey SB, Burr EC, et al. Evaluation of infectivity of a canine lineage H3N8 influenza A virus in ponies and in primary equine respiratory epithelial cells. Am J Vet Res 2011;72(8):1071–8.
18. Jeoung H-Y, Lim S-I, Shin B-H, et al. A novel canine influenza H3N2 virus isolated from cats in an animal shelter. Vet Microbiol 2013;165(3–4):281–6.
19. Lei N, Yuan Z-G, Huang S-F, et al. Transmission of avian-origin canine influenza viruses A (H3N2) in cats. Vet Microbiol 2012;160(3–4):481–3.
20. Lyoo K-S, Na W, Yeom M, et al. Virulence of a novel reassortant canine H3N2 influenza virus in ferret, dog and mouse models. Arch Virol 2016;161(7):1915–23.
21. Abente EJ, Anderson TK, Rajao DS, et al. The avian-origin H3N2 canine influenza virus that recently emerged in the United States has limited replication in swine. Influenza Other Respir Viruses 2016;10(5):429–32.
22. Jang H, Jackson YK, Daniels JB, et al. Seroprevalence of three influenza A viruses (H1N1, H3N2, and H3N8) in pet dogs presented to a veterinary hospital in Ohio. J Vet Sci 2017;18(S1):291–8.
23. Chen Y, Mo Y-N, Zhou H-B, et al. Emergence of human-like H3N2 influenza viruses in pet dogs in Guangxi, China. Virol J 2015;12:10.
24. Lyoo KS, Na W, Phan LV, et al. Experimental infection of clade 1.1.2 (H5N1), clade 2.3.2.1c (H5N1) and clade 2.3.4.4 (H5N6) highly pathogenic avian influenza viruses in dogs. Transbound Emerg Dis 2017. https://doi.org/10.1111/tbed.12731.
25. Na W, Lyoo K-S, Song E, et al. Viral dominance of reassortants between canine influenza H3N2 and pandemic (2009) H1N1 viruses from a naturally co-infected dog. Virol J 2015;12:134.
26. Lee IH, Le TB, Kim HS, et al. Isolation of a novel H3N2 influenza virus containing a gene of H9N2 avian influenza in a dog in South Korea in 2015. Virus Genes 2016; 52(1):142–5.
27. Pecoraro HL, Bennett S, Huyvaert KP, et al. Epidemiology and ecology of H3N8 canine influenza viruses in US shelter dogs. J Vet Intern Med 2014;28(2):311–8.
28. Newbury S, Godhardt-Cooper J, Poulsen KP, et al. Prolonged intermittent virus shedding during an outbreak of canine influenza A H3N2 virus infection in dogs in three Chicago area shelters: 16 cases (March to May 2015). J Am Vet Med Assoc 2016;248(9):1022–6.
29. Su S, Huang S, Fu C, et al. Identification of the IFN-β response in H3N2 canine influenza virus infection. J Gen Virol 2016;97(1):18–26.

Feline Panleukopenia
A Re-emergent Disease

Vanessa R. Barrs, BVSc(hons), PhD, MVetClinStud, FANZCVS

KEYWORDS

- Parvovirus • Canine • Feline • Panleukopenia • Enteritis • Shelter medicine
- Carnivore protoparvovirus

KEY POINTS

- Feline panleukopenia (FPL) is caused by Carnivore protoparvovirus 1. Feline parvovirus (FPV) causes 95% of cases, whereas 5% are caused by Canine parvovirus (CPV) variants, specifically CPV-2a, b, and c.
- Outbreaks of FPL occur in shelters from summer to autumn (median age at diagnosis 2–4 months) associated with a seasonal influx of kittens with waning or absent maternally derived antibodies.
- In Australia FPL has re-emerged to cause large-scale outbreaks among unvaccinated shelter cats with spill over to the owned cat population.
- In contrast to CPV enteritis of dogs, hemorrhagic diarrhea occurs in only 3% to 15% of cases of FPL. Lethargy, anorexia, and fever, the most prominent signs in some cats, precede vomiting and diarrhea.
- Even with treatment FPL has a high mortality rate of 50% to 80%. Poor prognostic indicators include low leukocyte or platelet counts or hypoalbuminaemia or hypokalemia at presentation.

INTRODUCTION

Feline panleukopenia (FPL) is the clinical disease syndrome caused by infection with Carnivore protoparvovirus 1. Both feline parvovirus (FPV; formerly FPL virus) and canine parvovirus (CPV) can cause FPL, although CPV infections in cats are uncommon.

The detection of endogenous parvovirus-like DNA sequences in the genomes of numerous carnivore species provides evidence that parvoviruses have likely been circulating in carnivores for millions of years.[1] Feline panleukopenia is the oldest known viral disease of cats. Several epizootics that decimated domestic cat

Disclosure Statement: The author has nothing to disclose.
Sydney School of Veterinary Science, Faculty of Science, and Marie Bashir Institute of Infectious Diseases & Biosecurity, University of Sydney, New South Wales 2006, Australia
E-mail address: vanessa.barrs@sydney.edu.au

Vet Clin Small Anim 49 (2019) 651–670
https://doi.org/10.1016/j.cvsm.2019.02.006
0195-5616/19/© 2019 Elsevier Inc. All rights reserved.

populations in the 1800s could have been caused by FPV.[2,3] In the first decade of the 1900s, multiple reports of an infectious enteritis in cats, with high mortality and seasonal incidence were published, and subsequently reviewed in 1934.[4] Feline panleukopenia was first identified to have a viral cause in 1928,[5] and cats were successfully vaccinated against FPV in 1934 using formalin-inactivated tissue extracts from infected cats.[4] A breakthrough in 1964 led to successful isolation of FPV in tissue culture,[6] which paved the way for the development of inactivated tissue culture vaccines and modified live virus (MLV) vaccines. With progressively increased uptake of primary kitten vaccinations by pet owners from ~18% in the UK in 1973 to ~82% in 2016,[7,8] FPL became an uncommon disease diagnosis in companion animal veterinary practice in several countries including the UK, Australia, New Zealand, and United States, except for sporadic outbreaks in shelters.

In some countries, such as Australia, there were no outbreaks of FPL reported even in shelters for over 30 years. In 2014, FPL re-emerged in Australia, in Victoria, primarily among shelter-housed cats. Since then, large-scale outbreaks have occurred in multiple shelters in Eastern Australia in New South Wales and Queensland, with spillover to the owned cat population. A "perfect storm" of events surrounds the re-emergence including the failure of many municipal and privately owned shelters to routinely vaccinate cats, wide geographic dissemination of kittens to shelters and foster-care networks aided by social media, and poor infection control practices and training.[9] In addition, trap-neuter-return schemes are uncommon in Australia, and increasing lengths of stay associated with the introduction of "no kill" policies or higher rehoming targets, has resulted in crowding and longer duration of stay for individual cats in some shelters, increasing the risk of exposure to pathogens.

Here, the causes, epidemiology, diagnosis, treatment, prognostic indicators, and management of FPL outbreaks in shelters are reviewed.

VIRAL CAUSES OF FELINE PANLEUKOPENIA

The virus family *Parvoviridae*, contains vertebrate parvoviruses (subfamily *Parvovirinae*), and invertebrate parvoviruses (subfamily *Densovirinae*).[10] Carnivore protoparvovirus 1 is a viral species in genus *Protoparvovirus*. Feline panleukopenia is the clinical disease syndrome caused by infection with Carnivore protoparvovirus 1 strains, including FPV (90%–95% of cases) and current circulating strains of CPV (<10% of cases) (**Table 1**).

Carnivore protoparvovirus 1 is a small, nonenveloped, linear, single-stranded DNA virus with a 5.1-kb genome encoding 2 major genes, the nonstructural (NS) and structural protein genes. The NS gene encodes the NS1 and NS2 proteins involved in DNA replication, capsid assembly, and intracellular transport, whereas the structural gene encodes capsid virus protein 1 (VP1) and VP2. The viral capsid is comprised of 60 protein subunit molecules (~10% VP1 and 90% VP2) arranged in an icosahedral symmetry.

The host range of FPV includes domestic and wild felids (suborder Feliformia) and some wild canids (suborder Caniformia), for example, raccoons and foxes, but not domestic dogs.[11,12] Although FPV can replicate in lymphoid tissues of dogs (thymus and bone marrow) after experimental inoculation, it cannot bind to the canine transferrin receptor (TfR), which is critical for efficient infection, and onward transmission of infection does not occur.[13–15]

Canine parvovirus emerged as a new pathogen in domestic dogs in the mid-1970s and caused a global panzootic in 1978.[16,17] The virus was initially named CPV-2 to distinguish it from an unrelated canine parvovirus, Canine minute virus,

Table 1
CPV isolates detected among fecal samples testing positive for FPV or CPV from clinically unwell cats

Year	Country	No. of CPV-Positive Isolates/ No. of Isolates Examined (%)	CPV Variants Detected
1985–1990[104]	United States	2/20 (10)	CPV-2b
1989–1991[24]	Japan	3/48 (6)	unknown
1993–1994[30]	Japan	1/34 (3)	CPV-2a
1993–1995[104]	Germany	3/39 (8)	CPV-2a (2) CPV-2b (1)
2000–2009[33]	Italy	2/25 (8)	CPV-2a CPV-2c
2001–2007[105]	Italy/UK	0/39 (0)	
2004–2014[106]	Bulgaria	1/18 (6)	CPV-2a
2011–2014[26]	India	1/4 (25)	CPV-2a
2010–2013[107]	China	2/16 (13)	CPV-2a
All years and countries.		15/243 (6)	

which has since been reclassified as a *Bocaparvovirus* (Canine bocavirus 1).[10] The new CPV differed from FPV by only 6 amino acid residues in the VP2 region that are critical for virus binding to the canine TfR, and for efficient infection of canine cells through clathrin-mediated endocytosis.[15] Thus, CPV-2 was unable to replicate in any tissues of cats in vivo,[18] although it was able to grow in feline cell cultures in vitro.[13]

Frequent cross-transmission of FPV-like and CPV-like viruses between wild carnivore species suggests that FPV and CPV may have evolved independently from an ancestral sylvatic parvovirus.[11,12] Previously, it was thought that CPV evolved from an FPV of domestic cats after cross-species transmission to wild carnivores, because viruses intermediate between FPV and CPV have been detected in wild red foxes.[19] However, the directionality of mutations was not considered. It has since been shown that the VP2 mutations present in these viral intermediates can be induced by passaging CPV-2 in fox cells in vitro.[12]

In 1979, shortly after the emergence of CPV-2, a new antigenic CPV variant emerged (CPV2-a) with 4 amino acid mutations (L87M, I101T, A300G, and D305Y), which could bind to canine and feline TfRs and cause disease in both host species.[20,21] It soon replaced CPV-2 in the wild and 2 other antigenic variants subsequently evolved with nonsynonymous mutations involving amino acids 426 and 555, being first detected in 1984 in the United States[22] (N426D, I555V termed CPV-2b) and then in 2000 in Italy (D426E, termed CPV-2c).[23] These variants cocirculate in varying proportions in different geographic regions around the world. All 3 antigenic variants have retained the feline host range.

CANINE PARVOVIRUS CAUSES CLINICAL AND SUBCLINICAL INFECTIONS IN CATS
Active Subclinical Infections

Canine parvovirus-2 antigenic variant strains have been detected by polymerase chain reaction (PCR) and virus isolation in the feces of healthy cats.[24–26] In the UK, fecal shedding of CPV was detected in more than a third of fecal samples collected from healthy cats from 2 mixed canine and feline shelters.[25] None of the cats were found to be shedding FPV. Weekly fecal testing was performed in 1 of the shelters, in which 46% of cats, but no dogs, shed CPV on at least 1 occasion over an 8-week period. Fecal samples were screened using conventional PCR to detect the VP2 region of FPV/CPV, and sequencing and virus isolation was performed on positive samples. The diversity of isolates detected, the time association of shedding with arrival to the shelter, and the lack of fecal shedding by any dogs in the shelter, suggested that cats were infected with CPV before their arrival. Around half of the feline CPV sequence types were identical to those obtained from sick dogs with CPV-associated diarrhea in a previous study.[27]

The high prevalence of CPV shedding in healthy shelter-housed cats raised concerns about the role of cats as reservoirs of infection for dogs, and has important implications for biosecurity, especially in mixed animal shelters housing both cats and dogs. More recently, healthy shelter-housed cats were tested for fecal shedding of CPV in 3 shelters in 2 states of Australia, using conventional PCR. Canine parvovirus was not detected in any sample, while 4% of samples were FPV positive.[28] Ongoing surveillance and quantitation of fecal viral loads is required to further understand the significance of CPV shedding by cats in different geographic regions.

Active Clinical Infections

All antigenic variants of CPV-2 have been detected among samples testing positive for parvoviruses from clinically unwell cats in many countries (see **Table 1**). In general, CPV is an uncommon cause of FPL, although only small numbers of isolates have been tested (see **Table 1**). Samples testing positive for CPV were from individual feline submissions to veterinary virology testing laboratories, and to date no large-scale outbreaks of FPL, for example in shelter-housed cats, have been confirmed to be caused by CPV.

Naturally occurring CPV infections with clinical signs indistinguishable to those caused by FPV, have been described in several cats.[29–31] In 1 case of a fatal CPV-2a infection in a 3-month-old Persian kitten, the source of infection was considered likely to be from 2 puppies with parvoviral enteritis that were infected with the same strain and cohoused with the cat in a pet shop.[31] Coinfections of CPV and FPV have also been detected in cats with clinical disease.[32,33] All CPV antigenic variants have been shown to cause clinical disease in experimental infections of cats.[34,35]

Latent Infections

Carnivore protoparvovirus 1 DNA persists for long periods in the tissues of animals that have recovered from infection, leaving behind a convenient molecular footprint of previous infection.[11,12] The virus can remain latent in peripheral blood mononuclear cells, as demonstrated by successful culture of FPV and CPV from the peripheral blood mononuclear cells of healthy cats with high virus-neutralizing titers.[36–38] Latency has been demonstrated for other parvoviruses, including B19 parvovirus of humans. The lifelong tissue persistence of B19 viral genomes, which are not re-shed, is termed the "bioportfolio."[39] Whether certain conditions such as immune-suppression could induce re-shedding of FPV or CPV in cats has not been investigated.

EPIDEMIOLOGY OF FELINE PANLEUKOPENIA
Age Susceptibility and Seasonality

Epidemiologic data from cases or outbreaks of FPL have been reported over many decades (**Table 2**).[40–43] Younger median age was apparent in reports involving shelter-housed cats compared with reports from veterinary hospitals.

Table 2
Epidemiologic data from FPV outbreaks in the United States, Europe, and Australia

Year	Country	No. of Cases	% of Cases Occurring in Cats <1 y of Age	Median Age at Diagnosis (mo)	Age Range of Affected Cats
1946–1948[40]	United States	574	66	7	–
1964–1971[41]	United States	185	70	5	–
1990–2007[42]	Germany	244	72	4	2 wk–15 y
2010	United States	79	83% <6 mo of age	2–3	2 wk–7 y
2011–2013[71]	Italy	133	71	3	2 mo–3 y
2014–2018	Australia	326	89	2.5	3 wk–8 y

Males were affected more commonly than females in 3 studies (57%–59.5%),[40–42] although in 2 of these studies from 1949 to 1976, males outnumbered females in hospital admissions overall, partially reflecting a tendency for male cats to be kept preferentially as pets at a time when desexing was not routinely practiced.[40]

Feline panleukopenia occurs most frequently in unvaccinated and incompletely vaccinated kittens. Age susceptibility is correlated with waning titers of maternally derived antibodies (MDAs) as well as "the immunity gap" in incompletely vaccinated kittens, when MDAs have waned below protective titers but are adequate to neutralize vaccine antigen (see vaccination below). After being ingested in colostrum, MDAs have a biological half-life of 10 to 11 days,[44] and generally remain at protective titers until 6 to 8 weeks of age.[45] In 2 studies, 50% and 67%, respectively, of kittens born to FPV-immune queens became susceptible to FPV challenge at 10 weeks of age, whereas 75% and 100% were susceptible by 12 weeks of age, and all were susceptible by 16 weeks of age.[46,47] In a retrospective case series of FPL, of affected kittens that been vaccinated at least once, none had received a vaccination in the primary kitten series after 12 weeks of age.[42]

Importantly, almost 50% of kittens sourced from healthy queens in rescue shelters and breeding catteries to investigate the effects of MDA on serologic responses to vaccination had no MDAs at 6 weeks of age, highlighting the susceptibility of kittens to infection among population groups in which queens are unlikely to be vaccinated or exposed to FPV.[48]

The likelihood of an unvaccinated cat developing immunity to FPV from exposure to field virus increases with age.[49] Overall, seroprevalence among adult cats varies widely among different populations tested (**Table 3**). The extent to which exposure to CPV provides cross-reacting protective serum neutralizing antibody titers in cats is not fully known. Oral inoculation of 3 cats with CPV-2c resulted in high serum neutralizing antibody titers against a commonly studied FPV strain (TU-1), whereas inoculation of 2 cats with CPV-2a resulted in a low anti-TU-1 antibody titer in 1 cat and a high titer in another.[50] In vitro testing of FPV and CPV against a panel of monoclonal antibodies produced against these viruses also demonstrated cross-reactivity because many antigenic epitopes are shared.[21,51,52]

Feline panleukopenia generally occurs from summer to early autumn coinciding with the onset of seasonal polyestrus and the corresponding influx of large numbers of kittens with progressively waning MDA levels into shelters.[41]

Table 3
Seroprevalence of FPV among populations adult cats that were unvaccinated or of unknown vaccination status

Year of Sampling	Country	Origin of Cats	No. of Cats Tested	FPV Seroprevalence (%)
1968[108]	New Zealand	Commercial suppliers	50	78
1981[109]	Australia	Unowned stray and feral cats	92	79
1998[36–38]	Vietnam	Animal markets	119	50
1998–2000[110]	Saudi Arabia	Feral cats	10	10
1998–2001[111]	Costa Rica	Owned cats	52[a]	93
2001[112]	Guatemala	Owned cats	24	38
2005[113]	United States	Feral cats	61[a]	33
2007[114]	France	Owned and unowned stray cats	469[a]	25
2010[49]	United States	New shelter admissions	111	55
2011–2012[115]	Germany	Owned cats	28[a]	29
2013[116]	Russian	Owned cats	60	45

[a] Some cats <1 year old were included in these data.

PATHOGENESIS

Carnivore protoparvovirus 1 is a highly contagious, resilient virus capable of persisting in infected premises such as shelters for at least 1 year.[53,54] It is also resistant to heating (80°C for 30 min) and low pH (3.0).[55] In infected cats, virus is shed in large quantities in all excretions including saliva, urine, feces, and vomitus.[56]

The major portals of infection are the gastrointestinal (GI) tract via orofecal transmission and, less commonly, the respiratory tract through inhalation of aerosolized virus. The latter route was confirmed by transmission experiments in the 1930s through intranasal inoculation of FPV.[4,57] In the field, transmission is predominantly indirect by fomites.[56] In 1 retrospective review of naturally occurring FPV infections, 62% of affected cats were housed exclusively indoors, and 15% had no contact with other cats.[42]

After infection, Carnivore protoparvovirus 1 binds to its cellular receptor, the TfR, a transmembrane protein that is expressed in many tissues.[15,58,59] Virions enter cells by clathrin-mediated endocytosis and colocalize with transferrin in endosomes before entering the cytoplasm to allow viral DNA to gain access to the nucleus.[60] Viral DNA is released from the capsid and replicates through double-stranded RNA intermediates in the nucleus of the cell. The virus does not possess its own DNA polymerase and must "hijack" that of the host for replication to occur. Since the virus can only replicate in actively diving S-phase cells, it has tropism for lymphoid tissue, bone marrow, intestinal crypt epithelium, and the tissues of neonates still undergoing active replication-FPV can replicate in the Purkinje cells of the cerebellum in neonates less than 10 days old.[56,61]

Viral replication in oropharyngeal lymphoid tissue occurs 18 to 24 h postinfection, and viremia can be detected within 2 to 7 days postinfection (DPI).[56] Clinical disease occurs in cats after 2 to 10 days incubation.[56] Shedding of virus in feces may occur in the absence of clinical signs (subclinical infections), or before clinical signs of disease are detected. In experimental infections, virus shedding, detected by virus isolation, occurred in urine for as long as 21 DPI and in feces for up to 6 weeks, although most cats stopped shedding virus in feces after 3 weeks.[56,62] Low-level shedding of virus, as detected by sensitive methodologies such as quantitative PCR may persist for greater than 6 weeks.

Transplacental infection can also occur, resulting in abortion, mummified fetuses or stillborn kittens (early gestation), or kittens born with central nervous system deficits (late gestation) (see clinical signs).[63]

CLINICAL PRESENTATION

Infection by FPV or CPV can be clinical or subclinical. High seroprevalence rates in some populations of unvaccinated adult cats (see **Table 3**) suggest that subclinical infections are common in young adult cats. Determinants of clinical disease include age, immune status, and coinfections with intestinal parasites, viruses, and bacteria.[64]

Disease can be peracute, resulting in sudden death from septic shock with no premonitory signs, especially in kittens less than 2 month old. The most common presentation is characterized by an acute course of disease over several days with high fever 104°F to 106°F (40°C –41°C),[4] lethargy, anorexia, vomiting, diarrhea, and severe dehydration. Only some of these signs may be present, vomiting usually precedes diarrhea, and, in contrast to dogs with CPV enteritis, hemorrhagic diarrhea is much less common, ranging from 3% to 15% of cats with FPL in 3 studies.[40,43,65] Hypersalivation from nausea may be present (**Fig. 1**), and was observed in 20% of cats with FPL in 1 shelter.[43] Abdominal palpation may be painful and reveal thickened intestinal loops and/or mesenteric lymph node enlargement (**Fig. 2**).

Myocarditis is a recognized complication of CPV infection in puppies, but convincing evidence to support a role for parvoviral infection in cats with myocarditis is lacking. Although parvoviral DNA has been amplified from the myocardium of kittens[66] and cats with myocarditis,[67] this could be reflect previous active infection, because in situ hybridization did not show any association with inflammatory foci.[66]

Depending on the stage of pregnancy at which infection occurs, infected queens can abort (early pregnancy) or give birth to kittens with central nervous system and ocular defects (late pregnancy), including cerebellar hypoplasia, hydrocephalus, hydranencephaly, retinal dysplasia, and optic nerve hypoplasia.[63,68,69] Clinical signs of parvovirus infection in queens range from absent (subclinical infection) to severe.

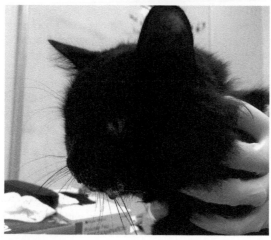

Fig. 1. FPV-infected cat with nausea-associated hypersalivation.

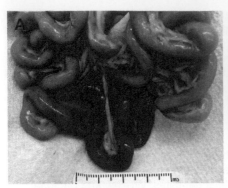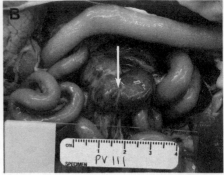

Fig. 2. (A) FPL causes severe enteritis, which is often segmental, affecting the jejunum, as shown here. Clinical signs on palpation may include thickened, painful intestinal loops or an abdominal mass associated with (B) mesenteric lymph node enlargement.

COMPLICATIONS OF FELINE PANLEUKOPENIA

Common complications that usually result in death include circulatory shock, septicemia, and disseminated intravascular coagulation (DIC). Cats with FPL are also susceptible to coinfections as a result of severe immunosuppression. In previous reports of disseminated fungal infections of cats, including aspergillosis and mucormycosis, 17% to 59% of cases had concurrent FPL.[70]

DIAGNOSIS
Hematology and Biochemistry

The onset of GI signs usually coincides with severe leukopenia (leukocyte counts 50–3000 cells/μL in severe cases; 3000–7000 cells/μL in less severe cases). Leukopenia is diagnosed in 65% to 75% of cases,[42,71] and is characterized by neutropenia and lymphopenia.[42] In 1 study 5 to 6 days after experimental inoculation, white blood cell counts were 350 to 500 cells/μL, but recovery was rapid and a rebound leukocytosis occurred within 2 to 3 days of the nadir.[72]

Thrombocytopenia, diagnosed in approximately 55% of cases,[42,71] results from megakaryocyte destruction or DIC. Anemia occurs in 50% of cases and is usually mild unless there is severe GI blood loss. The most common serum biochemical abnormalities are hypoalbuminemia (45%–52%), hypochloridemia (36%), hyponatremia (32%), hypoproteinemia (30%), and elevations of aspartate aminotransferase (27%).[42,71]

Neutralizing antibodies bind to the 3-fold spike regions of the viral capsid, the major antigenic site of FPV/CPV, and can be detected within 6 to 8 DPI.[56] Serologic detection of antibody is not used for diagnosis, because it does not distinguish between presence of MDAs or acquired humoral immunity to field or vaccine strains of virus.

Confirmatory Tests: Fecal Antigen Tests, Polymerase Chain Reaction, Virus Isolation

Cage-side fecal antigen enzyme-linked immunosorbent assay test kits designed to detect CPV in dogs can be used for diagnosis of FPL in cats, as they detect both CPV-2a-c and FPV antigen in feline feces. The sensitivity of these tests in 1 small study of 200 feline fecal samples, including 52 from cats with diarrhea, of which 10 were confirmed to have parvovirus infection on electron microscopy, ranged from 50% to 80% in 5 different commercial kits. Test specificity was high (94%–100%).[73] A diagnosis of FPL should never be ruled out based on a negative fecal antigen enzyme-linked immunosorbent assay test result; intermittent viral shedding or prevention of binding of monoclonal antibodies to viral epitopes by endogenous antibodies can negatively affect test sensitivity.

Vaccination against FPV using MLV vaccines can result in false-positive test fecal antigen results for at least 14 days after vaccination.[74] The specificity of CPV fecal antigen tests in recently vaccinated kittens was shown to vary widely depending on the brand of kit used (79.8%–98.4%).[75]

Polymerase chain reaction assays can be used to confirm the diagnosis of FPL in cases that test negative on point-of-care fecal antigen tests, but in which clinical presentation is suggestive of disease. Commercial PCR assays are usually quantitative PCR assays that will amplify and detect the DNA of carnivore protoparvovirus 1, but may not distinguish between feline (FPV) and canine (CPV) strains. False-positives can occur in recently vaccinated cats. Copy numbers of vaccine strains of CPV in dogs are generally 4- to 5-fold lower than those of dogs infected with field strains.[76,77] Whether the same is true in cats has not been determined.

Other confirmatory tests for diagnosis that have largely been superseded by the ready availability of fecal antigen tests and PCR include virus isolation, hemaglutination assays or detection of parvovirus particles using immuno-electron microscopy.

Necropsy

Gross postmortem findings range from minimal to extensive segmental enteritis with dilation, hyperemia, hemorrhage, and necrosis, and/or serosal petechial or ecchymotic hemorrhages (see **Fig. 2**). Lesions are most severe in the jejunum and ileum. Thickening of intestinal walls secondary to edema is also common. Mesenteric lymph nodes are often enlarged, hemorrhagic, and edematous.[4,57,61] On histology, intestinal crypts are dilated and distended, with mucus and sloughed necrotic cell debris.[78] Intranuclear inclusion bodies may be present in crypt enterocytes. Destruction of intestinal crypt epithelium results in mucosal collapse, with contraction and fusion of intestinal villi. In severe, acute disease, crypt epithelium can slough completely, leaving only the basement membrane. In addition to edema and hemorrhage, there is marked lymphocyte destruction in mesenteric lymph nodes. Lymphocytic infiltrates are absent from all tissues, and intestinal mucosal infiltration by inflammatory cells is mild, owing to the absence of leukocytes.

SEROLOGIC TESTING

Serology can be performed to identify cats at low risk of developing FPL after exposure to FPV. A point-of-care test (ImmunoComb Feline VacciCheck, Biogal), which requires minimal whole blood (10 µL), and tests up to 12 samples in parallel, was recently evaluated after modification by the manufacturers to increase its sensitivity.[79] Sera from 347 cats were tested and a hemagglutination inhibition assay was used as the reference method. Using a cutoff of ≥1:40 in the hemagglutination inhibition assay to define a protective titer, test sensitivity was 83%, specificity was 86%, and, given the overall antibody prevalence of 71%, the positive predictive value was 94% and the negative predictive value was 68%. Therefore, in the study population, a positive test result was very likely (94%) to indicate that the cat was protected against FPL, whereas a negative test result was much less likely (68%) to indicate lack of protection. For managing FPL in a shelter, the specificity of this serologic test is more critical than sensitivity, because the most likely consequence of a false-negative result is an unnecessary primary or booster vaccination. However, failure to identify a susceptible animal (false-positive result) confers a risk of fatal disease if the result is used to inform the decision whether to vaccinate the cat.

TREATMENT

Because of the high risk of contagion, any cat diagnosed with FPL and treated as an in-patient should be quarantined in isolation, and barrier-nursed using strict hygiene to prevent fomite transmission.

Fluid, Electrolyte, and Glucose Supplementation

Dehydration is often profound, and is a major contributor to mortality. Fluid, acid-base, and electrolyte imbalances should be monitored and restored. Blood glucose should be monitored in kittens. Parenteral glucose supplementation may be required in addition to intravenous crystalloid therapy. Hypoalbuminemic cats (albumin <20 g/L) require plasma, synthetic colloids (eg, hetastarch), or typed whole-blood transfusion if there is concurrent anemia. Plasma and heparin therapy are appropriate for treatment of DIC.

Antimicrobial Therapy and Anthelminthics

Antimicrobial therapy is essential, because overwhelming sepsis associated with translocation of GI tract bacteria and profound immunosuppression are a leading cause of death. Antimicrobials with efficacy against Gram-negative, Gram-positive and anaerobic bacteria should be chosen and given intravenously where possible. Other important considerations include patient factors such as age, hydration status, and renal function, as well as jurisdictional regulatory requirements for antimicrobial use. For example, amoxycillin-clavulanate, ampicillin-sulbactam, amoxicillin, or ampicillin could be combined with marbofloxacin, or, if the patient is rehydrated and there is no evidence of acute renal injury, with gentamicin. Others have recommended the combination of a potentiated penicillin with a third-generation cephalosporin.[80]

The use of anthelminthics (eg, milbemycin oxime-praziquantel, imidacloprid-moxidectin, or fenbendazole) is another important consideration, because intestinal parasitism is a common comorbidity, especially in shelter-housed cats. Oral anthelminthics should not be administered to vomiting cats.

Antiemetic and Gastroprotectants Therapy

Antiemetic therapy should be prescribed for vomiting cats. Early enteral nutrition with highly digestible diets is indicated as soon as emesis is controlled. Maropitant, a $5-HT_3$ receptor antagonist, is the antiemetic of choice,[71] and, when vomiting is intractable, it can be combined with ondansetron, another $5-HT_3$ receptor antagonist.[81] Mirtazapine, an antidepressant drug with serotonergic effects that is commonly used for appetite stimulation in cats, also has antinausea and antiemetic properties, mediated through $5-HT_3$ receptor antagonism.[82] However, caution should be exercised when using combinations of $5-HT_3$ receptor antagonists because serotonin syndrome is a possible adverse effect.[83] In addition, the safety of mirtazapine in kittens has not been evaluated. In cats with hematemesis or with severe intractable vomiting, and in which secondary reflux and esophagitis are of concern, parenteral GI protectants, such as proton pump inhibitors (eg, esomeprazole or pantoprazole) or H_2 receptor antagonists (eg, ranitidine or famotidine) may be indicated.

Recombinant Feline or Human Granulocyte Colony-Stimulating Factor Therapy

Prospective studies evaluating the efficacy of recombinant feline or human granulocyte colony-stimulating factor (rHuG-CSF) in cats with FPL are warranted. Bone marrow cultures derived from healthy cats were inoculated with FPV, resulting in loss of 80% to 90% of cells of myeloid lineage by 6 to 7 DPI.[84] Treatment of uninfected bone marrow cultures with rHuG-CSF, granulocyte macrophage-CSF, or macrophage-CSF stimulated growth of myeloid progenitor cells. However, myeloid progenitor cell proliferation was inhibited after inoculation of these cell cultures with FPV.[84] Treatment of clinical cases of FPL with rHuG-CSF did not increase leukocyte count.[85]

In dogs with parvoviral enteritis, 2 of 3 studies showed no effect of rHuG-CSF on neutrophil counts of CPV-infected dogs compared with controls.[85–87] Treatment of naturally occurring CPV infections in dogs using recombinant canine G-CSF was associated with a significant increase in neutrophil and white blood cell counts compared with controls, and with decreased hospitalization times.[88] However, mortality was significant higher in the treatment group, and 2 of the 4 dogs that died had DIC, raising questions about a possible adverse treatment effect.

Passive Immunotherapy

In some European countries, immune-serum raised in horses containing FPV antibodies is commercially available for treatment and prevention of infection in susceptible animals (Feliserin Plus, IDT Biologika GmbH, Germany). Treatment efficacy has not been evaluated in any prospective trials in cats. In 1 small retrospective study, the survival rate among 19 treated cats (68%), was significantly higher than in untreated cats (51%).[89] A prospective, randomized, placebo-controlled, double-masked study to evaluate its efficacy for treatment of CPV enteritis was performed in dogs, after establishing that the sera fully neutralized all antigenic variants of CPV in vitro.[90] No treatment benefit was demonstrated—there were no significant differences between treatment and placebo groups for clinical signs, laboratory parameters, survival, recovery time, or fecal viral loads. For information on passive immunization in shelter cats using homologous serum see "Shelter management of an FPL outbreak, *newly admitted cats.*"

PROGNOSIS

Feline panleukopenia has a high mortality rate; survival rates in 3 retrospective studies, in which all affected cats were given supportive treatment, were 20%, 34%, and 51%.[43,65,71] In 1 study, the risk of death was greater in cats with (vs without) lethargy, hypothermia (rectal temperature <100.2°F [37.9°C]), or low body weight at admission.[71] Treatment with any of the following—antibiotics (amoxicillin-clavulanic acid), antiparasiticides, or antiemetics (maropitant)—was associated with a lower risk of nonsurvival. Administration of a glucose infusion was statistically associated with death, and likely reflects the poor prognosis of cats with advanced sepsis. The administration of recombinant feline omega interferon (rFeIFN) at 1 MU/kg subcutaneously (SC) q24 h for 3 days was not associated with survival. The finding that treatment with rFeIFN did not confer an increased chance of survival contrasts with results of a report in which treatment of dogs experimentally infected with CPV was associated with improved clinical signs and reduced mortality.[91] In cats, further prospective investigations are warranted, because, in the retrospective feline study, the mortality rate was high (80%) and cats that died before completion of the 3-day course of therapy were included in the analyses.[71] In an in vitro study, treatment of feline cell cultures with rFeIFN before FPV infection had a strong antiviral effect.[92]

Other poor prognostic indicators for FPL include low leukocyte or platelet counts at presentation,[42] low leukocyte counts during hospitalization (days 3, 4, and 7),[71] or hypoalbuminaemia (albumin <30 g/L) or hypokalemia (<4 mmol/L) at presentation[42]

VACCINATION AGAINST FELINE PARVOVIRUS

In most kittens, MDAs have waned below concentrations that will cause vaccine interference by 8 to 12 weeks of age.[45] However, in some kittens MDAs may persist at interfering titers until 16 to 20 weeks of age,[48,93] especially if the queen has high antibody titers against FPV. The World Small Animal Veterinary Association (WSAVA) vaccination guidelines and the American Association of Feline Practitioners (AAFP) feline vaccination advisory panel report recommend a schedule of feline core vaccinations against FPV, feline calicivirus, and feline herpesvirus 1 commencing at 6 to 8 weeks of age, and then repeating vaccination every 2 to 4 weeks until ≥16 weeks of age.[45,94] The WSAVA guidelines also recommend consideration of bringing forward the "booster" vaccine, which aims to capture nonresponders to the primary series of kitten vaccines, from 12 to 6 months of age, to decrease the risk of exposure to field virus in unprotected individuals.[45]

For adult cats receiving their first vaccination, an initial series of 2 doses of an inactivated or MLV core vaccine, administered 2 to 4 weeks apart, is recommended to establish a protective immune-response to feline calicivirus and feline herpesvirus 1, although only a single dose of an MLV vaccine is required to establish a protective immune-response to FPV.[45] Modified live virus vaccines should be avoided in pregnant queens to prevent severe neurologic sequelae in developing fetuses.[69]

Vaccination against FPV induces a long-lasting humoral immunity in responders (approximately 7 years), and a triannual revaccination interval is recommended. However, for cats entering potentially high-stress, high-exposure environments such as boarding facilities, the AAFP guidelines recommend considering a booster 7 to 10 days before admission, particularly if the cat has not received a vaccination in the last 12 months.

In shelter environments the core vaccine schedule is as above, except that the first dose is recommended to be given as early as 4 weeks of age, but not later than 6 weeks of age.[45,94] Administration of MLV vaccines against FPV in kittens younger than 4 weeks of age is not recommended because of the risk of cerebellar hypoplasia.[94] Because of faster onset of action,[95] greater efficacy at overcoming MDAs,[48] and greater likelihood of a protective antibody titer occurring, MLV parenteral vaccines are recommended over inactivated vaccines.[45,94] Intranasal FPV vaccination is not recommended in shelters because it is inferior to FPV parenteral vaccines, and its use was associated with re-emergent outbreaks of FPV in shelters in the United States in the late 1990s and early 2000s.[96] In shelters where FPV exposure is likely to occur, vaccination of pregnant queens or queens of unknown pregnancy status, with MLV vaccines, with an inherent risk of fetal death or malformation, may be preferable to not vaccinating against FPV, which risks loss of both the queen and her offspring from FPL.[94]

SHELTER MANAGEMENT OF A FELINE PANLEUKOPENIA OUTBREAK
Diagnosis and Isolation

After confirmation of a suspected outbreak of FPL in a shelter (see confirmatory tests above), diagnosis of FPL in subsequent cases is often based on 1 or more of the following: consistent clinical signs in exposed cats, positive fecal antigen test results, and/or low white blood cell count on a peripheral blood smear. It is imperative that all sick cats with confirmed or suspected FPL are moved to an isolation area for treatment that is, ideally, physically separated from the rest of the shelter. Staff working in the isolation area should not enter other areas of the shelter.

Identification and Quarantine of Exposed Cats

In the face of an outbreak, all clinically healthy exposed and at-risk cats and kittens more than 4 weeks old should be vaccinated with MLV vaccines immediately and held in a separate quarantine area for 2 weeks. The quarantine area should only contain nonporous surfaces that are easy to clean and disinfect. Handling of cats should be kept to a minimum, to reduce stress and the risk of fomite transmission.

Serologic testing can be used to identify adult cats at low risk of infection and to reduce the number of cats requiring quarantine during an outbreak. Seropositive exposed cats are unlikely to develop FPL and can be adopted out of the shelter immediately, bypassing the need for quarantine during the incubation period, even if they have not been vaccinated or vaccination status is unknown. All kittens should be vaccinated regardless, since serologic tests do not differentiate MDAs from acquired humoral immunity. All seronegative animals are susceptible and should be vaccinated and subsequently retested to confirm seroconversion.

Biosecurity

Infection control practices including signage (eg, infectious disease hazard signs, handwashing, and disinfection posters), personal protective equipment (disposable gloves, gown, boots/shoe covers), and equipment, as well as infection control training procedures for shelter staff and volunteers, should be reviewed, to minimize the potential for fomite spread. Restriction of access of nonessential personnel to the shelter and closure to new intake should occur until the outbreak is controlled. Infection control training for all staff and volunteers (eg, workshops, on-line modules) is highly recommended.

Effective disinfectants against Carnivore protoparvovirus 1 include sodium hypochlorite (5%–6% household bleach diluted 1:30), accelerated hydrogen peroxide (eg, Accel or Rescue, Virox Technologies Inc.), and potassium peroxymonosulfate (eg, Trifectant, Virkon). Parvoviruses are resistant to quaternary ammonium compounds (QAC). Some disinfectants containing QAC/biguanide combinations (eg, F10, Trigene II) carry label claims of efficacy against parvoviruses in Europe, although independent, peer-reviewed, published efficacy trials are lacking. Since most disinfectants are inactivated by the presence of organic matter, cleaning with detergent before application of disinfection is essential. Disinfection of porous surfaces, such as carpets, is problematic because residual organic matter is likely to persist after cleaning. Also, using wet heat (eg, steam cleaning), a temperature of $\geq 90°C$ and minimum application time of 10 minutes, is required to inactivate parvoviruses.[97]

Alcohol-based hand sanitizers are ineffective against parvoviruses. Handwashing using liquid-soap or foaming handwash from dispensers is required to physically remove fomites.[98] Manufacturer guidelines for disinfectant dilutions, shelf-life once diluted, and contact times should be strictly observed. For example, diluted bleach solutions must be made-up fresh monthly and stored in light-proof containers to retain efficacy.[99] Rinse steps are also essential after contact times have been observed, because some disinfectants are corrosive (eg, bleach and potassium peroxymonosulfate) and/or cause caustic injury to cats after direct exposure to footpads, conjunctiva, and skin, as well as oral ulceration and esophagitis from inadvertent ingestion during grooming.[100]

Isolation and quarantine areas should each have their own dedicated equipment for cleaning and disinfection to prevent inadvertent fomite transmission to other parts of the shelter. Work flow, based on infection risk, is critical during an outbreak. Separate staff should care for each different cohort and, if possible, their movements to other parts of the shelter should be restricted. If staff numbers are limited, new admissions should be cleaned and fed first, followed by quarantine incumbent cats, then sick affected cats in isolation.

Protection of Newly Admitted Cats

All cats and kittens $\geq$4 weeks of age should be vaccinated against FPV using MLV vaccines and kittens should be revaccinated every 2 weeks, while they remain in the shelter, until 20 weeks of age.[45]

For exposed cats and kittens that are known to be unvaccinated or colostrum deprived, passive immunization using homologous serum from a recently immunized cat, or nonhomologous serum (eg, Feliserin Plus), can be used to confer rapid protection. Passive immunization of kittens using sera from cats recovered from recent FPV infection was practiced as early as 1949, and was found to confer protection against infection for 2 to 3 weeks.[40] A study in 2001 found that administration of 150 mL/kg of adult cat serum given SC or intraperitoneally (IP) to colostrum-deprived kittens achieved comparable concentrations with those ingested in colostrum.[101] For passive immunization against FPV, a dose of homologous serum from a recently vaccinated cat, of 2 mL/kitten SC or IP, has also been recommended.[102] Alternatively, plasma can be given intravenously. Because immunoglobulins can persist for up to 4 weeks, vaccination of passively immunized kittens must be delayed by 2 to 4 weeks.[103]

Documentation and Communication

Comprehensive daily records should be maintained, documenting all aspects of an FPL outbreak including case numbers, clinical presentation and disease course, mortality, methods of diagnosis, biosecurity and vaccination protocols, and husbandry practices before and after the outbreak, so that progress can be tracked. A communication strategy is essential to limit disease spread, and all stakeholders should be informed of the outbreak, including other shelters and veterinary hospitals in the same region, foster carers, shelter-volunteers, as well as shelter and veterinary associations.

SUMMARY

Feline panleukopenia, the oldest known viral disease of cats, is highly contagious. Despite the availability of highly effective vaccines against FPV, which also confer a long duration of immunity, the prevalence of exposure to FPV remains high worldwide. In some countries, such as Australia, FPL is a re-emerging disease. In addition, all current circulating canine parvoviruses can infect and cause disease in cats. Group-housed cats are highly susceptible to FPL outbreaks, which are most likely to occur from summer to autumn, in association with an influx of kittens with waning maternally derived immunity into shelters. To effectively combat outbreaks of FPL, knowledge of the characteristics of parvoviruses, disease epidemiology, diagnostics, optimal treatment, and infection control practices, as well as WSAVA- and AAFP-recommended vaccination strategies, is essential.

ACKNOWLEDGEMENTS

The author's research on FPL is generously funded by the Cat Protection Society of New South Wales, the Morris Animal Foundation (D18FE-001) and the Winn Feline Foundation (W18-006).

REFERENCES

1. Liu H, Fu Y, Xie J, et al. Widespread endogenization of densoviruses and parvoviruses in animal and human genomes. J Virol 2011;85(19):9863–76.
2. Fairweather J. Epidemic among cats in Delhi, resembling cholera. Lancet 1876; 2:115–7, 148-150.
3. Scott FW. Viral diseases - Panleukopenia. In: Holzworth J, editor. Diseases of the cat, vol. 1. Philadelphia: W. B. Saunders; 1987. p. 182–93.
4. Leasure EE, Lienardt HF, Taberner FR. Feline infectious enteritis. North Am Vet 1934;15(7):30–4.
5. Verge J, Cristoforoni N. La gastroenterite infectieuse des chats est elle due a un virus filtrable? Comptes rendus des seances de la Societe de biologie (Paris) 1928;99:312–4.
6. Johnson RH. Isolation of a virus from a condition simulating feline panleukopaenia in a leopard. Vet Rec 1964;76:1008–12.
7. Povey RC. Feline panleukopenia – which vaccine? J Small Anim Pract 1973; 14(7):399–406.
8. People's Dispensary for Sick Animals. PDSA Animal Wellbeing Report 2017. Telford (United Kingdom): PDSA; 2017. p. 27.
9. Barrs VR, Brailey J, Allison AB, et al. Re-emergence of feline panleukopenia in Australia. 27th ECVIM-CA Congress. St Julian's, Malta, September 14–16. 2017:ISCAID_0_4.
10. Cotmore SF, Agbandje-McKenna M, Chiorini JA, et al. The family Parvoviridae. Arch Virol 2014;159(5):1239–47.
11. Allison AB, Kohler DJ, Fox KA, et al. Frequent cross-species transmission of parvoviruses among diverse carnivore hosts. J Virol 2013;87(4):2342–7.
12. Allison AB, Kohler DJ, Ortega A, et al. Host-specific parvovirus evolution in nature is recapitulated by in vitro adaptation to different carnivore species. PLoS Pathog 2014;10(11):e1004475.
13. Truyen U, Parrish CR. Canine and feline host ranges of canine parvovirus and feline panleukopenia virus: distinct host cell tropisms of each virus in vitro and in vivo. J Virol 1992;66(9):5399–408.
14. Hoelzer K, Parrish CR. The emergence of parvoviruses of carnivores. Vet Res 2010;41(6):39.
15. Hueffer K, Parker JS, Weichert WS, et al. The natural host range shift and subsequent evolution of canine parvovirus resulted from virus-specific binding to the canine transferrin receptor. J Virol 2003;77(3):1718–26.
16. Parrish CR. Host range relationships and the evolution of canine parvovirus. Vet Microbiol 1999;69(1–2):29–40.
17. Allison AB, Parrish CR. Parvoviruses of carnivores. Their transmission and the variation of viral host range. In: Johnson N, editor. The role of animals in emerging viral diseases. Oxford, UK: Elsevier Science & Technology; 2014.
18. Truyen U, Agbandje M, Parrish CR. Characterization of the feline host range and a specific epitope of feline panleukopenia virus. Virology 1994;200(2):494–503.
19. Truyen U, Muller T, Heidrich R, et al. Survey on viral pathogens in wild red foxes (*Vulpes vulpes*) in Germany with emphasis on parvoviruses and analysis of a DNA sequence from a red fox parvovirus. Epidemiol Infect 1998;121(2):433–40.
20. Parrish CR, Have P, Foreyt WJ, et al. The global spread and replacement of canine parvovirus strains. J Gen Virol 1988;69(Pt 5):1111–6.
21. Parrish CR, O'Connell PH, Evermann JF, et al. Natural variation of canine parvovirus. Science 1985;230(4729):1046–8.

22. Parrish CR, Aquadro CF, Strassheim ML, et al. Rapid antigenic-type replacement and DNA sequence evolution of canine parvovirus. J Virol 1991;65(12): 6544–52.

23. Buonavoglia C, Martella V, Pratelli A, et al. Evidence for evolution of canine parvovirus type 2 in Italy. J Gen Virol 2001;82(Pt 12):3021–5.

24. Mochizuki M, Harasawa R, Nakatani H. Antigenic and genomic variabilities among recently prevalent parvoviruses of canine and feline origin in Japan. Vet Microbiol 1993;38(1–2):1–10.

25. Clegg SR, Coyne KP, Dawson S, et al. Canine parvovirus in asymptomatic feline carriers. Vet Microbiol 2012;157(1–2):78–85.

26. Mukhopadhyay HK, Nookala M, Thangamani NR, et al. Molecular characterisation of parvoviruses from domestic cats reveals emergence of newer variants in India. J Feline Med Surg 2017;19(8):846–52.

27. Clegg SR, Coyne KP, Parker J, et al. Molecular epidemiology and phylogeny reveal complex spatial dynamics in areas where canine parvovirus is endemic. J Virol 2011;85(15):7892–9.

28. Byrne P, Beatty JA, Slapeta J, et al. Shelter-housed cats show no evidence of faecal shedding of canine parvovirus DNA. Vet J 2018;239:54–8.

29. Miranda C, Parrish CR, Thompson G. Canine parvovirus 2c infection in a cat with severe clinical disease. J Vet Diagn Invest 2014;26(3):462–4.

30. Mochizuki M, Horiuchi M, Hiragi H, et al. Isolation of canine parvovirus from a cat manifesting clinical signs of feline panleukopenia. J Clin Microbiol 1996;34(9): 2101–5.

31. Decaro N, Buonavoglia D, Desario C, et al. Characterisation of canine parvovirus strains isolated from cats with feline panleukopenia. Res Vet Sci 2010; 89(2):275–8.

32. Battilani M, Balboni A, Giunti M, et al. Co-infection with feline and canine parvovirus in a cat. Vet Ital 2013;49(1):127–9.

33. Battilani M, Balboni A, Ustulin M, et al. Genetic complexity and multiple infections with more parvovirus species in naturally infected cats. Vet Res 2011;42: 43.

34. Nakamura K, Sakamoto M, Ikeda Y, et al. Pathogenic potential of canine parvovirus types 2a and 2c in domestic cats. Clin Diagn Lab Immunol 2001;8(3): 663–8.

35. Gamoh K, Shimazaki Y, Makie H, et al. The pathogenicity of canine parvovirus type-2b, FP84 strain isolated from a domestic cat, in domestic cats. J Vet Med Sci 2003;65(9):1027–9.

36. Ikeda Y, Miyazawa T, Nakamura K, et al. Serosurvey for selected virus infections of wild carnivores in Taiwan and Vietnam. J Wildl Dis 1999;35(3):578–81.

37. Miyazawa T, Ikeda Y, Nakamura K, et al. Isolation of feline parvovirus from peripheral blood mononuclear cells of cats in northern Vietnam. Microbiol Immunol 1999;43(6):609–12.

38. Nakamura K, Ikeda Y, Miyazawa T, et al. Comparison of prevalence of feline herpesvirus type 1, calicivirus and parvovirus infections in domestic and leopard cats in Vietnam. J Vet Med Sci 1999;61(12):1313–5.

39. Norja P, Hokynar K, Aaltonen LM, et al. Bioportfolio: lifelong persistence of variant and prototypic erythrovirus DNA genomes in human tissue. Proc Natl Acad Sci U S A 2006;103(19):7450–3.

40. Bentinck-Smith J. Feline panleukopenia (feline infectious enteritis) - a review of 574 cases. North Am Vet 1949;30:379–84.

41. Reif JS. Seasonality, natality and herd immunity in feline panleukopenia. Am J Epidemiol 1976;103(1):81–7.
42. Kruse BD, Unterer S, Horlacher K, et al. Prognostic factors in cats with feline panleukopenia. J Vet Intern Med 2010;24(6):1271–6.
43. Litster A, Benjanirut C. Case series of feline panleukopenia virus in an animal shelter. J Feline Med Surg 2014;16(4):346–53.
44. Crawford PC, Hanel RM, Levy JK. Evaluation of treatment of colostrum-deprived kittens with equine IgG. Am J Vet Res 2003;64(8):969–75.
45. Day MJ, Horzinek MC, Schultz RD, et al. WSAVA Guidelines for the vaccination of dogs and cats. J Small Anim Pract 2016;57(1):E1–45.
46. Scott F, Csiza CK, Gillespie JH. Maternally derived immunity to feline panleukopenia. J Am Vet Med Assoc 1970;156:439–53.
47. Scott FW. Comments on feline panleukopenia biologics. J Am Vet Med Assoc 1971;158:910–5.
48. Digangi BA, Levy JK, Griffin B, et al. Effects of maternally-derived antibodies on serologic responses to vaccination in kittens. J Feline Med Surg 2012;14(2): 118–23.
49. DiGangi BA, Levy JK, Griffin B, et al. Prevalence of serum antibody titers against feline panleukopenia virus, feline herpesvirus 1, and feline calicivirus in cats entering a Florida animal shelter. J Am Vet Med Assoc 2012;241(10):1320–5.
50. Nakamura K, Ikeda Y, Miyazawa T, et al. Characterisation of cross-reactivity of virus neutralising antibodies induced by feline panleukopenia virus and canine parvoviruses. Res Vet Sci 2001;71(3):219–22.
51. Parrish CR, Carmichael LE, Antczak DF. Antigenic relationships between canine parvovirus type 2, feline panleukopenia virus and mink enteritis virus using conventional antisera and monoclonal antibodies. Arch Virol 1982;72(4):267–78.
52. Parrish CR, Carmichael LE. Antigenic structure and variation of canine parvovirus type-2, feline panleukopenia virus, and mink enteritis virus. Virology 1983;129(2):401–14.
53. Johnson RH. Feline panleucopaenia virus. III. Some properties compared to a feline herpes virus. Res Vet Sci 1966;7:112–5.
54. Johnson RH. Feline panleucopaenia. Vet Rec 1969;84:338–40.
55. Goto H, Yachida S, Shirahata T, et al. Feline panleukopenia in Japan. I. Isolation and characterization of the virus. Nihon Juigaku Zasshi 1974;36(3):203–11.
56. Csiza CK, Scott FW, De Lahunta A, et al. Pathogenesis of feline panleukopenia virus in susceptible newborn kittens I. Clinical signs, hematology, serology, and virology. Infect Immun 1971;3(6):833–7.
57. Dalling T. Distemper of the cat. Vet Rec 1934;14(38):1137–48.
58. Hueffer K, Govindasamy L, Agbandje-McKenna M, et al. Combinations of two capsid regions controlling canine host range determine canine transferrin receptor binding by canine and feline parvoviruses. J Virol 2003;77(18): 10099–105.
59. Parker JS, Murphy WJ, Wang D, et al. Canine and feline parvoviruses can use human or feline transferrin receptors to bind, enter, and infect cells. J Virol 2001;75(8):3896–902.
60. Hueffer K, Palermo LM, Parrish CR. Parvovirus infection of cells by using variants of the feline transferrin receptor altering clathrin-mediated endocytosis, membrane domain localization, and capsid-binding domains. J Virol 2004; 78(11):5601–11.

61. Csiza CK, De Lahunta A, Scott FW, et al. Pathogenesis of feline panleukopenia virus in susceptible newborn kittens II. Pathology and immunofluorescence. Infect Immun 1971;3(6):838–46.
62. Csiza CK, Scott FW, de Lahunta A, et al. Immune carrier state of feline panleukopenia virus-infected cats. Am J Vet Res 1971;32(3):419–26.
63. Csiza CK, Scott FW, Gillespie JH, et al. Feline viruses. XIV. Transplacental infections in spontaneous panleukopenia of cats. Cornell Vet 1971;61(3):423–39.
64. Moschidou P, Martella V, Lorusso E, et al. Mixed infection by feline astrovirus and feline panleukopenia virus in a domestic cat with gastroenteritis and panleukopenia. J Vet Diagn Invest 2011;23(3):581–4.
65. Kruse BD, Unterer S, Horlacher K, et al. Feline panleukopenia - different course of disease in cats younger than versus older than 6 months of age? Tierarztl Prax Ausg K Kleintiere Heimtiere 2011;39(4):237–42 [in German].
66. McEndaffer L, Molesan A, Erb H, et al. Feline panleukopenia virus is not associated with myocarditis or endomyocardial restrictive cardiomyopathy in cats. Vet Pathol 2017;54(4):669–75.
67. Meurs KM, Fox PR, Magnon AL, et al. Molecular screening by polymerase chain reaction detects panleukopenia virus DNA in formalin-fixed hearts from cats with idiopathic cardiomyopathy and myocarditis. Cardiovasc Pathol 2000;9(2): 119–26.
68. Url A, Truyen U, Rebel-Bauder B, et al. Evidence of parvovirus replication in cerebral neurons of cats. J Clin Microbiol 2003;41(8):3801–5.
69. Sharp NJ, Davis BJ, Guy JS, et al. Hydranencephaly and cerebellar hypoplasia in two kittens attributed to intrauterine parvovirus infection. J Comp Pathol 1999; 121(1):39–53.
70. Ossent P. Systemic aspergillosis and mucormycosis in 23 cats. Vet Rec 1987; 120(14):330–3.
71. Porporato F, Horzinek MC, Hofmann-Lehmann R, et al. Survival estimates and outcome predictors for shelter cats with feline panleukopenia virus infection. J Am Vet Med Assoc 2018;253(2):188–95.
72. Riser WH. Infectious panleukopenia of cats. North Am Veterinarian 1943;24: 293–8.
73. Neuerer FF, Horlacher K, Truyen U, et al. Comparison of different in-house test systems to detect parvovirus in faeces of cats. J Feline Med Surg 2008;10(3): 247–51.
74. Patterson EV, Reese MJ, Tucker SJ, et al. Effect of vaccination on parvovirus antigen testing in kittens. J Am Vet Med Assoc 2007;230(3):359–63.
75. Meason-Smith C, Diesel A, Patterson AP, et al. Characterization of the cutaneous mycobiota in healthy and allergic cats using next generation sequencing. Vet Dermatol 2017;28(1):71–e17.
76. Decaro N, Desario C, Campolo M, et al. Clinical and virological findings in pups naturally infected by canine parvovirus type 2 Glu-426 mutant. J Vet Diagn Invest 2005;17(2):133–8.
77. Freisl M, Speck S, Truyen U, et al. Faecal shedding of canine parvovirus after modified-live vaccination in healthy adult dogs. Vet J 2017;219:15–21.
78. Machlachlan N, Dubovi EJ, Barthold SW, et al. Parvoviridae. In: Machlachlan N, Dubovi EJ, editors. Fenner's Veterinary Virology. London: Elsevier; 2016. p. 245–58.
79. Mende K, Stuetzer B, Truyen U, et al. Evaluation of an in-house dot enzyme-linked immunosorbent assay to detect antibodies against feline panleukopenia virus. J Feline Med Surg 2014;16(10):805–11.

80. Stuetzer B, Hartmann K. Feline parvovirus infection and associated diseases. Vet J 2014;201(2):150–5.
81. Quimby JM, Lake RC, Hansen RJ, et al. Oral, subcutaneous, and intravenous pharmacokinetics of ondansetron in healthy cats. J Vet Pharmacol Ther 2014; 37(4):348–53.
82. Quimby JM, Lunn KF. Mirtazapine as an appetite stimulant and anti-emetic in cats with chronic kidney disease: a masked placebo-controlled crossover clinical trial. Vet J 2013;197(3):651–5.
83. Quimby JM, Gustafson DL, Samber BJ, et al. Studies on the pharmacokinetics and pharmacodynamics of mirtazapine in healthy young cats. J Vet Pharmacol Ther 2011;34(4):388–96.
84. Kurtzman GJ, Platanias L, Lustig L, et al. Feline parvovirus propagates in cat bone marrow cultures and inhibits hematopoietic colony formation in vitro. Blood 1989;74(1):71–81.
85. Kraft W, Kuffer M. Treatment of severe neutropenias in dogs and cats with filgrastim. Tierarztl Prax 1995;23(6):609–13 [in German].
86. Mischke R, Barth T, Wohlsein P, et al. Effect of recombinant human granulocyte colony-stimulating factor (rhG-CSF) on leukocyte count and survival rate of dogs with parvoviral enteritis. Res Vet Sci 2001;70(3):221–5.
87. Rewerts JM, McCaw DL, Cohn LA, et al. Recombinant human granulocyte colony-stimulating factor for treatment of puppies with neutropenia secondary to canine parvovirus infection. J Am Vet Med Assoc 1998;213(7):991–2.
88. Duffy A, Dow S, Ogilvie G, et al. Hematologic improvement in dogs with parvovirus infection treated with recombinant canine granulocyte-colony stimulating factor. J Vet Pharmacol Ther 2010;33(4):352–6.
89. Wolfesberger B, Tichy A, Afenzeller N, et al. Clinical outcome of 73 cases with feline panleukopenia. Wien Tierarztl Monatsschr 2012;99:11–7.
90. Gerlach M, Proksch AL, Unterer S, et al. Efficacy of feline anti-parvovirus antibodies in the treatment of canine parvovirus infection. J Small Anim Pract 2017;58(7):408–15.
91. Martin V, Najbar W, Gueguen S, et al. Treatment of canine parvoviral enteritis with interferon-omega in a placebo-controlled challenge trial. Vet Microbiol 2002;89(2–3):115–27.
92. Mochizuki M, Nakatani H, Yoshida M. Inhibitory effects of recombinant feline interferon on the replication of feline enteropathogenic viruses in vitro. Vet Microbiol 1994;39(1–2):145–52.
93. Jakel V, Cussler K, Hanschmann KM, et al. Vaccination against feline panleukopenia: implications from a field study in kittens. BMC Vet Res 2012;8:62.
94. Scherk MA, Ford RB, Gaskell RM, et al. 2013 AAFP feline vaccination advisory panel report. J Feline Med Surg 2013;15(9):785–808.
95. Lappin MR. Feline panleukopenia virus, feline herpesvirus-1 and feline calicivirus antibody responses in seronegative specific pathogen-free kittens after parenteral administration of an inactivated FVRCP vaccine or a modified live FVRCP vaccine. J Feline Med Surg 2012;14(2):161–4.
96. Schultz RD. A commentary on parvovirus vaccination. J Feline Med Surg 2009; 11(2):163–4.
97. Boschetti N, Wyss K, Mischler A, et al. Stability of minute virus of mice against temperature and sodium hydroxide. Biologicals 2003;31(3):181–5.
98. Anderson ME. Contact precautions and hand hygiene in veterinary clinics. Vet Clin North Am Small Anim Pract 2015;45(2):343–60, vi.

99. Piskin B, Turkun M. Stability of various sodium hypochlorite solutions. J Endod 1995;21(5):253–5.
100. Addie DD, Boucraut-Baralon C, Egberink H, et al. Disinfectant choices in veterinary practices, shelters and households: ABCD guidelines on safe and effective disinfection for feline environments. J Feline Med Surg 2015;17(7):594–605.
101. Levy JK, Crawford PC, Collante WR, et al. Use of adult cat serum to correct failure of passive transfer in kittens. J Am Vet Med Assoc 2001;219(10):1401–5.
102. Greene CE. Feline enteric viral infections. In: Greene CE, editor. Infectious diseases of the dog and cat. Fourth edition. Philadelphia: Elsevier; 2011. p. 80–91 [Chapter 9].
103. Truyen U, Addie D, Belak S, et al. Feline panleukopenia. ABCD guidelines on prevention and management. J Feline Med Surg 2009;11(7):538–46.
104. Truyen U, Platzer G, Parrish CR. Antigenic type distribution among canine parvoviruses in dogs and cats in Germany. Vet Rec 1996;138(15):365–6.
105. Decaro N, Desario C, Miccolupo A, et al. Genetic analysis of feline panleukopenia viruses from cats with gastroenteritis. J Gen Virol 2008;89(Pt 9):2290–8.
106. Filipov C, Desario C, Patouchas O, et al. A ten-year molecular survey on parvoviruses infecting carnivores in Bulgaria. Transbound Emerg Dis 2016;63(4): 460–4.
107. Wu J, Gao XT, Hou SH, et al. Molecular epidemiological and phylogenetic analyses of canine parvovirus in domestic dogs and cats in Beijing, 2010-2013. J Vet Med Sci 2015;77(10):1305–10.
108. Fastier LB. Feline panleucopenia – a serological study. Vet Rec 1968;83(25): 653–4.
109. Coman BJ, Jones EH, Westbury HA. Protozoan and viral infections of feral cats. Aust Vet J 1981;57(7):319–23.
110. Ostrowski S, Van Vuuren M, Lenain DM, et al. A serologic survey of wild felids from central west Saudi Arabia. J Wildl Dis 2003;39(3):696–701.
111. Blanco K, Prendas J, Cortes R, et al. Seroprevalence of viral infections in domestic cats in Costa Rica. J Vet Med Sci 2009;71(5):661–3.
112. Lickey AL, Kennedy M, Patton S, et al. Serologic survey of domestic felids in the Peten region of Guatemala. J Zoo Wildl Med 2005;36(1):121–3.
113. Fischer SM, Quest CM, Dubovi EJ, et al. Response of feral cats to vaccination at the time of neutering. J Am Vet Med Assoc 2007;230(1):52–8.
114. Hellard E, Fouchet D, Santin-Janin H, et al. When cats' ways of life interact with their viruses: a study in 15 natural populations of owned and unowned cats (Felis silvestris catus). Prev Vet Med 2011;101(3–4):250–64.
115. Mende K, Stuetzer B, Sauter-Louis C, et al. Prevalence of antibodies against feline panleukopenia virus in client-owned cats in Southern Germany. Vet J 2014; 199(3):419–23.
116. Pavlova EV, Kirilyuk VE, Naidenko SV. Patterns of seroprevalence of feline viruses among domestic cats (Felis catus) and Pallas' cats (Otocolobus manul) in Daursky Reserve, Russia. Can J Zool 2015;93:849–55.

Diversity of the Lyme Disease Spirochetes and its Influence on Immune Responses to Infection and Vaccination

Jerilyn R. Izac, BS, Richard T. Marconi, PhD*

KEYWORDS

- Lyme disease • Canines • OspC • Ixodes ticks • Lyme vaccines • Borrelia
- Lyme diagnostics • OspA

KEY POINTS

- The Lyme spirochetes are a unique and genetically diverse group of bacteria.
- To complete the enzootic cycle, the Lyme spirochetes must adapt to the radically different environmental conditions encountered in ticks and mammals.
- Outer surface proteins A and C play distinctly different but critical roles in the biology and pathogenesis of Lyme disease.
- OspC is an immunodominant antigen produced during early infection. Antibody responses to diverse OspC proteins are OspC type specific and driven by variable domains of the protein.
- Understanding the diversity of the Lyme spirochetes and its surface proteins is essential for interpreting immune responses elicited by infection or vaccination.

THE DISCOVERY OF LYME DISEASE

Lyme disease (LD), as a clinical entity, was first described in the United States in the late 1970s (reviewed by Steere[1]). The path toward defining the basis of this debilitating infection began when concerned parents living in Lyme, Connecticut, contacted the Connecticut State Department of Health and reported an unusual clustering of juvenile rheumatoid arthritis cases in their area.[1] A joint investigation launched by the

Disclosure: R.T. Marconi has a financial relationship with Zoetis and Global Lyme Diagnostics.
Department of Microbiology and Immunology, School of Medicine, Virginia Commonwealth University Medical Center, 1112 East Clay Street, Room 101 McGuire Hall, PO Box 980678, Richmond, VA 23298-0678, USA
* Corresponding author.
E-mail address: richard.marconi@vcuhealth.org

Vet Clin Small Anim 49 (2019) 671–686
https://doi.org/10.1016/j.cvsm.2019.02.007
0195-5616/19/© 2019 The Authors. Published by Elsevier Inc. This is an open access article under the CC BY license (http://creativecommons.org/licenses/by/4.0/).

Connecticut State Department of Health and Yale University School of Medicine identified 51 cases of oligoarthritis of unknown cause in children and adults living in Lyme, Old Lyme, and East Haddam, Connecticut.[2] Approximately 25% of the affected individuals recalled developing an enlarging rash in the weeks before disease onset. The general characteristics of the rash were similar to a rash described in 1909 in Sweden by Arvid Afzelius that was referred to as erythema migrans (EM).[3]

Afzelius made several seminal contributions to our current day understanding of the epidemiology of LD, including the establishment of a connection between the bite of Ixodes ricinus ticks (a European I. species) and the development of EM.[4] It was not until 1976 that a connection was made between the bite of I. scapularis ticks (formerly classified as I. dammini) and the development of EM and Lyme arthritis in patients in the United States.[5] Shortly thereafter, researchers at the Rocky Mountain Laboratories (NIH) cultured a previously uncharacterized spirochete from I. scapularis ticks that was designated as Borrelia burgdorferi.[6] A direct link between B. burgdorferi and Lyme arthritis was established with its cultivation from the blood of patients with LD.[7,8] The first case of canine Lyme arthritis was diagnosed shortly thereafter.[9]

Lyme disease is the most common arthropod-borne disease of canines and humans. The Companion Animal Parasite Council (CAPC) reported that there were 319,000 positive LD antibody tests in canines in 2018; up from 160,000 in 2012 (www.capcvet.org). As explained by CAPC, these values are underestimates because data are collected for only ~30% of the tests that are run. The Centers for Disease Control and Prevention estimates that the probable number of clinician-diagnosed cases of human LD each year in the United States is ~329,000.[10] The incidence and endemic regions for LD and I. ticks are expanding in the United States, Canada, Europe, and Asia.[11–14]

CLASSIFICATION OF TICK-BORNE SPIROCHETES

Before the identification of the LD spirochetes, the genus Borrelia consisted primarily of species associated with tick-borne relapsing fever (TBRF). The TBRF is a spirochetal infection transmitted by the soft-bodied Ornithodoros ticks.[15] Ornithodoros ticks are anatomically distinct from the hard-bodied I. ticks that transmit LD. They also have different feeding strategies and developmental processes.[15] Ticks that transmit TBRF are nocturnal feeders that reside in nesting materials in caves, rustic (unmaintained) cabins, and other similar structures. They feed rapidly and can transmit spirochetes within minutes. A hallmark feature of TBRF is a high-grade relapsing fever that coincides with the appearance of a remarkable number of spirochetes in the blood (10^6 to 10^8 mL^{-1} blood) (**Fig. 1**A). The molecular basis of the cyclic spirochetemias can be traced to an elaborate antigenic variation system.[16,17] Tick-borne relapsing fever occurs in isolated pockets in the United States but is widespread in other parts of the world. Its health consequences in parts of Africa are staggering.[18]

Lyme disease is transmitted by tick species belonging to the genus Ixodes. I. scapularis and I. pacificus are the primary species that transmit LD in the United States and Canada, whereas I. ricinus and I. persulcatus are the primary vectors in Europe and Asia.[19] I. ticks inhabit wooded areas, unkept brush, tall grasses, and leaf litter. They feed over the course of several days with transmission of the LD spirochetes typically requiring a feeding period of 24 to 72 hours. Transmission time can vary depending on the strain of the LD spirochete, the health of the tick and inherent variation among hosts. In contrast to TBRF, high-density spirochetemias are not a characteristic of LD. A notable exception is B. myiamotoi, which can cause transient spirochetemias.[20]

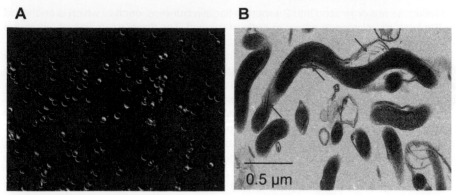

Fig. 1. The unique structure of spirochetes. (*A*) A dark-field microscopic image of *Borrelia hermsii*, a relapsing fever spirochete, in blood collected from an infected mouse. Mice were infected by needle inoculation and blood samples were collected 3 days after inoculation. The characteristic spiral morphology shared by all spirochetes is readily visible. Note, there is high-density spirochetemia. In contrast to relapsing fever, spirochetemias are not common in mammals infected with Lyme disease. (*B*) A transmission electron micrograph of the oral spirochete *Treponema denticola*. The endoflagella bundles that are unique to spirochetes are indicated by the arrows.

Although *B. myiamotoi* causes a TBRF-like illness, this species is transmitted by *I.* ticks and is more closely related to the LD spirochetes than it is to the TBRF spirochetes. Several reviews have detailed the biology, health toll, and pathogenesis of TBRF in humans and canines.[18,21,22]

Soon after the discovery of *B. burgdorferi*, comparative studies of LD spirochete isolates from North America, Europe, and Asia revealed significant genetic and antigenic diversity. Based on these analyses, *B. burgdorferi* was divided into 3 distinct species: *B. burgdorferi*, *B. garinii*, and *B. afzelii*.[23–25] *B. burgdorferi* is the primary species found in North America, whereas in Europe, all 3 species are present. Further exploration of the phylogenetic relationships among LD spirochete species and isolates led to the delineation of several additional species.[26–29] The potential significance of these species in veterinary and human health remains to be defined.

The genus *Borrelia* has been recently divided into 2 genera: *Borrelia* and *Borreliella*.[30] Consistent with taxonomic precedent, since the TBRF species were described first, they retain the *Borrelia* genus designation. The LD spirochetes and *B. myiamotoi* were assigned a new genus designation, *Borreliella*. Sharp differences of opinion exist concerning the practical implications of this reclassification.[31,32] Although the use of the designation *Borreliella* is voluntary, readers should be aware of this change because it has been fully applied in public databases and is beginning to appear in the literature.

UNIQUE FEATURES OF SPIROCHETES

Spirochetes are distinct from other bacteria in several fundamental and fascinating ways. A feature shared by all spirochetes is their unique flat wave or spirallike ultrastructure (see **Fig. 1**A).[33] This characteristic morphology results from the presence of endoflagella, which are found in all spirochetes. The flagella arrangement in *Treponema denticola*, the periodontal disease pathogen, is shown in **Fig. 1**B. The endoflagella are organized into 2 separate flagella bundles, each of which is anchored to the inner membrane at opposite ends of the cell. The flagella bundles sit within the periplasmic space and extend ~three-quarters of the length of the cell.[34]

Distinguishing features specifically of the LD and TBRF spirochetes include the composition of their cell wall and a unique genome arrangement (reviewed by Barbour and Hayes[21]). Like Gram-negative bacteria, they possess an inner and outer membrane, but lack lipopolysaccharide. Lipopolysaccharide is replaced by a diverse array of lipidated outer surface proteins (Osps) that play important roles in the host-pathogen interaction. Some of these Osps are described in detail below. The LD and TBRF spirochetes are distinct from all other bacteria, including other spirochetes, in that they possess a small, segmented genome consisting of a linear chromosome (0.9 Mb) and a series of linear and circular plasmids.[35] Linear DNA is rare in bacteria. The plasmids range in size from 9 to 200 kb and comprise nearly 40% of the total genome.[36] The total number and size of the plasmids carried by individual isolates can vary significantly.[37] Plasmid variation results from plasmid loss, acquisition and genetic rearrangement.[38] Some plasmids are dispensable,[39] whereas others are essential for infection or survival.[40] The unique properties of the LD spirochete genome are reviewed in.[41]

DEVELOPMENTAL STAGES OF *IXODES* TICKS

Lyme disease is maintained in nature in an enzootic cycle involving *I.* ticks and a diverse array of mammalian reservoir hosts.[42] The first developmental stage of a tick is the larva. Because transovarial transmission of the LD spirochetes in ticks does not occur, on emerging from the egg, larvae do not carry the LD spirochetes. *I.* ticks can only become infected by feeding on an infected mammal through a process referred to as acquisition. After taking their first and only bloodmeal, the 6-legged larvae detach from their feeding source and molt into 8-legged nymphs. This anatomic change has important implications for tick biology and feeding behavior, because it allows nymphs and adult ticks to climb up into brush where they gain better access to larger and more mobile mammals. Nymphs also feed just once and then molt into sexually differentiated adults. The body weight of an adult female tick may increase by as much as 500-fold after the bloodmeal. Because male ticks do not feed, they play no significant role in transmission of LD. Images of engorged adult female *I. scapularis* and *Amblyomma americanum* (lone star tick) ticks are presented in **Fig. 2**. Pets and their owners are merely accidental hosts, and as such, do not play a significant role in maintaining LD in nature.

ADAPTIVE RESPONSES AND THEIR IMPORTANCE IN THE ENZOOTIC CYCLE

The acquisition of spirochetes by ticks and their transmission to mammals are active processes that are dependent on tightly regulated adaptive responses.[43,44] Akins and colleagues[45] conducted a creative and pivotal study that provided insight into the nature of adaptive responses. They compared the protein content of laboratory grown spirochetes with that of host-adapted spirochetes. To accomplish this, cultures of LD spirochetes were placed in dialysis membrane chambers and implanted in the peritoneal cavity of rats. Spirochetes maintained in dialysis membrane chambers become host-adapted and thus, more closely resemble spirochetes during natural infection.[45] Comparison of the protein profiles of laboratory-cultivated and host-adapted spirochetes revealed significant differences in the production levels of OspA, OspB, and OspC (as well as other proteins). OspA and OspB were produced at high levels in laboratory-cultivated spirochetes but not host-adapted spirochetes.[45] In contrast,

A   **B**

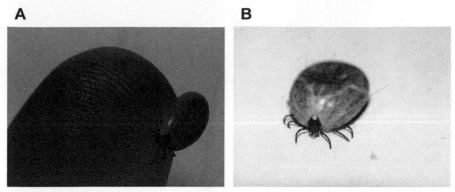

Fig. 2. Engorged adult female *Ixodes* and *Amblyomma* ticks. Images of engorged adult female *I. scapularis* and *Amblyomma americanum* ticks are shown in (*A*) and (*B*), respectively. The *I. scapularis* and *A americanum* ticks were found feeding on a cat and dog, respectively. Female *A americanum* ticks can be readily distinguished from *I. scapularis* ticks by the white dot on the dorsal shield. Both ticks were collected from pets at a single residential property in Midlothian, Virginia. *B. burgdorferi* was successfully cultured from the midgut of the *I. scapularis* tick shown in the image.

OspC production was low in laboratory spirochetes but high in host-adapted spirochetes (**Fig. 3**). The Akins study also proved central in shaping our understanding of humoral immune responses during infection. The Osp production patterns they reported are consistent with the development of a strong and early antibody response to OspC in mammals and the absence of a response to OspA and OspB.[46] Low-level production of OspC during cultivation is well documented in the literature.[47,48] Oliver and colleagues[47] demonstrated that only 10% of the individual cells in a laboratory culture produce detectable amounts of OspC.

Adaptation to the distinctly different environmental conditions present in unfed ticks, fed ticks, and mammals also requires changes in Osp production.[49] In an unfed tick, spirochetes residing in the nutrient-poor, midgut environment, produce high levels of OspA. Intake of a bloodmeal quickly changes the environment triggering a transition from OspA to OspC production.[50] The upregulation of OspC at the tick-host interface is consistent with studies that have demonstrated that OspC is required for transmission and the establishment of an active infection in mammals. Strains that have been modified to not produce a functional OspC are unable to infect mammals.[51–53]

OUTER SURFACE PROTEIN VARIATION: INFLUENCE ON VACCINE AND DIAGNOSTIC ASSAY DEVELOPMENT

The LD spirochetes produce a diverse array of Osps and the subset produced at any given time is controlled by environmental conditions. A comprehensive review of properties and functions of characterized Osps is beyond the scope of this report. Although several Osps have been investigated for use in vaccine or diagnostic assay development (reviewed by Earnhart and Marconi[54]), the discussion here is focused on OspC. OspC is a lipoprotein that varies in molecular weight (20–24 kDa) among isolates.[55] The *ospC* gene is carried by a highly stable circular plasmid of 26 kDa[56] referred to as cp26.[53] An individual LD isolate produces only a single OspC protein variant. The antigenic diversity of OspC among LD spirochete isolates is well documented and has been intensively studied.[57–59]

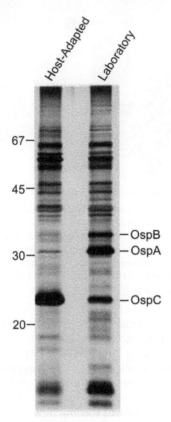

Fig. 3. Adaptive responses of Lyme disease spirochetes. The protein profiles of spirochetes cultivated in the laboratory or host-adapted spirochetes that were grown in dialysis membrane chambers implanted within the peritoneal cavity of rats are shown. The proteins were fractionated by gel electrophoresis (SDS-PAGE) and visualized by staining with Coomassie blue. Note, the significant differences in the production levels of OspA, OspB, and OspC. Molecular weight standards are shown on the left. (*Courtesy of* Dr. Darrin Akins, The University of Oklahoma Health Sciences Center, Oklahoma City, OK.)

Before our current understanding of OspC phylogenetics, sequence variation seemed an insurmountable hurdle to overcome in efforts to use OspC as a vaccine or diagnostic antigen.[60] It was assumed that *ospC* variation arises through mutation during infection with subsequent immune selection allowing for the emergence of new antigenic variants. However, OspC is genetically stable during infection.[61] Numerous distinct and stable variants of OspC, referred to as OspC types, have been identified. OspC types are differentiated by a letter or other appropriate designation (reviewed by Marconi and Earnhart[60]). OspC proteins of a given OspC type are conserved with percent amino acid identity values of ~95% or greater. Identity values between OspC types can be as low as 65%. For example, Earnhart and Marconi[57] compared the sequences of 55 OspC type A proteins and found that amino acid identity values among these proteins were greater than 97%.

Studies by Brisson and colleagues[62,63] have provided significant insight into the biological rationale for the existence and maintenance of multiple, stable *ospC* types in nature. Although an individual LD spirochete strain produces only a single OspC type, ticks commonly carry a heterogenous population of strains that as a whole can produce many different OspC proteins.[64] The existence of multiple OspC types in a given tick may help to ensure that upon feeding, at least a subset of the strains can infect an animal that has been immunologically primed by previous exposure to other OspC types. It has been hypothesized that OspC type identity may also influence mammalian host compatibility.[62] Certain OspC types may facilitate infection of specific mammals. Rhodes and colleagues[65] reported that the most common OspC type detected in infected canines was OspC type F. This is striking, because there have been no reports of the isolation of an OspC type F producing strain from humans. Although more research is required to address the biological rationale for the maintenance of distinct OspC types in nature, OspC diversity is critical to consider when assessing host immune responses to this immunodominant early antigen.

ANTIBODY RESPONSES TO OspC DURING INFECTION AND ON IMMUNIZATION

Evidence that antibody responses to OspC are type specific came from studies in which mice were inoculated with individual LD strains producing different OspC types.[66] Immunoblot analyses of the infection serum collected from these mice revealed that IgG responses are OspC type specific. Rabbits immunized with purified recombinant OspC proteins also developed type-specific IgG responses.[47] The lack of antibody cross-reactivity with different OspC types is intriguing because segments of sequence are shared by all OspC proteins (ie, are conserved). The specificity of the antibody response suggests that variable regions of OspC are presented to the immune system.[47]

OspC type-specific antibody responses have also been demonstrated in naturally infected canines.[47] Serum from dogs confirmed to be LD positive reacted with only a limited subset of OspC proteins in immunoblot analyses. The observed specificity of the OspC antibody response is consistent with epitope mapping studies that identified 2 dominant but variable epitopes of OspC.[67] The regions corresponding to these antigenic domains were designated as the L5 and H5 epitopes. Although the sequences of these epitopes vary among OspC proteins, they are highly conserved among proteins of an individual OspC type.[57,67,68] The immunodominance of the L5 and H5 epitopes likely explains the basis for type-specific nature of the OspC antibody response.

It has been reported in some studies that a conserved motif of OspC drives antibody responses.[69–71] This suggestion is difficult to reconcile in light of the type-specific responses detailed above. This motif, referred to as either the C7, C10, or pepC10 motif, is proline rich and comprises the last 10 C-terminal residues of OspC.[55] If a conserved sequence common to OspC types (ie, C10) constitutes a dominant epitope, then antibody to OspC should bind to all OspC proteins. In this report, potential immune responses to C10 were further investigated. All methods used in the experiments presented below have been described previously.[47] Recombinant OspC proteins (types I, F, and T) were generated with or without the C10 motif (OspC-IΔC10, OspC-FΔC10, and OspC-TΔC10), purified and screened with serum from representative LD-positive horses (animal ID number, 1026) and dogs (TF1286). Serum from dog TF1286 bound to OspC type T but not to type F (**Fig. 4**). Infection serum from horse number 1026 bound to OspC type F but OspC type I. Furthermore, OspC proteins that lack the C10 motif were readily detected by antibody in infection serum. These observations support the contention that the C10 motif is not a dominant epitope and that it is the variable domains of OspC that drive antibody responses.

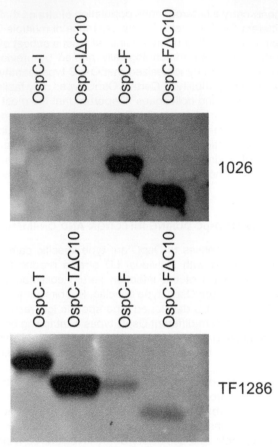

Fig. 4. Specificity of the antibody response to OspC in infected dogs and horses. Recombinant OspC proteins (types I, F, and T) with or without the putative C10 epitope were produced, purified, and transferred onto membranes for immunoblot analysis. The membranes were screened with serum from an infected dog (ID number, TF1286; top panel) or an infected horse (ID number, 1026; bottom panel), and IgG binding to each protein was assessed using the appropriate secondary antibody and chemiluminescence. Note that although antibody to OspC was detected, the antibody was not cross-reactive with the different OspC types. In addition, deletion of the C10 motif from each protein had no discernible impact on the level of antibody binding.

DOES INFECTION WITH THE LYME DISEASE SPIROCHETES ELICIT PROTECTIVE IMMUNITY?

It is common knowledge among veterinarians who practice in LD endemic areas that a significant percentage of dogs will develop repeated LD infections. This phenomenon is well documented in humans. In 1 study, 15% of patients with LD living in a Lyme endemic area developed 1 or more follow-up infections within 5 years.[72] To add to our understanding of LD and protective immunity, we sought to determine if infection of mice with clonal populations of LD spirochetes results in broad, or strain-specific, bactericidal antibody responses. In this report, separate groups of mice were infected with *B. burgdorferi* B31, N40, and 297 and *B. afzelii* PKo using previously detailed methods.[51] Sera harvested from the mice were then tested for bactericidal activity against each strain using in vitro assays.[73] Representative data are presented in **Fig. 5**. Serum from mice infected with *B. burgdorferi* B31 efficiently killed B31 but did not kill *B. burgdorferi* N40, 297, or *B. afzelii* PKo (see **Fig. 5**). Conversely, serum from mice infected with *B. afzelii* PKo efficiently killed PKo but not *B. burgdorferi* B31, N40, or 297. To determine if killing is complement dependent, 1 set of reactions were run with heat-inactivated complement or no complement added. Guinea pig serum served as the exogenous complement source. No killing was observed unless active complement was included in the assay. The data indicate that serum-mediated killing occurs through an antibody-mediated, complement-dependent mechanism. More importantly, it can be concluded that infection with a given LD spirochete does not induce broadly protective antibody responses.

PREVENTION: THE KEY TO TACKLING THE LYME DISEASE PROBLEM

Vaccination is widely considered to be the most cost-effective approach for prevention of infectious diseases. Concerns about accurate diagnosis and appropriate treatment strategies for LD could be alleviated to some degree through aggressive

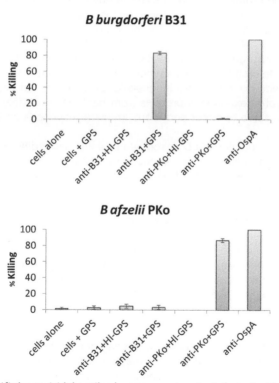

Fig. 5. Strain-specific bactericidal antibody responses in mice infected with Lyme disease spirochetes. As detailed in the text, sera from mice infected with *B. burgdorferi* B31 or *B. afzelii* PKo were assessed for bactericidal activity. The infection sera were incubated with each strain with or without complement preserved guinea pig serum. Bactericidal activity was measured by determining the percentage of spirochetes that were killed as a result of exposure to the infection serum (% killing). Note that the antibody-mediated killing was strain specific and occurred through a complement-dependent mechanism. It can be concluded that infection with an individual Lyme disease spirochete strain does not elicit a broadly protective antibody response.

vaccination. Several licensed LD vaccines are available and approved for use in canines.[54] These vaccines are of 2 general types: bacterin and subunit. Currently available bacterin vaccines are NovibacLyme (Merck), LymeVax (Zoetis) and Ultra Durammune Lyme (Elanco). Available subunit vaccines are VANGUARD crLyme (Zoetis) and Recombitek Lyme (Boehringer Ingleheim).

LYME DISEASE BACTERIN VACCINES

The composition of subunit and bacterin vaccines are inherently different. Lyme disease subunit vaccines consist of highly purified recombinant proteins (OspA and or OspC), whereas bacterin vaccines consist of lysates of 2 laboratory-cultivated LD spirochete strains.[74,75] The identity of the strains that comprise each commercially available bacterin vaccine is information that is not in the public domain. Because LD bacterin vaccines are generated from cell lysates, they contain a large number of proteins and other cellular constituents. In fact, genome sequencing and proteome analyses have demonstrated that the LD spirochetes can produce in excess of 1600 different proteins.[76,77] Most of these proteins are produced during laboratory cultivation.[78] The precise proteins that are present in any given bacterin vaccine have not been reported. Importantly, most of the proteins produced by bacteria under any growth scenario are localized within the cell and function in metabolic pathways and other important cellular processes.[79,80] Although intracellular proteins can elicit an antibody response on vaccination with a cell lysate–based bacterin formulation, they are not likely to elicit productive antibody (ie, antibody that contributes to protective immunity), because in live cells intracellular proteins are not accessible to antibody. The removal of extraneous proteins from bacterins is conceptually beneficial because it would serve to direct and focus immune responses on immunologically relevant proteins.

The differential production of LD spirochete proteins under different environmental conditions[81] may also influence the composition and antigenic content of subunit vaccines. Because bacterins are made from cultivated bacteria, they may lack potentially protective antigens that are produced by the LD spirochetes only during residence in mammals.[45] Similarly, there are additional proteins that are not produced during culture or in mammals that are selectively produced in ticks.[82] Antigens that are produced during infection in mammals or ticks would intuitively be those that are most desirable for inclusion in an LD vaccine. In this context, subunit vaccines offer some advantages in that they are composed of carefully chosen antigens with known production patterns. In addition, subunit vaccines lack extraneous proteins that are not involved in triggering protective immunity.[54]

LYME DISEASE SUBUNIT VACCINES

Recombitek Lyme is a subunit vaccine consisting of lipidated OspA. Anti-OspA antibody inhibits transmission from ticks to mammals by targeting spirochetes in the tick midgut.[83] OspA was also the sole component of LYMErix (SmithKline Beecham), the only human vaccine to have made it to market.[84] LYMErix was introduced in 1998 but then voluntarily removed in 2001. There were many factors that contributed to its demise and detailed assessments of its rise and fall can be found in several excellent reviews.[85,86] Leaving the more controversial issues aside, LYMErix was compromised by low efficacy (49%) after a 2-dose series. A 3-dose series increased efficacy to 76%.[87] The requirement for multiple boosts is because OspA-mediated protection is strictly dependent on high circulating antibody titers.[87] If titers drop below a critical threshold level, spirochetes are able to transit into a vaccinated animal.[88] Because

OspA is not produced by the LD spirochetes in mammals,[89] the spirochetes cannot be targeted by anti-OspA antibody after entering an OspA-vaccinated mammal.

VANGUARD crLyme (Zoetis), the newest canine LD vaccine to be approved by the United States Department of Agriculture, is a subunit vaccine consisting of OspA and a recombinant chimeric OspC epitope-based protein referred to as a chimeritope. OspC chimeritopes consist of linear epitopes derived from several antigenically distinct OspC proteins that are joined together in a single recombinant protein.[90] The rationale behind the development of OspC chimeritopes was to generate a protein that can elicit antibody that can target OspC proteins produced by diverse strains. The conceptual rationale for chimeritope proteins has been decribed in detail in earlier reviews and hence is not discussed further in this report.[54,60] Antibody elicited by OspC chimeritope vaccine antigens can target spirochetes during the process of transmission and during early infection in mammals. A vaccine that induces antibody that can kill spirochetes in both ticks and mammals has the potential to use 2 synergistic mechanisms of protection and thus be less dependent on the maintenance of high circulating antibody titers.

WHERE DO WE GO FROM HERE?

The Lyme spirochetes are a fascinating and remarkably diverse group of bacteria with unique biological properties. In this report, we have focused our discussion on the importance of understanding environmentally regulated protein production, the genetic and antigenic diversity of the LD spirochetes and how that diversity influences immune responses to infection and vaccination. There are many topics not addressed here that are equally worthy of discussion. As we move forward, our ability to critically assess and interpret the results of past and future studies focused on LD will directly affect how successful we are in addressing this important veterinary and human health concern.

REFERENCES

1. Steere AC. Lyme disease. N Engl J Med 2001;345:115–25.
2. Steere AC, Malawista SE, Snydman DR, et al. Lyme arthritis: an epidemic of oligoarticular arthritis in children and adults in three Connecticut communities. Arthritis Rheum 1977;20:7–17.
3. Dammin GJ. Erythema migrans: a chronicle. Rev Infect Dis 1989;11:142–51.
4. Afzelius A. Verhandlungen der dermatologischen Gesellschaft zu. Arch Dermatol Syph 1910;101:104.
5. Steere AC, Broderick TF, Malawista SE. Erythema chronicum migrans and Lyme arthritis: epidemiologic evidence for a tick vector. Am J Epidemiol 1978;108: 312–21.
6. Barbour AG. Isolation and cultivation of Lyme disease spirochetes. Yale J Biol Med 1984;57:521–5.
7. Benach JL, Bosler EM, Hanrahan JP, et al. Spirochetes isolated from the blood of two patients with Lyme disease. N Engl J Med 1983;308:740–2.
8. Steere AC, Grodzicki RL, Kornblatt AN, et al. The spirochetal etiology of Lyme disease. N Engl J Med 1983;308:733–40.
9. Lissman BA, Bosler EM, Camay H, et al. Spirochete-associated arthritis (Lyme disease) in a dog. J Am Vet Med Assoc 1984;185:219–20.
10. Nelson CA, Saha S, Kugeler KJ, et al. Incidence of clinician-diagnosed Lyme disease, United States, 2005-2010. Emerg Infect Dis 2015;21:1625–31.

11. Eisen RJ, Eisen L, Beard CB. County-scale distribution of Ixodes scapularis and Ixodes pacificus (acari: ixodidae) in the continental United States. J Med Entomol 2016;53:349–86.
12. Heyman P, Cochez C, Hofhuis A, et al. A clear and present danger: tick-borne diseases in Europe. Expert Rev Anti Infect Ther 2018;8:33–50.
13. Levy S. Northern Trek: the spread of Ixodes scapularis into Canada. Environ Health Perspect 2017;125:074002.
14. Sykes RA, Makiello P. An estimate of Lyme borreliosis incidence in Western Europe. J Public Health (Oxf) 2017;39(1):74–81.
15. Felsenfeld O. Borrelia. Strains, vectors, human and animal borreliosis. St Louis (MO): Warren H. Green, Inc.; 1971.
16. Barbour AG. Antigenic variation of a relapsing fever Borrelia species. Annu Rev Microbiol 1990;44:155–71.
17. Stoenner HG, Dodd T, Larsen C. Antigenic variation of Borrelia hermsii. J Exp Med 1982;156:1297–311.
18. Cutler SJ. Relapsing fever Borreliae: a global review. Clin Lab Med 2015;35: 847–65.
19. Keirans JE, Hutcheson HJ, Durden LA, et al. Ixodes (Ixodes) scapularis (Acari:Ixodidae): redescription of all active stages, distribution, hosts, geographical variation, and medical and veterinary importance. J Med Entomol 1996;33:297–318.
20. Fukunaga M, Takahashi Y, Tsuruta Y, et al. Genetic and phenotypic analysis of Borrelia miyamotoi sp. nov., isolates from the Ixodid tick Ixodes persulcatus, the vector for Lyme disease in Japan. Int J Syst Bacteriol 1995;45:804–10.
21. Barbour AG, Hayes SF. Biology of Borrelia species. Microbiol Rev 1986;50: 381–400.
22. Piccione J, Levine GJ, Duff CA, et al. Tick-borne relapsing fever in dogs. J Vet Intern Med 2016;30:1222–8.
23. Baranton G, Postic D, Saint Girons I, et al. Delineation of Borrelia burgdorferi sensu stricto, Borrelia garinii sp. nov., and group VS461 associated with Lyme borreliosis. Int J Syst Bacteriol 1992;42:378–83.
24. Marconi RT, Garon CF. Identification of a third genomic group of Borrelia burgdorferi through signature nucleotide analysis and 16S rRNA sequence determination. J Gen Microbiol 1992;138:533–6.
25. Postic D, Edlinger C, Richaud C, et al. Two genomic species in Borrelia burgdorferi. Res Microbiol 1990;141:465–75.
26. Marconi RT, Liveris D, Schwartz I. Identification of novel insertion elements, restriction fragment length polymorphism patterns, and discontinuous 23S rRNA in Lyme disease spirochetes: phylogenetic analyses of rRNA genes and their intergenic spacers in Borrelia japonica sp. nov. and genomic group 21038 (Borrelia andersonii sp. nov.) isolates. J Clin Microbiol 1995;33:2427–34.
27. Margos G,S, Vollmer A, Cornet M, et al. A new Borrelia species defined by multilocus sequence analysis of housekeeping genes. Appl Environ Microbiol 2009; 75:5410–6.
28. Postic D, Belfazia J, Isogai E, et al. A new genomic species in Borrelia burgdorferi sensu lato isolated from Japanese ticks. Res Microbiol 1993;144:467–73.
29. Pritt BS, Mead PS, Johnson DK, et al. Identification of a novel pathogenic Borrelia species causing Lyme borreliosis with unusually high spirochaetaemia: a descriptive study. Lancet Infect Dis 2016;16(5):556–64.
30. Adeolu M, Gupta RS. A phylogenomic and molecular marker based proposal for the division of the genus Borrelia into two genera: the emended genus Borrelia

containing only the members of the relapsing fever Borrelia, and the genus Borreliella gen. nov. containing the members of the Lyme disease Borrelia (*Borrelia burgdorferi* sensu lato complex). Antonie Van Leeuwenhoek 2014;105:1049–72.

31. Barbour AG, Adeolu M, Gupta RS. Division of the genus Borrelia into two genera (corresponding to Lyme disease and relapsing fever groups) reflects their genetic and phenotypic distinctiveness and will lead to a better understanding of these two groups of microbes (Margos et al. (2016) There is inadequate evidence to support the division of the genus Borrelia. Int. J. Syst. Evol. Microbiol. doi: 10.1099/ijsem.0.001717). Int J Syst Evol Microbiol 2017;67:2058–67.

32. Stevenson B, Fingerle V, Wormser GP, et al. Public health and patient safety concerns merit retention of Lyme borreliosis-associated spirochetes within the genus Borrelia, and rejection of the genus novum Borreliella. Ticks Tick Borne Dis 2018; 10(1):1–4.

33. Charon NW, Greenberg EP, Koopman MB, et al. Spirochete chemotaxis, motility, and the structure of the spirochetal periplasmic flagella. Res Microbiol 1992;143: 597–603.

34. Charon NW, Goldstein SF, Marko M, et al. The flat-ribbon configuration of the periplasmic flagella of *Borrelia burgdorferi* and its relationship to motility and morphology. J Bacteriol 2009;191:600–7.

35. Barbour AG. Plasmid analysis of *Borrelia burgdorferi*, the Lyme disease agent. J Clin Microbiol 1988;26:475–8.

36. Xu Y, Kodner C, Coleman L, et al. Correlation of plasmids with infectivity of *Borrelia burgdorferi* sensu stricto type strain B31. Infect Immun 1996;64:3870–6.

37. McDowell JV, Sung SY, Labandeira-Rey M, et al. Analysis of mechanisms associated with loss of infectivity of clonal populations of *Borrelia burgdorferi* B31MI. Infect Immun 2001;69:3670–7.

38. Qiu WG, Schutzer SE, Bruno JF, et al. Genetic exchange and plasmid transfers in *Borrelia burgdorferi* sensu stricto revealed by three-way genome comparisons and multilocus sequence typing. Proc Natl Acad Sci U S A 2004;101:14150–5.

39. Dulebohn DP, Bestor A, Rego RO, et al. *Borrelia burgdorferi* linear plasmid 38 is dispensable for completion of the mouse-tick infectious cycle. Infect Immun 2011;79:3510–7.

40. Casjens SR, Gilcrease EB, Vujadinovic M, et al. Plasmid diversity and phylogenetic consistency in the Lyme disease agent *Borrelia burgdorferi*. BMC Genomics 2017;18:165.

41. Casjens S. Evolution of the linear DNA replicons of the *Borrelia* spirochetes. Curr Opin Microbiol 1999;2:529–34.

42. Hovius JW, van Dam AP, Fikrig E. Tick-host-pathogen interactions in Lyme borreliosis. Trends Parasitol 2007;23:434–8.

43. Iyer R, Caimano MJ, Luthra A, et al. Stage-specific global alterations in the transcriptomes of Lyme disease spirochetes during tick feeding and following mammalian host adaptation. Mol Microbiol 2015;95:509–38.

44. Schwan TG, Piesman J. Vector interactions and molecular adaptations of Lyme disease and relapsing fever spirochetes associated with transmission by ticks. Emerg Infect Dis 2002;8:115–21.

45. Akins DR, Bourell KW, Caimano MJ, et al. A new animal model for studying Lyme disease spirochetes in a mammalian host-adapted state. J Clin Invest 1998;101: 2240–50.

46. Wilske B, Preac-Mursic V, Jauris S, et al. Immunological and molecular polymorphisms of OspC, an immunodominant major outer surface protein of *Borrelia burgdorferi*. Infect Immun 1993;61:2182–91.

47. Oliver LD Jr, Earnhart CG, Virgina-Rhodes D, et al. Antibody profiling of canine IgG responses to the OspC protein of the Lyme disease spirochetes supports a multivalent approach in vaccine and diagnostic assay development. Vet J 2016;218:27–33.

48. Xiang X, Yang Y, Du J, et al. Investigation of ospC expression variation among *Borrelia burgdorferi* strains. Front Cell Infect Microbiol 2017;7:131.

49. de Silva AM, Fikrig E. Arthropod- and host-specific gene expression by *Borrelia burgdorferi*. J Clin Invest 1997;99:377–9.

50. Schwan TG, Piesman J. Temporal changes in outer surface proteins A and C of the Lyme disease-associated spirochete, *Borrelia burgdorferi*, during the chain of infection in ticks and mice. J Clin Microbiol 2000;38:382–8.

51. Earnhart CG, Leblanc DV, Alix KE, et al. Identification of residues within ligand-binding domain 1 (LBD1) of the *Borrelia burgdorferi* OspC protein required for function in the mammalian environment. Mol Microbiol 2010;76:393–408.

52. Earnhart CG, Rhodes DV, Smith AA, et al. Assessment of the potential contribution of the highly conserved C-terminal motif (C10) of *Borrelia burgdorferi* outer surface protein C in transmission and infectivity. Pathog Dis 2014;70:176–84.

53. Tilly K, Casjens S, Stevenson B, et al. The *Borrelia burgdorferi* circular plasmid cp26: conservation of plasmid structure and targeted inactivation of the ospC gene. Mol Microbiol 1997;25:361–73.

54. Earnhart C, Marconi RT. Lyme disease. In: Barrett AD, Stanberry LR, editors. Vaccines for biodefense and emerging and neglected diseases. 1st edition. London: Elsevier; 2009. p. 1032–60.

55. Fuchs R, Jauris S, Lottspeich F, et al. Molecular analysis and expression of a *Borrelia burgdorferi* gene encoding a 22 kDa protein (pC) in *Escherichia coli*. Mol Microbiol 1992;6:503–9.

56. Marconi RT, Samuels DS, Garon CF. Transcriptional analyses and mapping of the ospC gene in Lyme disease spirochetes. J Bacteriol 1993;175:926–32.

57. Earnhart CG, Marconi RT. OspC phylogenetic analyses support the feasibility of a broadly protective polyvalent chimeric Lyme disease vaccine. Clin Vaccin Immunol 2007;14:628–34.

58. Jauris-Heipke S, Fuchs R, Motz M, et al. Genetic heterogenity of the genes coding for the outer surface protein C (OspC) and the flagellin of *Borrelia burgdorferi*. Med Microbiol Immunol 1993;182:37–50.

59. Theisen M, Frederiksen B, Lebech AM, et al. Polymorphism in ospC gene of *Borrelia burgdorferi* and immunoreactivity of OspC protein: implications for taxonomy and for use of OspC protein as a diagnostic antigen. J Clin Microbiol 1993;31:2570–6.

60. Marconi RT, Earnhart C. Lyme disease vaccines. In: Samuels DS, Radolf J, editors. Borrelia: molecular biology, host interaction and pathogenesis. Norfolk (United Kingdom): Caister Academic Press; 2010. p. 467–86.

61. Stevenson B, Bockenstedt LK, Barthold SW. Expression and gene sequence of outer surface protein C of *Borrelia burgdorferi* reisolated from chronically infected mice. Infect Immun 1994;62:3568–71.

62. Brisson D, Dykhuizen DE. ospC diversity in *Borrelia burgdorferi*: different hosts are different niches. Genetics 2004;168:713–22.

63. Brisson D, Vandermause MF, Meece JK, et al. Evolution of northeastern and midwestern *Borrelia burgdorferi*, United States. Emerg Infect Dis 2010;16:911–7.

64. Di L, Wan Z, Akther S, et al. Genotyping and quantifying Lyme pathogen strains by deep sequencing of the outer surface protein C (ospC) locus. J Clin Microbiol 2018;56 [pii:e00940-18].

65. Rhodes DV, Earnhart CG, Mather TN, et al. Identification of *Borrelia burgdorferi* ospC genotypes in canine tissue following tick infestation: implications for Lyme disease vaccine and diagnostic assay design. Vet J 2013;198:412–8.

66. Earnhart CG, Buckles EL, Dumler JS, et al. Demonstration of OspC type diversity in invasive human Lyme disease isolates and identification of previously uncharacterized epitopes that define the specificity of the OspC murine antibody response. Infect Immun 2005;73:7869–77.

67. Buckles EL, Earnhart CG, Marconi RT. Analysis of antibody response in humans to the type A OspC loop 5 domain and assessment of the potential utility of the loop 5 epitope in Lyme disease vaccine development. Clin Vaccine Immunol 2006;13:1162–5.

68. Earnhart CG, Buckles EL, Marconi RT. Development of an OspC-based tetravalent, recombinant, chimeric vaccinogen that elicits bactericidal antibody against diverse Lyme disease spirochete strains. Vaccine 2007;25:466–80.

69. Jobe DA, Lovrich SD, Schell RF, et al. C-terminal region of outer surface protein C binds borreliacidal antibodies in sera from patients with Lyme disease. Clin Diagn Lab Immunol 2003;10:573–8.

70. Lovrich SD, La Fleur RL, Jobe DA, et al. Borreliacidal OspC antibody response of canines with Lyme disease differs significantly from that of humans with Lyme disease. Clin Vaccin Immunol 2007;14:635–7.

71. Rousselle JC, Callister SM, Schell RF, et al. Borreliacidal antibody production against outer surface protein C of *Borrelia burgdorferi*. J Infect Dis 1998;178:733–41.

72. Khatchikian CE, Nadelman RB, Nowakowski J, et al. Evidence for strain-specific immunity in patients treated for early Lyme disease. Infect Immun 2014;82:1408–13.

73. Izac JR, Oliver LD Jr, Earnhart CG, et al. Identification of a defined linear epitope in the OspA protein of the Lyme disease spirochetes that elicits bactericidal antibody responses: implications for vaccine development. Vaccine 2017;35:3178–85.

74. Chu HJ, Chavez LG Jr, Blumer BM, et al. Immunogenicity and efficacy study of a commercial *Borrelia burgdorferi* bacterin. J Am Vet Med Assoc 1992;201:403–11.

75. LaFleur RL, Dant JC, Wasmoen TL, et al. Bacterin that induces anti-OspA and anti-OspC borreliacidal antibodies provides a high level of protection against canine Lyme disease. Clin Vaccin Immunol 2009;16:253–9.

76. Barbour AG, Jasinskas A, Kayala MA, et al. A genome-wide proteome array reveals a limited set of immunogens in natural infections of humans and white-footed mice with *Borrelia burgdorferi*. Infect Immun 2008;76:3374–89.

77. Fraser CM, Casjens S, Huang WM, et al. Genomic sequence of a Lyme disease spirochaete, *Borrelia burgdorferi*. Nature 1997;390:580–6.

78. Ojaimi C, Brooks C, Casjens S, et al. Profiling of temperature-induced changes in *Borrelia burgdorferi* gene expression by using whole genome arrays. Infect Immun 2003;71:1689–705.

79. Schutzer SE, Fraser-Liggett CM, Casjens SR, et al. Whole-genome sequences of thirteen isolates of *Borrelia burgdorferi*. J Bacteriol 2011;193:1018–20.

80. Schutzer SE, Fraser-Liggett CM, Qiu WG, et al. Whole-genome sequences of *Borrelia bissettii*, *Borrelia valaisiana*, and *Borrelia spielmanii*. J Bacteriol 2012;194:545–6.

81. Gilmore RD Jr, Mbow ML, Stevenson B. Analysis of *Borrelia burgdorferi* gene expression during life cycle phases of the tick vector *Ixodes scapularis*. Microbes Infect 2001;3:799–808.

82. Caimano MJ, Dunham-Ems S, Allard AM, et al. Cyclic di-GMP modulates gene expression in Lyme disease spirochetes at the tick-mammal interface to promote spirochete survival during the blood meal and tick-to-mammal transmission. Infect Immun 2015;83:3043–60.
83. Fikrig E, Telford SR 3rd, Barthold SW, et al. Elimination of *Borrelia burgdorferi* from vector ticks feeding on OspA-immunized mice. Proc Natl Acad Sci U S A 1992; 89:5418–21.
84. Parenti D. Lyme disease vaccine–LYMErix. Conn Med 1999;63:570.
85. Nigrovic LE, Thompson KM. The Lyme vaccine: a cautionary tale. Epidemiol Infect 2007;135:1–8.
86. Zundorf I, Dingermann T. Death of a vaccine – the fall of LYMErix. Pharm Unserer Zeit 2008;37:38–9 [in German].
87. Steere AC, Sikand VK, Meurice F, et al. Vaccination against Lyme disease with recombinant *Borrelia burgdorferi* outer-surface lipoprotein A with adjuvant. Lyme Disease Vaccine Study Group. N Engl J Med 1998;339:209–15.
88. de Silva AM, Zeidner NS, Zhang Y, et al. Influence of outer surface protein A antibody on *Borrelia burgdorferi* within feeding ticks. Infect Immun 1999;67:30–5.
89. Schwan TG. Temporal regulation of outer surface proteins of the Lyme-disease spirochaete *Borrelia burgdorferi*. Biochem Soc Trans 2003;31:108–12.
90. Earnhart CG, Marconi RT. An octavalent Lyme disease vaccine induces antibodies that recognize all incorporated OspC type-specific sequences. Hum Vaccin 2007;3:281–9.

Feline Vector-Borne Diseases in North America

Barbara Qurollo, MS, DVM

KEYWORDS

- Feline • Bartonella • Cytauxzoon • Anaplasma • Ehrlichia • Borrelia • Hepatozoon
- Rickettsia

KEY POINTS

- Many of the same vector-borne pathogens that infect dogs can infect cats.
- In North America, cats are routinely parasitized by ticks and exposed to tick-borne pathogens.
- Using both molecular and serologic vector-borne disease diagnostic modalities can improve identification of feline vector-borne disease.

INTRODUCTION

In North America, with the exceptions of *Bartonella henselae* and *Cytauxzoon felis,* feline vector-borne diseases (FVBDs) have been minimally studied in domestic cats. Vector-borne pathogens, including *Anaplasma, Babesia, Borrelia, Ehrlichia, Hepatozoon, Leishmania, Rickettsia,* and *Trypanosoma* species remain poorly defined in cats. Potential factors contributing to this include less exposure to outdoor environments, grooming habits that may remove the disease-transmitting ectoparasites, and limited availability and use of feline vector-borne disease diagnostics due to presumptions of less frequent tick-borne disease when compared with dogs.

In addition to providing an overview on diagnostic approaches, treatment, and prevention of FVBDs, this review focuses on recent findings related to commonly recognized FVBDs, such as bartonellosis and cytauxzoonosis, and highlights less frequently documented FVBDs, such as anaplasmosis, ehrlichiosis, borreliosis, rickettsiosis, and hepatozoonosis.

FELINE VECTOR-BORNE DISEASE DIAGNOSTICS
Serology

Serology is a diagnostic modality that can be used to identify exposure to or infection with vector-borne pathogens. Antibodies made in response to pathogens can take

Dr. Qurollo is a co-director of the NC State-CVM-VBDDL and IDEXX Laboratories, Inc funds a portion of her salary.
Department of Clinical Sciences, College of Veterinary Medicine, North Carolina State University, Research Building, Office 464, 1060 William Moore Drive, Raleigh, NC 27606, USA
E-mail address: Barbara_qurollo@ncsu.edu

Vet Clin Small Anim 49 (2019) 687–702
https://doi.org/10.1016/j.cvsm.2019.02.012
0195-5616/19/© 2019 Elsevier Inc. All rights reserved.

several weeks postexposure to become detectable, thus serology is not appropriate for the diagnosis of acute disease. Immunofluorescent antibody (IFA) assays detect and quantify antibodies that cross react with whole-cell vector-borne pathogens. IFA assays can be performed on cats, provided the fluorescent-labeled secondary antibody conjugate is specific for feline antibodies. Individual diagnostic laboratories may perform different serial dilutions of the serum, and thus establish different endpoint titers to indicate positive or negative results. Because of this, it is recommended to use the same diagnostic laboratory when comparing IFA results from acute and convalescent samples. When comparing acute and convalescent antibody titers, a fourfold increase in the convalescent titer indicates an active infection. Detection of antibodies at a single point in time may represent a past exposure or an active infection.

Commercially available point-of-care (POC) assays designed to detect antibodies seroreactive to tick-borne diseases are licensed only for use in dogs. However, several recent studies report seroreactivity to peptides specific to *Anaplasma* spp, *Ehrlichia* spp, and *Borrelia burgdorferi* using feline sera with a POC assay, licensed only for use in dogs.[1–4] Clinicians who may choose to use serologic tests not licensed for use in cats should do so with the understanding that the feline sera may not consistently react with small peptides validated for canine seroreactivity, potentially generating inaccurate results.

Polymerase Chain Reaction

Molecular diagnostic polymerase chain reaction (PCR) is commonly used to detect the presence of pathogen DNA. PCR assays are not host-specific and can be applied to almost any animal and most specimen types (eg, whole blood, tissue, cerebrospinal fluid, urine). Although PCR is a highly sensitive method for the detection of pathogen DNA, false-negative results may occur if the pathogen load is below the limit of detection or it is not in the specimen submitted for testing. For example, *B burgdorferi* (Lyme disease) DNA is rarely detected in whole blood but more frequently PCR-amplified from tissue near the site of tick attachment.[5] Clinicians should not consider a negative diagnostic PCR result as conclusive evidence for the absence of an infection, but rather that the pathogen DNA was not detected in a particular sample at a particular point in time. Furthermore, the stage of infection can impact pathogen load. For example, FVBD pathogen DNA is typically more readily detected in whole blood sampled during the acute phase of an infection, whereas antibodies are more commonly detected during a later stage. As is the case with many canine vector-borne diseases, combining molecular and serologic modalities can improve the likelihood of obtaining a diagnosis for FVBD.[6]

FELINE VECTOR-BORNE DISEASE TREATMENT AND PREVENTION

In general, most FVBDs are treated with antibiotics or antiprotozoal therapies similar to those used for canine vector-borne diseases, as well as elimination of any ectoparasite infestation. Specific therapies are addressed for each FVBD within the respective sections of this review. Most FVBDs are transmitted by fleas and ticks, and prevention of disease relies primarily on prevention of ectoparasite infestation. Long-acting ectoparasiticides that are safe for cats and effective against fleas only include imidacloprid, selamectin, spinetoram, spinosad, dinotefuran, and metaflumizone[7,8]; and those effective against fleas and ticks include imidacloprid/flumethrin, fipronil, and isoxazolines.[9–13] Isoxazolines are a relatively new class of ectoparasiticide and include afoxolaner, fluralaner, sarolaner, and lotilaner.[11–13] Ectoparasiticides with permethrin, deltamethrin, and amitraz cannot be used in cats, and topical preventives with these compounds should not be used on pets that cohabitate with cats.

BARTONELLOSIS
Transmission and Prevalence

Bartonella are intracellular bacteria transmitted by fleas, among other arthropod vectors. Inside the mammalian host, *Bartonella* invades erythrocytes, macrophages, endothelial cells, and pericytes, often establishing persistent infections.[14] Many different *Bartonella* spp infect cats (**Table 1**).[15–20] Cats are reservoirs for *Bartonella*; thus, demonstrating *Bartonella* exposure or infection in the face of disease may support a diagnosis or only be an incidental finding. Clinical illness likely depends on the immune status of the animal, the species or strain of *Bartonella,* and the presence of coinfections, including multiple species or strains of *Bartonella*.[20,21]

Clinical Signs

Experimental *Bartonella* infection studies have been performed in cats.[16,22–26] Comparisons made between these studies can be challenging due to varying inoculation protocols. Common among all experimental infections was the development of bacteremia. In 3 *B henselae* experimental infections using various strains, doses, and routes of inoculation, none of the cats developed clinical disease, and cats experimentally infected with *Bartonella koehlerae* or *Bartonella clarridgeiae* did not develop clinical disease but all became bacteremic.[16,23,25] Clinicopathological abnormalities identified across other *B henselae* experimental infections were nonspecific and included transient fever, lethargy, decreased appetite, peripheral lymphadenopathy, mild central nervous system abnormalities, reproductive failure, inflammatory leukogram, transient anemia, and eosinophilia. Fever has commonly been reported in cats experimentally and naturally infected with *Bartonella* spp, but significant associations were not demonstrated.[27,28]

Statistical correlations between some clinical abnormalities in cats and natural *Bartonella* infection or exposure have been shown.[27,29–33] Cats with antibodies to *B henselae* were more likely to have hyperglobulinemia than *Bartonella*-seronegative cats.[29] Gingivostomatitis was associated with cats positive for *Bartonella* by blood-culture but not by seroreactivity.[30] A recent retrospective study assessed a large diagnostic database for associations between select complete blood count abnormalities and cats infected with *Bartonella*, based on PCR-positive blood.[31] Results showed cats with *Bartonella* bacteremia were slightly more likely to have thrombocytopenia but less likely to be anemic. These results support a previous case-control study reporting anemia was not associated with feline bartonellosis.[32] When clinicopathological abnormalities in cats with acute-onset fever were compared between *Bartonella*-infected and uninfected cats, neutrophilia was significantly associated with *B henselae* infections.[27] Another study reported associations between feline bartonellosis and neutrophilia and monocytosis.[33] Different clinical presentations in naturally infected cats occur and could be due to differences in strain pathogenicity, coinfections, or the immune status of the cat.

Cardiac disease in cats naturally infected with *Bartonella* have been reported.[21,26,34] *Bartonella* was amplified by PCR more frequently in cardiac tissue from cats with endomyocarditis-left ventricular endocardial fibrosis than in cats with hypertrophic cardiomyopathy, and it was not amplified from cats without cardiac disease.[21] Other case reports have identified endocarditis and myocarditis in cats with bartonellosis.[26,34]

Table 1
Feline vector-borne disease pathogens, diagnostic modalities, clinical signs and treatment recommendations

Disease	Pathogens Detected by PCR in Cats	Diagnostics	Potential Clinical Abnormalities	Recommended Treatment*
Bartonellosis	Bartonella henselae, Bartonella clarridgeiae, Bartonella bovis, Bartonella koehlerae, Bartonella quintana, Bartonella vinsonii berkoff	PCR, ePCR, IFA, Western blot, culture	Asymptomatic, transient fever, lethargy, lymphadenopathy, mild CNS signs, inflammatory leukogram, thrombocytopenia, hyperglobulinemia, neutropenia, eosinophilia, anemia	Doxycycline (10 mg/kg PO, q12 h) and Pradofloxacin (5–10 mg/kg PO q 12 h or q24 h) for 28–42 d; or Pradofloxacin (7.5 mg/kg PO, q12 h)
Cytauxzoonosis	Cytauxzoon felis	PCR, tissue or blood cytology	Fever, anorexia, lethargy, icterus, dyspnea and generalized pain, pancytopenia, hyperbilirubinemia, neurologic abnormalities, hypothermia, asymptomatic	Atovaquone (15 mg/kg PO q8 h) and Azithromycin (10 mg/kg PO q24 h) for 10 days, aggressive supportive care
Anaplasmosis	Anaplasma phagocytophilum, Anaplasma platys, Anaplasma platys-like, Anaplasma bovis	PCR, ELISA, IFA, blood cytology	Fever, anorexia, dehydration, lethargy, abdominal pain, swollen joints, epistaxis, thrombocytopenia, anemia, asymptomatic	Doxycycline (10 mg/kg PO q24 or 5mg/kg PO q12 for 28 days)
Ehrlichiosis	Ehrlichia canis, Ehrlichia canis-like, Ehrlichia chaffeensis, Ehrlichia ewingii	PCR, ELISA, IFA, blood cytology	Fever, lethargy, joint pain, splenomegaly, lymphadenomegaly, epistaxis, anemia, hyperglobulinemia, hypoalbuminemia, thrombocytopenia, lymphopenia, monocytosis,	
Borreliosis	Borrelia burgdorferi (LB), Borrelia miyamotoi (RFB), Borrelia persica (RFB)	PCR, ELISA, IFA, Western blot, culture, blood cytology (RFB)	Asymptomatic, LB (lethargy, inappetence, lameness, fever, ataxia), RFB (fever, lethargy, anemia, thrombocytopenia)	
Rickettsiosis	Rickettsia felis, Rickettsia conorii, Rickettsia massiliae, Rickettsia typhi	PCR, IFA	Fever, asymptomatic	
Hepatozoonosis	Hepatozoon canis, Hepatozoon americanum-like, Hepatozoon felis, Hepatozoon silvestris, Hepatozoon spp	PCR, blood cytology, muscle histology	Fever, lymphadenopathy, myocarditis, thrombocytopenia, hyperglobulinemia, neutropenia, hyperbilirubinemia, elevated SLD, elevated CK, asymptomatic	Unknown

Abbreviations: CK, creatinine kinase; CNS, central nervous system; ELISA, enzyme-linked immunosorbent assay; ePCR, Bartonella alpha proteobacterium growth medium enrichment PCR; IFA, immunofluorescent antibody; LB, Lyme borrelia; PCR, polymerase chain reaction; PO, by mouth; q, every; RFB, relapsing fever borrelia; SLD, serum lactate dehydrogenase.
* To avoid esophagitis, use drugs with suspension or perform water flush after administering each oral dose.

Diagnosis

Modalities used to diagnose bartonellosis in cats include PCR, *Bartonella* alphaproteobacterium growth medium enrichment PCR (ePCR), culture, and detection of antibodies against *Bartonella* spp antigens using IFA assays or Western blot analysis. Serology should not be used to speciate an infection, as there is likely some degree of crossreactivity among the different *Bartonella* spp. PCR can often detect *Bartonella* infections in cats due to high bacteremic loads; however, fluctuating pathogen loads can generate false-negative results. Greater PCR sensitivity has been demonstrated when blood samples were tested by ePCR.[35]

Treatment

Clinically ill cats that are *Bartonella*-PCR positive should be treated after other etiologies have been ruled out. It may not be necessary to treat asymptomatic, PCR-positive cats, or cats that are only *Bartonella* seropositive, because cats are *Bartonella* reservoirs. Clinicians should consider treating asymptomatic *Bartonella*-infected cats that live with immunocompromised people due to the possible risk of zoonosis.

Treatment consists of using 1 or a combination of 2 antibiotics. *Bartonella* resistance has been induced in vitro by azithromycin, enrofloxacin, pradofloxacin, and rifampicin.[36] Resistance has not been reported with doxycycline, so it may be an option for single drug therapy. Using a combination of 2 drugs may mitigate antibiotic resistance; thus, a recommended treatment protocol for feline bartonellosis includes doxycycline (10 mg/kg by mouth [PO], every 12 hours, followed immediately by food or water to avoid esophagitis) and pradofloxacin (5–10 mg/kg PO every 12 hours or every 24 hours).[37,38] A recent study assessed the safety and efficacy of high-dose pradofloxacin (7.5 mg/kg PO, every 12 hours) for the elimination of *B henselae* in 8 experimentally infected cats.[38] All cats were bacteremic and eliminated the infection after 28 days of treatment. All cats were *Bartonella*-PCR negative at 10 weeks posttreatment and after immunosuppression. Historically, it has been difficult to document clearance of *Bartonella* due to relapsing bacteremia in naturally infected cats.

CYTAUXZOONOSIS
Transmission and Prevalence

C felis is a tick-transmitted, protozoal parasite that infects felids. The primary reservoir host of *C felis* is the bobcat, and natural vectors are *Amblyomma americanum* and *Dermacentor variabilis*.[39,40] Following the bite of *A americanum,* transmission of *C felis* can occur in approximately 36 hours.[39] Transmission can happen inadvertently through a blood transfusion with infected blood, but has not been demonstrated through ingestion of the pathogen, cat-to-cat contact, or vertically.[39,41]

C felis is most prevalent in the southern and mid-Atlantic United States, and evidence supports a risk of infection for cats in the northeastern United States.[42–46] Recent *C felis* PCR prevalence rates reported from cats in the south and southeastern United States ranged from 0.3% to 30% (identified in a higher-risk population).[42–44] In domestic cats, natural infections are more common between the months of April and September.[46]

Clinical Signs

Although cats infected with *C felis* can develop clinical signs ranging in severity up to acute death, some are asymptomatically infected. Variables dictating the degree of illness likely include the route of infection, pathogen stage and genotype, and the host response. Most domestic cats infected with sporozoites or schizonts, either via a tick bite or experimental infection, develop severe clinical signs due to thrombi formation from schizont-laden macrophages. Initial signs of infection include fever, anorexia, lethargy, icterus, dyspnea, and generalized pain, with onset usually occurring approximately 1 to 2 weeks after infection.[40,46–48] Pancytopenia and hyperbilirubinemia are the most common hematologic abnormalities. As the disease progresses, cats may develop neurologic abnormalities and hypothermia and die from multiorgan failure within a week. Cats that survive cytauxzoonosis may be protected from later infections.[41] Naturally and experimentally infected cats may develop only mild disease or remain asymptomatic.[43,44,46,49] For example, cats inoculated using piroplasm-infected blood did not develop disease, despite maintaining parasitemia.[41] The detection of mildly symptomatic or asymptomatic C felis–infected cats may increase as PCR panels with C felis testing are more routinely performed and PCR surveys are conducted.

Diagnosis

Cytauxzoonosis is diagnosed using blood or tissue samples evaluated for C felis by microscopy or PCR. Monocyte or macrophage-laden schizonts and intraerythrocytic piroplasms can be visualized in blood or tissue smears using light microscopy (**Fig. 1**). Because piroplasms are released after schizont formation, their visualization is rare in early disease onset. Schizonts may be present in blood smears, typically seen at the feathered edge. Because schizonts are more prominent in tissues such as spleen, liver, or lymph nodes, a fine-needle tissue aspirate could be more sensitive for microscopic diagnosis. PCR is the most sensitive method for C felis detection.

Treatment

Effective treatment evaluated against C felis is a combination of atovaquone (15 mg/kg PO every 8 hours) and azithromycin (10 mg/kg PO every 24 hours)

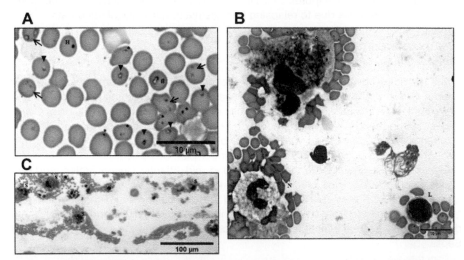

Fig. 1. *Cytauxzoon felis* piroplasms and schizonts in blood smear under light microscopy. (*A*) Intraerythrocytic piroplasms as signet rings (*arrowhead*), multiple organisms in one erythrocyte (*arrow*), dividing piroplasm (*Hash*), and other morphologies (*asterisk*). Howell-Jolly bodies (H). (*B*) *C felis* schizont-infected leukocyte (S) near neutrophil (N) and lymphocyte (L). (*C*) Schizont-infected cells (S) on feathered edge of blood smear. (*Courtesy of* Megan Schreeg, DVM, PhD, North Carolina State University, Raleigh, NC.)

(AA), administered for 10 days; a 60% survival rate was obtained with AA when compared with treatment with imidocarb dipropionate (26%).[50] Equally important is aggressive supportive care, including intravenous fluid therapy, blood transfusion, anticoagulants, enteral feeding, antiemetics, and pain management. Before obtaining a *C felis* diagnosis, AA therapy should be considered in cats presenting with clinical signs of cytauxzoonosis that have exposure to ticks or that live in *C felis*–endemic regions. Furthermore, all cats living in *C felis*–endemic regions, regardless of outdoor access, should be on acaricides due to the high mortality of cytauxzoonosis. The application of an imidacloprid/flumethrin collar can prevent the attachment of ticks and transmission of *C felis*.[9]

ANAPLASMOSIS AND EHRLICHIOSIS
Anaplasma Transmission and Prevalence

Anaplasma are tick-transmitted, intracellular pathogens that infect hematopoietic cells. Natural *Anaplasma* infections in cats have been documented worldwide by PCR and/or visualization of morulae in neutrophils or platelets (see **Table 1**).[1,51–54] *Anaplasma phagocytophilum*, transmitted by *Ixodes* spp ticks, is the most common species detected in cats.[1,4,51,52,55–58] Currently, there is a lack of knowledge regarding feline anaplasmosis from infections with *Anaplasma* spp other than *A phagocytophilum*.

A North American–wide feline serosurvey using *A. phagocytophilum* whole-cell IFA or species-specific SNAP enzyme-linked immunosorbent assay (ELISA) test (IDEXX Laboratories, Westbrook, ME) reported a seroprevalence of 4.3% and 1.8%, respectively, in client-owned cats undergoing vector-borne disease testing.[1,59] Most of the seropositive cats resided in the northeastern and mid-Atlantic states. Other recent feline serosurveys report even higher seroprevalences in northeastern populations (3.6%–15.4%).[2,3,58]

Anaplasmosis Clinical Signs

Studies that reported *A. phagocytophilum* infections in cats describe nonspecific clinical findings, including fever, anorexia, dehydration, and lethargy.[1,3,4,56,58] Abdominal pain, polyarthropathy, and epistaxis were infrequently documented, and several cats were asymptomatic. *Ixodes scapularis* ticks were found on many naturally infected cats. The most common hematologic abnormality was thrombocytopenia and moderate anemia. Serum biochemistry abnormalities were infrequently detected.

Ehrlichia Transmission and Prevalence

Ehrlichia spp. are tick-transmitted, intracellular bacteria that primarily infect neutrophils and monocytes. Although infrequently diagnosed, evidence for feline ehrlichiosis is supported by reports of cats infected with various *Ehrlichia* spp (see **Table 1**).[1,57,60–62] Most *Ehrlichia* are transmitted by *A. americanum* and *Rhipicephalus sanguineus* (*sensu lato*). Cats can be parasitized by both of these tick species, lending support for tick transmission of *Ehrlichia* to cats.

Few feline ehrlichiosis surveys have been reported in cats in North America. A study including cats being tested for vector-borne disease used an *Ehrlichia* species–specific SNAP ELISA test to report a seroprevalence of 0.14%, with reactivity primarily to *Ehrlichia canis* peptides.[1] The same study detected *Ehrlichia* DNA, including *E canis*, *E. chaffeensis*, and *E. ewingii*, in 1.8% of cats. South America and Europe report higher feline *Ehrlichia* infection rates at 9.4% and 5.4%, respectively.[57,63]

Ehrlichiosis Clinical Signs

Clinical disease has been reported in cats naturally infected with *Ehrlichia*.[1,60–62] The most frequently reported abnormalities were nonspecific and included fever, lethargy, joint pain, nonregenerative anemia, hyperglobulinemia, thrombocytopenia, lymphopenia, and monocytosis.

Diagnosis of Feline Anaplasmosis and Ehrlichiosis

Feline anaplasmosis and ehrlichiosis are diagnosed using IFA, ELISA, or PCR. Cytologic examination of blood or joint fluid smears infrequently reveal morulae in neutrophils, platelets, lymphocytes, or monocytes. *Anaplasma* and *Ehrlichia* spp DNA can be PCR-amplified from blood and tissue. Although not licensed for use in cats, commercially available ELISA kits have been shown to detect feline antibodies made against *Anaplasma* spp and *Ehrlichia* spp peptides.[1–4]

Treatment for Anaplasmosis and Ehrlichiosis

Tetracyclines and supportive care resolved clinical signs linked to feline anaplasmosis and ehrlichiosis.[56,60] Doxycycline (10 mg/kg PO, every 24 hours, followed immediately by food or water, for 28 days), is recommended.[64] Although not reported for use in feline anaplasmosis or ehrlichiosis, minocycline is effective for most rickettsial infections in dogs and people.[65]

BORRELIOSIS
Transmission and Prevalence

Borrelia spp. are spirochete bacteria transmitted primarily by ticks or lice.[66] *B burgdorferi* (Lyme borreliosis), transmitted by *Ixodes* spp., is transiently in the blood before localizing to collagen-rich tissues.[67] Relapsing fever borrelia (RFB), caused by various *Borrelia* spp., is transmitted by ticks (hard and soft) or lice, and remain in the blood with relapsing episodes of bacteremia.[66]

Serosurveys indicate cats are commonly exposed to *B burgdorferi*.[3,4,68,69] A North American–wide feline serosurvey reported *B burgdorferi* as the most seroprevalent tick-borne pathogen at 5.5% when compared with *Anaplasma* and *Ehrlichia*.[1] Most cats seropositive for *B burgdorferi* were from the northeastern and mid-Atlantic states, regions with a high prevalence of *Ixodes* ticks. Higher seroprevalence rates were reported in cats in Maine (18%–20%) and Maryland (36%).[3,69]

RFB has infrequently been detected in cats. *Borrelia miyamotoi* DNA was amplified by PCR in 2 asymptomatic cats in Maryland.[69] *B miyamotoi* is responsible for RFB in people and is commonly transmitted by *Ixodes* spp., sharing the same regional prevalence as Lyme disease. A recent study identified RFB, *Borrelia persica*, in 5 cats in Israel.[70] Another study was unable to amplify RFB DNA from 84 cats with acute-onset fever in the United States.[27] Based on limited studies, RFB does not appear to be a common disease in cats; however, it is likely infrequently tested for and may be underdiagnosed in cats.

Clinical Signs

Overall, studies report a lack of clinical disease in cats with borreliosis. Although cats are commonly exposed to *B burgdorferi* and experimental inoculation studies demonstrate they are susceptible to infection, clinical disease is infrequently attributed to *B burgdorferi*.[3,4,68,69] In limited cases in which cats with Lyme borreliosis developed clinical signs, other FVBDs were not consistently ruled out.[4,68,69] A recent study highlighted disease in cats seropositive for *B burgdorferi*, but seronegative for *A phagocytophilum*. Common clinical abnormalities included lethargy and inappetence; some cats had gait abnormalities, ataxia, lameness, or fever. Most of the clinical signs resolved following treatment with doxycycline.[3] Five cats from Israel with RFB developed lethargy, fever, anemia, and thrombocytopenia.[70]

Diagnosis

Methods used to diagnose Lyme borreliosis and RFB are different. Serologic or culture modalities are more commonly used to diagnose Lyme borreliosis. Although not licensed for use in cats, commercially available ELISA kits have been shown to detect feline antibodies made against *B burgdorferi* C6 antigen.[1–4] *B burgdorferi* DNA has been PCR-amplified from tissue (at the site of tick attachment), joint fluid, or cerebrospinal fluid, but rarely from blood.[5,71] RFB is diagnosed by visualization of spirochetemia during microscopic examination of stained blood smears, or by PCR amplification from blood.

Treatment

There is little evidence documenting the best treatment for feline borreliosis. Treatment recommendations for dogs include a variety of antibiotics, with doxycycline (10 mg/kg PO every 24 hours or 5 mg/kg PO every 12 hours, followed immediately by food or water, for 30 days) most commonly used.[72] Clinical signs resolved in 5 *B burgdorferi*–seropositive cats following treatment with doxycycline (40–50 mg/cat every 24 hours, followed immediately by food or water, for 28 days).[3] Efficacy of an injectable, long-lasting cephalosporin against *B burgdorferi* has been demonstrated in dogs.[5]

RICKETTSIOSIS
Transmission and Prevalence

Rickettsia spp are flea-transmitted and tick-transmitted, intracellular bacteria that infect endothelial cells. *Rickettsia* are categorized as spotted-fever group rickettsia (SFGR) vectored primarily by ticks, or typhus group (TG) vectored by fleas or lice. PCR has confirmed natural feline *Rickettsia* infections, worldwide (see **Table 1**).[27,73–75] Studies reported feline seroreactivity by IFA for SFGR whole-cell antigens, including *Rickettsia rickettsii*, *Rickettsia japonica*, *Rickettsia typhi*, *Rhipicephalus massiliae*, *Rickettsia conorii*, and *Rhipicephalus felis*.[74–77]

Clinical Signs

Feline rickettsioses is infrequently linked to clinical illness in cats. Significant associations between disease and *Rickettsia* seropositivity or infection have not been established; however, a wide range of nonspecific clinical signs, including fever, have been documented in cats seropositive for *R conorii*, *R massiliae,* or *R rickettsii*, and 1 *R felis* PCR-positive cat was febrile.[27,73–76] Overall, data supporting clinical disease in cats exposed to or infected with *Rickettsia* are lacking; however, cats may play a role as reservoir hosts for ectoparasites harboring and transmitting rickettsial disease to other animals and humans.

Diagnosis

PCR and IFA serology are the most common modalities used for diagnosing rickettsioses. Most *Rickettsia* infect endothelial cells and are only transiently in the blood of mammalian hosts. DNA can be PCR-amplified from blood collected during acute stages of disease. Sera screened against a specific *Rickettsia* sp should be interpreted as exposure to *Rickettsia* within the respective SFGR or TG. Paired acute and convalescent samples with a fourfold or greater titer increase lend support for an active infection with the specific *Rickettsia* sp used in the IFA test.

Treatment

There is little evidence documenting the best treatment for feline rickettsioses. Doxycycline and fluoroquinolones have been used successfully to treat rickettsioses in dogs and people; thus, clinicians may consider these drugs when treating feline rickettsioses.[78]

HEPATOZOONOSIS
Transmission and Prevalence

Hepatozoon spp are protozoal parasites that infect an extensive range of vertebrate hosts, including reptiles, amphibians, birds, and mammals.[79] In carnivores, vectors are primarily ticks, including *R sanguineus* s.l., and *Amblyomma maculatum*.[80,81] The transmission route for most *Hepatozoon* infections is unclear; however, experimental infection of *Hepatozoon americanum* and *Hepatozoon canis* through the ingestion of vectors or infected vertebrates has been demonstrated.[80,81] Vertical transmission may also be possible.[82] Once ingested, *Hepatozoon* undergo merogony in various organs before disseminating to leukocytes and muscles (cardiac and striated). Vectors, transmission routes, and *Hepatozoon* spp. that cause feline infections are unclear.

Cats infected with *Hepatozoon* spp. are reported worldwide, but rarely in the United States (see **Table 1**).[27,83–86] A *Hepatozoon* prevalence of 2.4% was identified in 84 cats in the United States with acute-onset fever. Rates reported in cats in Europe ranged from 1.6% to 5.1%.[27,83–85] *Hepatozoon felis* is the most common *Hepatozoon* spp. detected in cats, worldwide. An *H americanum*-like species was identified in a domestic cat from Oklahoma, and 2 bobcats from Georgia were infected with a *Hepatozoon* sp similar to a species in cats in Spain.[86] One cat from Virginia and 1 from New Jersey were infected with *H felis* and a *Hepatozoon* spp. similar to one identified in Georgia bobcats, respectively.[27]

Clinical Signs

Many cats with hepatozoonosis are asymptomatic, but clinical illness may be linked to some *Hepatozoon* infections.[83,87,88] Significant associations have been reported between feline hepatozoonosis and clinical abnormalities, including anemia and elevated serum creatinine.[52,84] One report describes a cat with granulomatous cholangiohepatitis infected with a *Hepatozoon* sp.[87] Seven cats infected with *Hepatozoon* developed a range of nonspecific clinical signs, including increased serum lactate dehydrogenase and creatine kinase.[88] One cat infected with *Hepatozoon silvestris* died from severe lympho-plasmacytic and histiocytic myocarditis; no other cause of disease was identified.[83] Fever, neutropenia, thrombocytopenia, and bilirubinemia were reported in a cat in the United States infected with *H felis* and negative for other FVBDs.[27] A second *Hepatozoon*-infected cat was febrile, thrombocytopenic, hyperglobulinemic with pyogranulomatous lymphadenitis, and developed a fluid-filled mass over the heart; the cat was coinfected with *Mycoplasma haemominutum* and was *B burgdorferi* seropositive. Combined, these studies suggest hepatozoonosis may play a bigger role in feline clinical disease than previously realized.

Diagnosis

Hepatozoonosis is diagnosed primarily by histology, cytology, or PCR. In cats, cytologic examination of blood smears infrequently reveal *Hepatozoon* gamonts inside leukocytes. PCR of blood or buffy coat is sensitive at detecting *Hepatozoon* spp; however, different PCR targets and protocols can significantly affect sensitivity.[89]

Treatment

There is little evidence documenting effective treatments for feline hepatozoonosis.[90] Resolution of clinical signs occurred in one cat using a combination of oxytetracycline and primaquine.[91]

SUMMARY

In North America, cats are exposed to a wide range of FVBDs with varying degrees of prevalence and clinical manifestations. Many FVBDs are linked to nonspecific clinical abnormalities and may not be routinely considered by clinicians in differential diagnoses. FVBD diagnostics are underused by veterinarians likely due, in part, to reduced availability and reduced awareness of FVBD by owners and clinicians. Between 2008 and 2018, the North Carolina State Vector-borne Disease Diagnostic Laboratory sample submissions were approximately 90% canine and 10% feline (unpublished data Qurollo, 2018). Veterinarians may be more likely to associate tick-borne diseases with dogs, rather than cats; however, cats in North America are routinely exposed to ticks.[27,69,92] Veterinarians should consider ectoparasite prevention for all feline patients, especially those products that are effective against fleas and ticks.

REFERENCES

1. Hegarty BC, Qurollo BA, Thomas B, et al. Serological and molecular analysis of feline vector-borne anaplasmosis and ehrlichiosis using species-specific peptides and PCR. Parasit Vectors 2015;8:320.
2. Hoyt K, Chandrashekar R, Breitschwerdt E. Anaplasma phagocytophilum and *Borrelia burgdorferi* antibodies in naturally exposed cats in Maine. ACVIM Forum Research Abstracts Program. J Vet Intern Med 2014;28:1068.
3. Hoyt K, Chandrashekar R, Beall M, et al. Evidence for clinical anaplasmosis and borreliosis in cats in Maine. Top Companion Anim Med 2018;33(2):40–4.
4. Lappin MR, Chandrashekar R, Stillman B, et al. Evidence of *Anaplasma phagocytophilum* and *Borrelia burgdorferi* infection in cats after exposure to wild-caught adult *Ixodes scapularis*. J Vet Diagn Invest 2015;27(4):522–5.
5. Wagner B, Johnson J, Garcia-Tapia D, et al. Comparison of effectiveness of cefovecin, doxycycline, and amoxicillin for the treatment of experimentally induced early Lyme borreliosis in dogs. BMC Vet Res 2015;11(1):163.
6. Maggi RG, Birkenheuer AJ, Hegarty BC, et al. Comparison of serological and molecular panels for diagnosis of vector-borne diseases in dogs. Parasit Vectors 2014;7:127.
7. Siak M, Burrows M. Flea control in cats: new concepts and the current armoury. J Feline Med Surg 2013;15(1):31–40.
8. Paarlberg T, Winkle J, Rumschlag AJ, et al. Effectiveness and residual speed of flea kill of a novel spot on formulation of spinetoram (Cheristin®) for cats. Parasit Vectors 2017;10(1):59.
9. Reichard MV, Thomas JE, Arther RG, et al. Efficacy of an imidacloprid 10%/flumethrin 4.5% Collar (Seresto (R), Bayer) for preventing the transmission of cytauxzoon felis to domestic cats by *Amblyomma americanum*. Parasitol Res 2013;112(1):11–20.
10. Kilp S, Ramirez D, Allan MJ, et al. Comparative pharmacokinetics of fluralaner in dogs and cats following single topical or intravenous administration. Parasit Vectors 2016;9(1):296.

11. Cavalleri D, Murphy M, Seewald W, et al. A randomized, controlled field study to assess the efficacy and safety of lotilaner (Credelio™) in controlling fleas in client-owned cats in Europe. Parasit Vectors 2018;11(1):410.

12. Meadows C, Guerino F, Sun F. A randomized, blinded, controlled USA field study to assess the use of fluralaner topical solution in controlling feline flea infestations. Parasit Vectors 2017;10(1):37.

13. Wright I. Lotilaner-a novel formulation for cats provides systemic tick and flea control. Parasit Vectors 2018;11(1):407. BioMed Central.

14. Breitschwerdt EB, Kordick DL. Bartonella species and vascular pathology. Vascular responses to pathogens. Cambridge (MA): Elsevier; 2016. p. 61–74.

15. Droz S, Chi B, Horn E, et al. Bartonella koehlerae sp. nov., isolated from cats. J Clin Microbiol 1999;37(4):1117–22.

16. Yamamoto K, Chomel BB, Kasten RW, et al. Experimental infection of specific pathogen free (SPF) cats with two different strains of Bartonella henselae type I: a comparative study. Vet Res 2002;33(6):669–84.

17. Breitschwerdt EB, Maggi RG, Sigmon B, et al. Isolation of Bartonella quintana from a woman and a cat following putative bite transmission. J Clin Microbiol 2007;45(1):270–2.

18. Koehler JE, Glaser CA, Tappero JW. Rochalimaea henselae infection: a new zoonosis with the domestic cat as reservoir. JAMA 1994;271(7):531–5.

19. La VD, Tran-Hung L, Aboudharam G, et al. Bartonella quintana in domestic cat. Emerg Infect Dis 2005;11(8):1287.

20. Kordick DL, Brown TT, Shin K, et al. Clinical and pathologic evaluation of chronic Bartonella henselae or Bartonella clarridgeiae infection in cats. J Clin Microbiol 1999;37(5):1536–47.

21. Donovan T, Balakrishnan N, Barbosa IC, et al. Bartonella spp. as a possible cause or cofactor of feline endomyocarditis–left ventricular endocardial fibrosis complex. J Comp Pathol 2018;162:29–42.

22. O'Reilly KL, Bauer RW, Freeland RL, et al. Acute clinical disease in cats following infection with a pathogenic strain of Bartonella henselae (LSU16). Infect Immun 1999;67(6):3066–72.

23. Abbott RC, Chomel BB, Kasten RW, et al. Experimental and natural infection with Bartonella henselae in domestic cats. Comp Immunol Microbiol Infect Dis 1997; 20(1):41–51.

24. Chomel BB, Kasten RW, Floyd-Hawkins K, et al. Experimental transmission of Bartonella henselae by the cat flea. J Clin Microbiol 1996;34(8):1952–6.

25. Regnery R, Rooney J, Johnson A, et al. Experimentally induced Bartonella henselae infections followed by challenge exposure and antimicrobial therapy in cats. Am J Vet Res 1996;57(12):1714–9.

26. Bradbury CA, Lappin MR. Evaluation of topical application of 10% imidacloprid–1% moxidectin to prevent Bartonella henselae transmission from cat fleas. J Am Vet Med Assoc 2010;236(8):869–73.

27. Qurollo B, Walsh E, Lemler E, et al. Feline vector-borne disease in cats with acute-onset fever. 2018. Available at: https://www.vin.com/acvim/2018. Accessed September 17, 2018.

28. Lappin MR, Breitschwerdt E, Brewer M, et al. Prevalence of Bartonella species antibodies and Bartonella species DNA in the blood of cats with and without fever. J Feline Med Surg 2009;11(2):141–8.

29. Whittemore J, Hawley J, Radecki S, et al. Bartonella species antibodies and hyperglobulinemia in privately owned cats. J Vet Intern Med 2012;26(3):639–44.

30. Sykes JE, Westropp JL, Kasten RW, et al. Association between *Bartonella* species infection and disease in pet cats as determined using serology and culture. J Feline Med Surg 2010;12(8):631–6.

31. Lappin MR, LC, Braff J, et al. Assessment for associations between *Bartonella* spp. and select complete blood cell count abnormalities. 2018. Available at: https://www.vin.com/acvim/2018. Accessed September 17, 2018.

32. Ishak AM, Radecki S, Lappin MR. Prevalence of *Mycoplasma haemofelis*, 'Candidatus Mycoplasma haemominutum', *Bartonella* species, *Ehrlichia* species, and *Anaplasma phagocytophilum* DNA in the blood of cats with anemia. J Feline Med Surg 2007;9(1):1–7.

33. Hassan U, Dhaliwal G, Watanabe M, et al. Feline bartonellosis associated with some clinico-pathological conditions in a veterinary hospital in Selangor, Malaysia. Trop Biomed 2017;34(1):174–9.

34. Perez C, Hummel JB, Keene BW, et al. Successful treatment of *Bartonella henselae* endocarditis in a cat. J Feline Med Surg 2010;12(6):483–6.

35. Drummond MR, Lania BG, de Paiva Diniz PPV, et al. Improvement of *Bartonella henselae* DNA detection in cat blood samples by combining molecular and culture methods. J Clin Microbiol 2018;56(5) [pii:e01732-17].

36. Rolain JM, Maurin M, Bryskier A, et al. In vitro activities of telithromycin (HMR 3647) against *Rickettsia rickettsii, Rickettsia conorii, Rickettsia africae, Rickettsia typhi, Rickettsia prowazekii, Coxiella burnetii, Bartonella henselae, Bartonella quintana, Bartonella bacilliformis,* and *Ehrlichia chaffeensis.* Antimicrobial Agents Chemother 2000;44(5):1391–3.

37. Breitschwerdt E. Bartonellosis of the cat and dog. Plumb's therapeutic brief 2015. Available at: https://www.cliniciansbrief.com/article/bartonellosis-cat-dog. Accessed September 9, 2018.

38. Lappin MR, FR. Pradofloxacin for treatment of *Bartonella henselae* in experimentally inoculated cats. 2018. Available at: https://www.vin.com/acvim/2018. Accessed September 17, 2018.

39. Thomas JE, Ohmes CM, Payton ME, et al. Minimum transmission time of *Cytauxzoon felis* by *Amblyomma americanum* to domestic cats in relation to duration of infestation, and investigation of ingestion of infected ticks as a potential route of transmission. J Feline Med Surg 2018;20(2):67–72.

40. Reichard MV, Edwards AC, Meinkoth JH, et al. Confirmation of *Amblyomma americanum* (Acari: Ixodidae) as a vector for *Cytauxzoon felis* (Piroplasmorida: Theileriidae) to domestic cats. J Med Entomol 2010;47(5):890–6.

41. Motzel S, Wagner J. Treatment of experimentally induced cytauxzoonosis in cats with parvaquone and buparvaquone. Vet Parasitol 1990;35(1–2):131–8.

42. Rizzi TE, Reichard MV, Cohn LA, et al. Prevalence of *Cytauxzoon felis* infection in healthy cats from enzootic areas in Arkansas, Missouri, and Oklahoma. Parasit Vectors 2015;8:13.

43. Haber MD, Tucker MD, Marr HS, et al. The detection of *Cytauxzoon felis* in apparently healthy free-roaming cats in the USA. Vet Parasitol 2007;146(3–4):316–20.

44. Brown HM, Lockhart JM, Latimer KS, et al. Identification and genetic characterization of *Cytauxzoon felis* in asymptomatic domestic cats and bobcats. Vet Parasitol 2010;172(3–4):311–6.

45. Birkenheuer AJ, Marr HS, Warren C, et al. *Cytauxzoon felis* infections are present in bobcats (*Lynx rufus*) in a region where cytauxzoonosis is not recognized in domestic cats. Vet Parasitol 2008;153(1–2):126–30.

46. Birkenheuer AJ, Le JA, Valenzisi AM, et al. *Cytauxzoon felis* infection in cats in the mid-Atlantic states: 34 cases (1998-2004). J Am Vet Med Assoc 2006;228(4): 568–71.

47. Greene C, Latimer K, Hopper E, et al. Administration of diminazene aceturate or imidocarb dipropionate for treatment of cytauxzoonosis in cats. J Am Vet Med Assoc 1999;215(4):497–500, 482.

48. Kier A, Wagner J, Kinden D. The pathology of experimental cytauxzoonosis. J Comp Pathol 1987;97(4):415–32.

49. Meinkoth J, Kocan AA, Whitworth L, et al. Cats surviving natural infection with *Cytauxzoon felis*: 18 cases (1997–1998). J Vet Intern Med 2000;14(5):521–5.

50. Cohn LA, Birkenheuer AJ, Brunker JD, et al. Efficacy of atovaquone and azithromycin or imidocarb dipropionate in cats with acute cytauxzoonosis. J Vet Intern Med 2011;25(1):55–60.

51. Lima M, Soares P, Ramos C, et al. Molecular detection of *Anaplasma platys* in a naturally-infected cat in Brazil. Braz J Microbiol 2010;41(2):381–5.

52. Attipa C, Papasouliotis K, Solano-Gallego L, et al. Prevalence study and risk factor analysis of selected bacterial, protozoal and viral, including vector-borne, pathogens in cats from Cyprus. Parasit Vectors 2017;10(1):130.

53. Oliveira AC, Luz MF, Granada S, et al. Molecular detection of *Anaplasma bovis, Ehrlichia canis* and *Hepatozoon felis* in cats from Luanda, Angola. Parasit Vectors 2018;11(1):167.

54. Qurollo BA, Balakrishnan N, Cannon CZ, et al. Co-infection with *Anaplasma platys, Bartonella henselae, Bartonella koehlerae* and 'Candidatus Mycoplasma haemominutum' in a cat diagnosed with splenic plasmacytosis and multiple myeloma. J Feline Med Surg 2014;16(8):713–20.

55. Lappin MR, Breitschwerdt EB, Jensen WA, et al. Molecular and serologic evidence of *Anaplasma phagocytophilum* infection in cats in North America. J Am Vet Med Assoc 2004;225(6):893–6.

56. Savidge C, Ewing P, Andrews J, et al. *Anaplasma phagocytophilum* infection of domestic cats: 16 cases from the northeastern USA. J Feline Med Surg 2016; 18(2):85–91.

57. Spada E, Proverbio D, Galluzzo P, et al. Molecular study on selected vector-borne infections in urban stray colony cats in Northern Italy. J Feline Med Surg 2014; 16(8):684–8.

58. Galemore ER, Labato MA, O'Neil E. Prevalence of *Anaplasma phagocytophilum* infection in feral cats in Massachusetts. JFMS Open Rep 2018;4(1). 2055116917753804.

59. Billeter SA, Spencer JA, Griffin B, et al. Prevalence of *Anaplasma phagocytophilum* in domestic felines in the United States. Vet Parasitol 2007;147(1–2):194–8.

60. Breitschwerdt EB, Abrams-Ogg AC, Lappin MR, et al. Molecular evidence supporting *Ehrlichia canis*-like infection in cats. J Vet Intern Med 2002;16(6):642–9.

61. Braga IA, dos Santos LG, Melo AL, et al. Hematological values associated to the serological and molecular diagnostic in cats suspected of *Ehrlichia canis* infection. Rev Bras Parasitol Vet 2013;22(4):470–4.

62. Bouloy R, Lappin M, Holland C, et al. Clinical ehrlichiosis in a cat. J Am Vet Med Assoc 1994;204(9):1475–8.

63. Braga IA, dos Santos LG, de Souza Ramos DG, et al. Detection of *Ehrlichia canis* in domestic cats in the central-western region of Brazil. Braz J Microbiol 2014; 45(2):641–5.

64. Neer TM, Breitschwerdt EB, Greene RT, et al. Consensus statement on ehrlichial disease of small animals from the infectious disease study group of the ACVIM. J Vet Intern Med 2002;16(3):309–15.
65. Jenkins S, Ketzis J, Dundas J, et al. Efficacy of minocycline in naturally occurring nonacute ehrlichia canis infection in dogs. J Vet Intern Med 2018;32(1):217–21.
66. Halperin JJ, García-Moncó JC. The human borreliosis: Lyme neuroborreliosis and relapsing fever. CNS Infections. New York: Springer; 2018. p. 233–49.
67. Straubinger RK. PCR-based quantification of *Borrelia burgdorferi* organisms in canine tissues over a 500-day postinfection period. J Clin Microbiol 2000;38(6): 2191–9.
68. Magnarelli LA, Bushmich SL, IJdo JW, et al. Seroprevalence of antibodies against *Borrelia burgdorferi* and *Anaplasma phagocytophilum* in cats. Am J Vet Res 2005;66(11):1895–9.
69. Shannon AB, Rucinsky R, Gaff HD, et al. *Borrelia miyamotoi*, other vector-borne agents in cat blood and ticks in Eastern Maryland. Ecohealth 2017;14(4):816–20.
70. Baneth G, Nachum-Biala Y, Halperin T, et al. Borrelia persica infection in dogs and cats: clinical manifestations, clinicopathological findings and genetic characterization. Parasit Vectors 2016;9(1):244.
71. Exner MM, Lewinski MA. Isolation and detection of Borrelia burgdorferi DNA from cerebral spinal fluid, synovial fluid, blood, urine, and ticks using the Roche MagNA Pure system and real-time PCR. Diagnostic microbiology and infectious disease 2003;46(4):235–40.
72. Littman MP, Gerber B, Goldstein RE, et al. ACVIM consensus update on Lyme borreliosis in dogs and cats. J Vet Intern Med 2018;32(3):887–903.
73. Lappin MR, Hawley J. Presence of *Bartonella* species and *Rickettsia* species DNA in the blood, oral cavity, skin and claw beds of cats in the United States. Vet Dermatol 2009;20(5-6):509–14.
74. Nogueras MM, Pons I, Ortuño A, et al. Molecular detection of *Rickettsia typhi* in cats and fleas. PloS One 2013;8(8):e71386.
75. Segura F, Pons I, Miret J, et al. The role of cats in the eco-epidemiology of spotted fever group diseases. Parasit Vectors 2014;7(1):353.
76. Bayliss DB, Morris AK, Horta MC, et al. Prevalence of *Rickettsia* species antibodies and *Rickettsia* species DNA in the blood of cats with and without fever. J Feline Med Surg 2009;11(4):266–70.
77. Tabuchi M, Sakata Y, Miyazaki N, et al. Serological survey of *Rickettsia japonica* infection in dogs and cats in Japan. Clin Vaccine Immunol 2007;14(11):1526–8.
78. Breitschwerdt E, Papich M, Hegarty B, et al. Efficacy of doxycycline, azithromycin, or trovafloxacin for treatment of experimental Rocky Mountain spotted fever in dogs. Antimicrob Agents Chemother 1999;43(4):813–21.
79. Smith TG. The genus Hepatozoon (Apicomplexa: Adeleina). J Parasitol 1996;82: 565–85.
80. Mathew J, Ewing S, Panciera R, et al. Experimental transmission of *Hepatozoon americanum* Vincent-Johnson et al., 1997 to dogs by the Gulf Coast tick, *Amblyomma maculatum* Koch. Vet Parasitol 1998;80(1):1–14.
81. Baneth G, Samish M, Alekseev E, et al. Transmission of *Hepatozoon canis* to dogs by naturally-fed or percutaneously-injected *Rhipicephalus sanguineus* ticks. J Parasitol 2001;87(3):606–11.
82. Baneth G, Sheiner A, Eyal O, et al. Redescription of *Hepatozoon felis* (Apicomplexa: Hepatozoidae) based on phylogenetic analysis, tissue and blood form morphology, and possible transplacental transmission. Parasit Vectors 2013; 6(1):102.

83. Kegler K, Nufer U, Alic A, et al. Fatal infection with emerging apicomplexan parasite *Hepatozoon silvestris* in a domestic cat. Parasit Vectors 2018;11(1):428.
84. Díaz-Regañón D, Villaescusa A, Ayllón T, et al. Molecular detection of *Hepatozoon* spp. and *Cytauxzoon* sp. in domestic and stray cats from Madrid, Spain. Parasit Vectors 2017;10(1):112.
85. Giannelli A, Latrofa MS, Nachum-Biala Y, et al. Three different *Hepatozoon* species in domestic cats from southern Italy. Ticks Tick Borne Dis 2017;8(5):721–4.
86. Allen KE, Yabsley MJ, Johnson EM, et al. Novel *Hepatozoon* in vertebrates from the southern United States. J Parasitol 2011;97(4):648–53.
87. Ewing G. Granulomatous cholangiohepatitis in a cat due to a protozoan parasite resembling *Hepatozoon canis*. Feline Practice 1977;7:37–40.
88. Baneth G, Aroch I, Tal N, et al. *Hepatozoon* species infection in domestic cats: a retrospective study. Vet Parasitol 1998;79(2):123–33.
89. Li Y, Wang C, Allen KE, et al. Diagnosis of canine *Hepatozoon* spp. infection by quantitative PCR. Vet Parasitol 2008;157(1–2):50–8.
90. Lloret A, Addie DD, Boucraut-Baralon C, et al. Hepatozoonosis in cats: ABCD guidelines on prevention and management. J Feline Med Surg 2015;17(7):642–4.
91. Van Amstel S. Hepatozoonose in n' Kat. J S Afr Vet Med Assoc 1979;50(3):215–6.
92. Little SE, Barrett AW, Nagamori Y, et al. Ticks from cats in the United States: patterns of infestation and infection with pathogens. Vet Parasitol 2018;257:15–20.

Optimal Vector-borne Disease Screening in Dogs Using Both Serology-based and Polymerase Chain Reaction–based Diagnostic Panels

Linda Kidd, DVM, PhD

KEYWORDS

• PCR • Antibody • Serology • Tick • Flea • Rickettsial • Piroplasm

KEY POINTS

- Vector-borne disease and idiopathic immune-mediated disease present similarly. Ruling out infection is important.
- Comprehensive diagnostic panels that include multiple organisms help detect infection and identify coinfections.
- Consider breed, lifestyle, geographic locale, and clinical presentation to determine which organisms to include in a panel for an individual dog.
- Panels that combine polymerase chain reaction (PCR) and serology should be used in initial screening of clinically unwell dogs to maximize sensitivity.
- Repeat testing using PCR is warranted in dogs at high risk of infection with organisms that circulate in blood in low numbers or intermittently.
- Convalescent serologic testing can the facilitate diagnosis of acute infection.

INTRODUCTION

Vector-borne disease is an important cause of morbidity and mortality in companion animals. In addition to causing acute illness, many vector-borne disease agents cause chronic subclinical infections that can recrudesce. Importantly, the clinical and laboratory abnormalities associated with vector-borne disease, such as vasculitis, hemolytic anemia, thrombocytopenia, and proteinuria, also occur in dogs with idiopathic immune-mediated disease. In addition, a few vector-borne disease agents may cause

Disclosure: Dr L. Kidd has been a paid speaker for IDEXX laboratories and has received reduced assay costs from Antech Diagnostics for research. Research supported by Canine Health Foundation Grant 02285-A: Investigation of Association between Thrombocytopenia and Occult Vector BorneDisease in Greyhound Dogs with and without a History of Racing and Western University of Health Sciences College of Veterinary Medicine Grant Matching Program.
Western University of Health Sciences College of Veterinary Medicine, 309 East Second Street, Pomona, CA 91766, USA
E-mail address: lkidd@westernu.edu

Vet Clin Small Anim 49 (2019) 703–718
https://doi.org/10.1016/j.cvsm.2019.02.011
0195-5616/19/© 2019 Elsevier Inc. All rights reserved.

immune-mediated disease, such as immune-mediated hemolytic anemia (IMHA), immune-mediated thrombocytopenia, and immune-complex glomerulonephritis.[1–14] Like vector-borne disease, the incidence of idiopathic immune-mediated disease can be seasonal.[15,16] Furthermore, occult vector-borne disease has been documented in dogs diagnosed with idiopathic immune-mediated disease.[17] Because immunosuppression is the mainstay of treatment of immune-mediated disease, overlooking infection may significantly affect morbidity and mortality.

The diagnosis of vector-borne disease has been greatly facilitated by advances in molecular biology and the availability of tick panels or vector-borne disease panels from major diagnostic commercial and university laboratories (**Table 1**). These panels test for multiple organisms using polymerase chain reaction (PCR) to directly detect the organism and/or serology to detect antibodies that indicate an immune response against an organism. Although the umbrella term tick panel is commonly used to refer to them all, it is important to recognize that the panels differ in which organisms are included, how many are included, and whether PCR or serology, or a combination of these methodologies, are used for each organism (see **Table 1**). This article discusses how to consider the pathophysiology and epidemiology of the organisms and presents information to facilitate panel selection and recognize when more aggressive, additional testing for an organism is warranted.

WHICH ORGANISMS SHOULD BE INCLUDED IN VECTOR-BORNE DISEASE SCREENING?

Considering geographic locale, lifestyle, breed, and specific clinical and laboratory findings helps determine which organisms should be included in a panel for an individual dog.

Geographic Locale

The distribution of vector-borne diseases generally follows the distribution of vectors. Although fleas and mosquitos are widely distributed, knowledge of which ticks are common in a given geographic locale informs which vector-borne diseases should be screened for in an individual dog. For example, *Anaplasma phagocytophilum* and *Borrelia burgdorferi* are primarily distributed in the north east, Midwest, and Pacific coast because of the distribution of *Ixodes scapularis* and *Ixodes pacificus* ticks.[18] *Ehrlichia ewingii* and *Ehrlichia chaffeensis* are common in the southern and mid-Atlantic states because of the distribution of *Amblyomma americanum*.[18,19] *Rhipicephalus sanguineus* is a ubiquitously distributed tick but is particularly well adapted to hot climates.[20,21] It is the confirmed or suspected vector for numerous vector-borne disease agents, including *Ehrlichia canis*, *Babesia canis*, *Anaplasma platys*, *Babesia conradae*, *Bartonella* species, hemotropic *Mycoplasma*, and spotted fever group (SFG) *Rickettsia*.[22–29] Accordingly, dogs the southwestern and southern United States are commonly infected with these organisms.[17,24,26,30,31] This tick is also responsible for the expanding geographic distribution of Rocky Mountain spotted fever (RMSF) in the United States.[25,27,32] Historically, the distribution of RMSF followed the distribution of its *Dermacentor* tick vectors in the United States, *Dermacentor variabilis* and *Dermacentor andersoni*. The southeastern United States accounts for most cases. However, a recent outbreak of RMSF with associated mortality occurred in a nonendemic area of Arizona. Retrospectively it was shown that infection existed in the dog population before the fatal outbreak in people, and the vector was *Rh sanguineus*.[27] This epidemic shows how the geographic distribution of vector-borne diseases is expanding. There are also focal differences in the prevalence of infectious

Table 1
Examples of canine vector-borne disease diagnostic panels available at some diagnostic laboratories in the United States

Laboratory Name	Panel Name	Methodology	Organisms
Antech Diagnostics	Fastpanel PCR Canine Tick Borne Profile with Lyme Serology	PCR	*Anaplasma phagocytophilum, Anaplasma platys, Babesia canis, Babesia* spp *Coco, Babesia conradae, Babesia gibsoni, Bartonella henselae, Bartonella vinsonii, Ehrlichia canis, Ehrlichia chaffeensis, Ehrlichia ewingii, Mycoplasma haemocanis, Mycoplasma haemotoparvum, Neorickettsia risticii, Rickettsia rickettsii*
		Serology	*Borrelia burgdorferi*
Antech Diagnostics	Accuplex 4	Serology	*Ehrlichia canis, Anaplasma phagocytophilum, Dirofilaria immitis* (antigen), *Borrelia burgdorferi*
Colorado State University Specialized Infectious Diseases Laboratory	Canine Fever/Blood Donor Panel	PCR	• *Bartonella* spp • *Ehrlichia* spp • *Hemoplasma* spp • *Rickettsia* spp
IDEXX	Tick Panel	Serology	*Ehrlichia canis,* Rocky Mountain spotted fever screen, and Lyme titer by IFA
IDEXX	Tick RealPCR Panel	PCR	*Anaplasma* spp and *Ehrlichia* spp RealPCR test
IDEXX	Tick/Vector Comprehensive RealPCR Panel with Lab 4Dx Plus Test-Canine	PCR	*Anaplasma* spp, *Babesia* spp, *Bartonella* spp, canine hemotropic *Mycoplasma, Ehrlichia* spp, *Hepatozoon* spp, *Leishmania* spp quantitative, *Neorickettsia risticii,* and Rocky Mountain spotted fever (*Rickettsia rickettsii*) RealPCR tests
		Serology	*Borrelia burgdorferi, Anaplasma* spp, *Ehrlichia* spp and *Dirofilaria immitis* (antigen)
IDEXX	Tick/Vector Comprehensive RealPCR Panel-Canine	PCR	*Anaplasma* spp, *Babesia* spp, *Bartonella* spp, canine hemotropic *Mycoplasma, Ehrlichia* spp, *Hepatozoon* spp, *Leishmania* spp quantitative, *Neorickettsia risticii,* and Rocky Mountain spotted fever (*Rickettsia rickettsii*) RealPCR tests

(continued on next page)

Table 1 (continued)			
Laboratory Name	Panel Name	Methodology	Organisms
IDEXX	Tick/Vector Comprehensive RealPCR Panel with Comprehensive Serology - Canine	PCR	Canine Tick/Vector Comprehensive RealPCR Panel (*Anaplasma* spp, *Babesia* spp, *Bartonella* spp, canine hemotropic *Mycoplasma*, *Ehrlichia* spp, *Hepatozoon* spp, *Leishmania* spp quantitative, *Neorickettsia risticii*, and Rocky Mountain spotted fever (*Rickettsia ricketsii*) RealPCR tests
		Serology	*Babesia canis*, *Babesia gibsoni*, *Bartonella henselae*, *Bartonella koehlerae*, *Bartonella vinsonii*, and Rocky Mountain spotted fever antibodies by IFA; SNAP 4Dx Plus (ELISAs for heartworm antigen, *Anaplasma phagocytophilum*, *Anaplasma platys*, *Ehrlichia canis*, *Ehrlichia ewingii*, and Lyme C6 antibodies)
Michigan State University Veterinary Diagnostic Laboratory	Tick-borne disease antibody screen	Serology (IFA)	*Babesia canis*, *Ehrlichia canis*, *Anaplasma phagocytophilum*, *Borrelia burgdorferi*, *Rickettsia rickettsii*
NCSU CVM VBDDL	Canine Comprehensive Panel	PCR	*Babesia*, *Bartonella*, *Anaplasma*, *Ehrlichia*, *Rickettsia*, and hemotropic *Mycoplasma*
		Serology (IFA)	*Babesia canis*, *Babesia gibsoni*, *Ehrlichia canis*, *Rickettsia rickettsii*, *Bartonella henselae*, *Bartonella vinsonii*, *Bartonella koehlerae*
		Serology (SNAP 4Dx Plus)	*Borrelia burgdorferi*, *Anaplasma* spp, *Ehrlichia* spp, and *Dirofilaria immitis* (antigen)
University of California Davis Real-time PCR Research and Diagnostics Core Facility	Canine vector-borne panel	PCR	*Anaplasma phagocytophilum*, *Anaplasma platys*, *Bartonella* spp, *Ehrlichia canis*, *Rickettsia* spp, *Borrelia burgdorferi*, *Babesia* spp, *Mycoplasma haemocanis*. The laboratory notes: whole blood not recommended for *Borrelia burgdorferi* testing by qPCR

This is not a comprehensive list of laboratories or their available tests. The intent of the table is to conceptually show differences between PCR and serologic panels available at diagnostic laboratories that test for more than 1 vector-borne agent.

All panel listings accessed November and December 2018.

Abbreviations: ELISA, enzyme-linked immunosorbent assay; IFA, immunofluorescent assay; NCSU CVM VBDDL, North Carolina State University College of Veterinary Medicine Vector Borne Disease Diagnostic Laboratory; PCR, polymerase chain reaction; qPCR, quantitative polymerase chain reaction.

Courtesy of Linda Kidd, DVM, PhD, Pomona, CA.

agents carried by ticks.[33] For example, *B conradae*, which may be transmitted by *Rh sanguineus*, seems to currently have a focal geographic distribution, with most cases being reported in California.[24,34,35] In addition to possible transmission by *Rh sanguineus*, exposure to coyotes and bite transmission may also play a role.[35] General summaries of geographic distributions of arthropod vectors and the infectious agents that parasitize them are available to help guide testing for individual dogs.[36] Useful epidemiologic information regarding vector-borne disease prevalence and the distribution of their associated vectors is available from several online resources, including the Companion Animal Parasite Council (capcvet.org), the Companion Vector Borne Disease Web site (CVBD.org), the Centers for Disease Control and Prevention (cdc.gov), Show Us Your Ticks (https://www.showusyourticks.org/let-us-show-you-our-ticks/), and local county veterinary public health Web sites.

Given that the geographic distribution of vector-borne disease is expanding, comprehensive testing can help identify novel infections and disease emergence. Comprehensive screening also helps identify coinfections, which are common because of simultaneous transmission of multiple agents from 1 vector, or exposure to multiple tick species.[17,19,30] This is important, because undetected coinfection can have clinical implications. For example, if a dog with thrombocytopenia and anemia is found to be infected with *E canis*, because of coexposure risk, the dog should also be screened for *B canis*.[16]

Lifestyle and Breed

Considering lifestyle and breed can also help determine which agents should be included in diagnostic panels. For example, studies suggest that hunting or outdoor dogs are at increased risk for some vector-borne diseases, such as RMSF and Lyme nephritis.[37,38] Retired racing greyhounds and other dogs with heavy exposure to *Rh sanguineus* are commonly infected with organisms found in that tick, in particular *B canis*, hemotropic *Mycoplasma*, and *E canis*[30,39-41] (Kidd, unpublished data, 2019). As mentioned earlier, coyote-hunting greyhounds and greyhound mixes seem to be at increased risk of infection with *B conradae*.[35] Pit bull breeds are commonly infected with *Babesia gibsoni*, likely because of vertical transmission and transmission through fighting and dog-to-dog bites.[39,42] The clinical implications of these lifestyle and breed-associated risks are that careful screening is warranted in at-risk dogs with clinical signs of vector-borne disease. For example, finding thrombocytopenia or hemolytic anemia, hyperglobulinemia, or proteinuria in pit bull breeds warrants combined PCR and serologic testing followed by repeated PCR testing for *B gibsoni* if initial tests are negative. Ruling out *B canis* and *E canis* in a thrombocytopenic, proteinuric retired racing greyhound is prudent, and dogs living in California and coyote-hunting dogs should be specifically screened for *B conradae*. Being familiar with the geographic distribution and breed risks of diseases, and taking a complete lifestyle and travel history, can inform which organisms should be included on the diagnostic panel.

Clinical and Laboratory Abnormalities

Common clinical signs and laboratory abnormalities associated with vector-borne diseases include nonspecific gastrointestinal signs, lethargy, arthralgia, myalgia, spinal pain, neurologic abnormalities, vasculitis, fever, thrombocytopenia, anemia, hyperglobulinemia, and proteinuria. Although there is overlap among agents, some abnormalities are commonly or specifically associated with a few agents. Knowing which agents have been associated with a particular clinical abnormality can prompt the clinician to include them in testing. For example, although IMHA has been associated with several vector-borne disease agents, the strongest evidence for a causative association exists for *Babesia* species.[14] Therefore, a negative result for a tick panel that tests for antibodies to *B burgdorferi*, *Rickettsia rickettsii*, and *E canis* would not rule out vector-borne diseases as a cause for the IMHA.[14] Similarly, because SFG *Rickettsia* infect endothelial cells, these organisms cause vasculitis.[43–46] *E canis* and *Bartonella* species have also been associated with clinical findings consistent with vasculitis.[47,48] Therefore, signs of increased vascular permeability, such as peripheral edema, petechiation, retinal hemorrhages, and uveitis should prompt clinicians to include these organisms in the diagnostic investigation. Careful consideration of which organisms to include in screening is especially important with serologic testing, because most serologic panels are not as comprehensive as PCR panels. In addition, comprehensive testing using panels that include multiple organisms can be helpful, regardless of geographic locale, breed, and major clinical signs. Combining PCR with serology and repeated testing increases diagnostic sensitivity and helps ensure infection is not overlooked (discussed later).[17,49]

WHICH TESTING METHODOLOGY SHOULD BE USED: POLYMERASE CHAIN REACTION, SEROLOGY, OR BOTH?
General Concepts

Peripheral blood is the most commonly used diagnostic sample to detect infection with, or exposure to, vector-borne disease agents. Many, but not all, vector-borne disease agents circulate in peripheral blood during certain stages of infection; therefore, depending on the organism, cytologic examination, culture, and PCR can be used to directly detect their presence.

Cytology

In general, PCR is more sensitive and specific than cytologic examination to identify vector-borne disease agents that are visible in peripheral blood.[50–54] However, cytologic examination of peripheral blood smears should be a part of routine testing for any animal with suspected vector-borne disease. Red cell morphology should be assessed for the presence of immune-mediated destruction (spherocytosis), oxidative damage, or other morphologic abnormalities, and the presence or absence of regeneration. Platelet counts can be estimated, and any large platelets should be noted. Toxic changes to neutrophils can also be evaluated. All of these findings are potentially helpful from diagnostic, prognostic, and treatment standpoints.

Although less sensitive than PCR, cytologic examination of blood films can also directly show some organisms that circulate in peripheral blood. For example, *Babesia* species can be observed in infected red blood cells, *Ehrlichia* species in monocytes or neutrophils, and *Anaplasma* species in neutrophils or platelets. Cytologic examination is also the only way to directly detect *Borrelia* species that can cause tick-borne relapsing fever, because there is no commercial PCR assay currently available.[55] The sensitivity of cytologic examination of blood smears depends on the pathophysiology of the organism, phase of infection, and the skill of the cytologist. Some organisms cannot be visualized. For example, *R rickettsii* infects endothelial cells, and *B burgdorferi* is primarily found in solid connective tissues when clinical signs manifest. Thus cytologic demonstration in peripheral blood is not feasible. It is also important to remember that even if organisms infect circulating cells in high numbers, direct demonstration is not necessarily easy. In general, organisms that infect peripheral blood cells do so most abundantly during the acute phase of infection. Thus, screening a canine blood smear for the presence of *E canis* or *E chaffeensis* in monocytes; *E ewingii* or *A phagocytophilum* in neutrophils; or *B gibsoni*, *B conradae*, or *B canis* in red blood cells has transiently heightened sensitivity shortly after infection.

In contrast, infecting organisms are less commonly observed in peripheral blood smears from chronically infected dogs. Of note, cytologic examination does not allow speciation of organisms, because morulae from different infecting species can be indistinguishable. For example, a morula in a neutrophil in a blood smear from a dog from a mid-Atlantic state could likely represent either *A phagocytophilum* or *E ewingii*.

Culture
The presence of active infection can also be shown by positive culture for many (but not all) vector-borne disease agents. However, culture is rarely performed to document infection with vector-borne disease agents, because most require cell culture and specialized techniques and equipment. For some organisms, culture poses significant biological risk to laboratory workers, requiring specialized containment facilities (eg, *R rickettsii*). Culture is also, in general, a less sensitive diagnostic technique than PCR. For these reasons, culture is seldom used outside of research settings for the detection of infection with vector-borne disease agents.

Polymerase chain reaction
PCR directly shows the presence of an organism by detecting the DNA or, in the case of reverse transcriptase PCR, RNA of the organism. PCR has revolutionized diagnostic testing for several infectious disease agents. Recently, advances in molecular biology have made PCR panels easy to perform and widely available. Advanced technology makes it possible to directly detect multiple organisms with high sensitivity and specificity. This high sensitivity and specificity assumes appropriate primer design and assay optimization, use of appropriate positive and negative controls, and physical and procedural protocols to minimize contamination.

The absolute sensitivity of a PCR refers to how many copies of the DNA target it can reliably detect in a test sample with a known amount of DNA template. Many PCRs have very high absolute sensitivity and can detect the presence of very few organisms reliably. However, it is very important for clinicians to understand that absolute sensitivity does not necessarily translate into clinical sensitivity. Clinical sensitivity refers to whether infection can be detected in an infected dog.[56] Importantly, the organism must be present in the blood sample for it to be detected by PCR.

Although many factors affect the clinical sensitivity of a PCR assay, organism pathophysiology is arguably the most important. This factor determines the likelihood of the organism being in a blood sample at the time of sampling. As mentioned previously, organisms generally circulate in the highest copy number during the acute phase of infection (**Fig. 1**).[52,57–60] However, some organisms never circulate in high numbers in the peripheral blood.[56] Moreover, organisms commonly circulate intermittently during chronic infection (see **Fig. 1**).[53,60,61] Therefore, PCR is also intermittently negative. Testing for antibodies using serology combined with repeated testing using PCR can facilitate diagnosis.[17,49,58] In addition to the pathophysiology of the organism, host factors, such as previous antimicrobial treatment, may also decrease circulating copy number, contributing to a negative PCR test during active infection. Although PCR is highly sensitive, a negative result does not rule out active infection, so a negative result should be interpreted as no organism detected rather than uninfected.

Assay design can affect both the sensitivity and the specificity of an assay. From a clinical perspective, this means that clinicians must select assays that target organisms at the genus level rather than at the species level, because such assays are designed to detect all relevant species within that genus. Most laboratories post

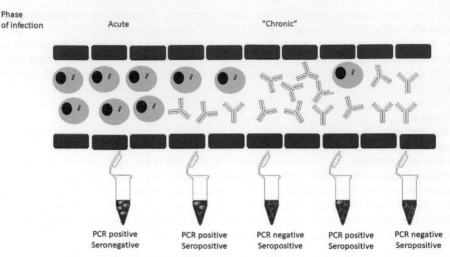

Fig. 1. Theoretical results of PCR and serologic testing for an organism that causes both acute and chronic infection. (*Courtesy of* Linda Kidd, DVM, PhD, Pomona, CA.)

information on their Web sites regarding which species genera-specific assays detect. The laboratory is responsible for ensuring specificity; that is, that the assay amplifies DNA only from the organism of interest. Using reputable laboratories that use validated assays is critically important.

Serology

Serologic testing detects antibodies that are produced by the immune system in response to the presence of an infectious disease agent. The presence of a serologic response indicates previous or recent exposure, and seroconversion (the demonstration of a 4-fold change in antibody titer within 4 weeks) indicates active infection (because it takes about 2–4 weeks after infection for antibodies to be detectable). Immunoassays such as indirect immunofluorescent assays (IFAs) and enzyme-linked immunosorbent assays (ELISAs) are commonly used to detect antibodies. Basically, if antibodies are present in a serum sample, they bind to target antigen fixed to a glass slide (IFA) or microtiter plate (ELISA), and are detected with a secondary antibody conjugated to a fluorescent (IFA) or enzyme-based (ELISA) label. Modifications of these traditional assays include mounting antigens on spinning silicon discs, membrane filters, colloidal gold particles, or fluorescent beads.[a,b,c,d] Along with other advances in molecular biology, testing for multiple organisms simultaneously using small sample volumes is possible. Note that immunoassays can also be used to detect antigen.

Historically, serologic testing to detect antibodies has been the mainstay of diagnostic testing for vector-borne disease because of the technical difficulties associated with isolating and culturing organisms from clinical specimens. PCR has overcome

---

[a] Accuplex 4 BioCD System Antech Diagnostics.

[b] Lyme Disease Canine Multiplex Assay, Cornell University College of Veterinary Medicine Animal Health Diagnostic Center.

[c] IDEXX SNAP 4Dx Plus.

[d] Abaxis VETSCAN FLEX4 Rapid Test.

difficulties associated with culture, but serology still plays an important role in the diagnosis of vector-borne disease, not only for routine in-clinic screening but as a means to identify infection when organisms are circulating in numbers below the limit of detection for PCR.

In general, serologic testing is sensitive if performed after seroconversion has occurred. This property is particularly valuable from a diagnostic standpoint during chronic infection, when PCR can be negative. However, serology may be falsely negative if a dog is presented for evaluation before seroconversion. Because the phase of infection is rarely known in natural infections, combining PCR with serology or demonstration of seroconversion using convalescent serologic testing facilitates the diagnosis of acute infections.

For some organisms, such as *Bartonella* species, it seems that some dogs do not develop detectable antibodies even after seroconversion should have occurred.[62] Puppies or immunocompromised dogs also may not have detectable antibodies.[63] Therefore, as with PCR, a negative serologic test does not necessarily rule out infection with a vector-borne disease agent.

Plasma cells that produce antibodies can be long lived. Therefore, a positive antibody test suggests previous exposure, but not necessarily active infection. It can be difficult to determine whether clinical signs are attributable to infection in dogs seropositive for some agents, particularly in endemic areas, where exposure is common in healthy dogs. It is also important to remember that antibodies can cross react between shared epitopes among members of the same genus and sometimes between genera. Therefore, the species responsible for the clinical signs cannot always be assumed based on the species of organism that is used in the assay. Exposure to nonpathogenic endosymbionts of ticks can also result in cross-reacting antibody formation against some pathogens, which occurs commonly in dogs and humans exposed to nonpathogenic SFG *Rickettsia*.[64,65] It is also important to note that serologic cross reactivity between all species of a given genus does not always occur. Therefore, a negative serologic test for one member of a genus does not rule out infection with other members of that genus.

APPLYING THESE CONCEPTS IN THE CLINICAL SETTING
What is the Significance of a Negative Result?

Polymerase chain reaction
As mentioned earlier, although PCR is very sensitive and has revolutionized diagnostic testing for vector-borne disease, in order for PCR to be positive, the organism has to be present in the sample. Therefore, a negative PCR test does not rule out infection. Considering the pathophysiology of an organism can help determine whether a false-negative PCR result is likely. If organisms are circulating in blood in high numbers at the time they cause clinical signs, it is very likely that a PCR test will detect the organism. However, some organisms do not circulate in high copy numbers when clinical signs of illness are present. For example, *R rickettsii* infects endothelial cells and primarily causes acute illness in naturally infected dogs. Because of its endotheliotropic nature, PCR of peripheral blood is often negative in an actively infected, clinically affected dog. Repeating PCR on the same or additional samples can facilitate diagnosis.[56] Because *R rickettsii* causes acute illness, antibodies may not yet be detectable at presentation. Thus, serology may also be falsely negative at the time of presentation. Combined testing using PCR and serology on acute samples can increase sensitivity. In these cases, treatment based on clinical suspicion is indicated,

and showing a 4-fold change in titer by repeating sampling during convalescence may be necessary to confirm the clinical diagnosis.

During chronic infection, organisms may circulate in low copy number. For example:

- *Ehrlichia* species often circulate in monocytes in peripheral blood in low copy numbers and/or intermittently during chronic infection; thus, PCR can sometimes be negative despite active infection.[53,66,67] Therefore, simultaneous serologic testing facilitates the diagnosis of chronic ehrlichiosis. Repeat testing using PCR can also be helpful.
- *Babesia* species infect circulating red blood cells. Therefore, PCR of peripheral blood is useful in diagnosing active *Babesia* infection. However, as with *Ehrlichia* species, *Babesia* species may also circulate intermittently or in low numbers in the chronic phase of infection.[1,58,60,68] Although PCR is a sensitive method to detect *Babesia* in peripheral blood, test results may be negative during infection.[17,58,60] Therefore, repeated testing using PCR and combining PCR with serology is recommended to increase sensitivity.[14,50]
- *Bartonella* species may also circulate only intermittently or in low copy numbers during chronic infection in dogs.[62] Although serologic testing may facilitate diagnosis, seroconversion may not occur in up to 50% of dogs.[62] Whole-blood samples collected using a sterile technique can be grown in enrichment media to increase copy number before PCR, thereby increasing sensitivity.
- Clinical signs of Lyme borreliosis do not occur in experimentally infected dogs until 2 to 6 months after tick exposure and organisms do not circulate in peripheral blood in high numbers.[69] Consequently, serologic testing rather than PCR is routinely used to document exposure to *B burgdorferi* using peripheral blood samples.

These examples show how the pathophysiology of the organism can dictate whether or not organisms are detectable in blood samples during infection.

PCR may also be negative because the infecting species within a genus is not targeted by primers. Primers that target genus rather than species facilitate testing for a broad range of species in an individual dog, but it is important to verify with the laboratory that a particular species of interest is amplified by the primers for that genus.

Serology

As mentioned earlier, serologic testing can be negative despite active infection. Dogs that present acutely, before antibodies are detectable, test seronegative. For example, serologic testing is sometimes negative in dogs acutely infected with agents such as *R rickettsii*, *E canis*, *Babesia* species, and *A phagocytophilum* because clinical abnormalities can manifest before seroconversion.[52,58,65,68,70,71] A recent study showed that 44% of clinically ill dogs naturally infected with *A phagocytophilum* were seronegative at the time of presentation.[72] Convalescent testing documenting seroconversion, or adding PCR to the diagnostic regimen, helps confirm active infection. As mentioned earlier, for some organisms, including *Bartonella* species and possibly *Babesia* species, and in puppies or immunosuppressed dogs, antibodies may not be detectable.[62,63,70] PCR can facilitate diagnosis in these cases.

Sensitivity can also differ among different types of serologic assay testing for the same organism. For example, on rare occasions, dogs actively infected with *E canis* can test seropositive using IFA and seronegative using ELISA. This discrepancy may be related to differences in the nature of antigens used in the respective assays.[17,73]

In addition, antibodies cannot be detected for some organisms simply because a commercial assay is not available. Examples include hemotropic *Mycoplasma* and *B conradae*. PCR or microscopic examination of blood smears is required to detect infection with these agents.

What is the Significance of a Positive Result?

Polymerase chain reaction

Assuming appropriate laboratory controls are in place, a positive PCR result indicates active infection or the presence of circulating dead organisms. Response to appropriate antimicrobial therapy helps to determine whether presenting clinical signs can be attributed to infection or whether coinfection or other underlying disease should also be considered. False-positive results caused by cross reactivity of primers to homologous DNA shared by multiple organisms or host DNA are usually eliminated by appropriate assay design, but they are possible. Considering whether or not infection with a specific agent makes sense given the signalment, clinical signs, and geographic locale is helpful. If the PCR results do not make sense in an individual dog, consulting the laboratory and further testing, including DNA sequencing to verify the infecting species, could be considered.

Serology

When considering the significance of a positive serologic titer on a single sample it is again useful to consider the pathophysiology of the organism, because a positive serologic test may indicate exposure and not necessarily active infection. For example, *R rickettsii* and *A phagocytophilum* cause acute rather than chronic disease in naturally infected dogs. However, previous infection may result in long-lived antibody titers.[52,74] Therefore, if serologic testing is positive for these agents and clinical abnormalities have been present for many months, previous exposure, but not active infection, is possible. In these cases, coinfection with other vector-borne agents, the presence of cross-reacting antibodies, or the presence of other underlying disease should be considered.

Serologic cross reactivity among species within a genus and between genera also affects the interpretation of a positive serologic test. As is the case with PCR, considering whether or not infection with the specific agent is consistent with the signalment, clinical findings, and geographic locale is helpful. For example, there is extensive serologic cross reactivity among SFG *Rickettsia*.[75] In general, the species of infecting *Rickettsia* has been presumed based on geographic locale, so if a dog from the southeastern United States seroconverts to *R rickettsii*, RMSF becomes the presumptive diagnosis. However, other species of SFG *Rickettsia* that infect humans are present in the United States and it is also likely that these organisms infect dogs and induce disease.[26,64,76] Furthermore, exposure to nonpathogenic SFG *Rickettsia*, some of which are common endosymbionts in ticks, may be a common cause of positive titers, particularly low and persistent titers, to *R rickettsii* in dogs.[65,77] Serologic cross reactivity with SFG *Rickettsia* also seems to occur in dogs infected with *Bartonella henselae*.[78] Therefore, a single positive titer to *R rickettsii* may not represent infection with that organism. PCR testing on banked acute EDTA (ethylenediaminetetraacetic acid) samples can facilitate species verification, and acute PCR and convalescent serology can help confirm the presence of active infection in seropositive dogs.[56]

When interpreting results of positive serologic assays in individual canine patients, clinicians should also keep in mind that infection with novel species and expanding geographic distribution of known species occurs, because this phenomenon is responsible for outbreaks of emerging infectious disease. For example, the geographic distribution of RMSF in the United States has increased beyond the distribution of its primary tick vectors, *D variabilis* and *D andersoni*. In addition, *Rh sanguineous* recently caused an outbreak of RMSF with associated mortality in a nonendemic area of Arizona.[28] It was shown retrospectively that infection existed in the dog population before the fatal outbreak in people.[27] This example shows how a positive titer in a nonendemic region does not necessarily represent a false-positive result and may represent disease emergence.

Testing the same sample initially using both PCR and serology, repeating PCR on the same or additional samples, and testing convalescent samples with serology increases diagnostic sensitivity.[17,49]

THE IMPORTANCE OF BANKING SAMPLES

In order to enable appropriate testing using PCR and serology, both serum and whole blood in EDTA should be obtained at initial presentation. Based on the presenting scenario, a decision can be made to determine whether initial testing using serology, PCR, or both, is the most appropriate. Both serology and PCR are recommended whenever possible. If initial PCR or serologic testing is negative, and both testing methodologies were not used, the alternative methodology can be used to test banked samples. Convalescent serologic testing can be considered in order to confirm active infection, particularly when there is an acute history of illness. Repeating PCR on initial or additional samples may also be advantageous in some cases.

SUMMARY

The epidemiology, clinical findings, and pathophysiology of vector-borne disease agents are helpful in determining which organisms to test for and which methodologies should be used for a given presentation. Comprehensive screening that includes multiple organisms and combination testing using PCR and serology may be necessary to accurately diagnose infection with vector-borne agents. Most importantly, clinicians should remember that a negative panel using either serology or PCR does not necessarily rule out the presence of underlying vector-borne disease in a dog with clinical signs of immune-mediated disease, and retesting should be considered, based on case context.

REFERENCES

1. Wozniak EJ, Barr BC, Thomford JW, et al. Clinical, anatomic, and immunopathologic characterization of Babesia gibsoni infection in the domestic dog (Canis familiaris). J Parasitol 1997;83(4):692–9.
2. Morita T, Saeki H, Imai S, et al. Reactivity of anti-erythrocyte antibody induced by Babesia gibsoni infection against aged erythrocytes. Vet Parasitol 1995;58(4):291–9.
3. Adachi K, Tateishi M, Horii Y, et al. Reactivity of serum anti-erythrocyte membrane antibody in Babesia gibsoni-infected dogs. J Vet Med Sci 1994;56(5):997–9.
4. Adachi K, Tateishi M, Horii Y, et al. Elevated erythrocyte-bound IgG value in dogs with clinical Babesia gibsoni infection. J Vet Med Sci 1994;56(4):757–9.
5. Otsuka Y, Yamasaki M, Yamato O, et al. The effect of macrophages on the erythrocyte oxidative damage and the pathogenesis of anemia in Babesia gibsoni-infected dogs with low parasitemia. J Vet Med Sci 2002;64(3):221–6.
6. Adachi K, Makimura S. Changes in anti-erythrocyte membrane antibody level of dogs experimentally infected with Babesia gibsoni. J Vet Med Sci 1992;54(6):1221–3.

7. Grindem CB, Breitschwerdt EB, Perkins PC, et al. Platelet-associated immuno-globulin (antiplatelet antibody) in canine Rocky Mountain spotted fever and ehrlichiosis. J Am Anim Hosp Assoc 1999;35(1):56–61.
8. Bexfield NH, Villiers EJ, Herrtage ME. Immune-mediated haemolytic anaemia and thrombocytopenia associated with Anaplasma phagocytophilum in a dog. J Small Anim Pract 2005;46(11):543–8.
9. Cortese L, Terrazzano G, Piantedosi D, et al. Prevalence of anti-platelet antibodies in dogs naturally co-infected by Leishmania infantum and Ehrlichia canis. Vet J 2011;188(1):118–21.
10. Smith RD, Ristic M, Huxsoll DL, et al. Platelet kinetics in canine ehrlichiosis: evidence for increased platelet destruction as the cause of thrombocytopenia. Infect Immun 1975;11(6):1216–21.
11. Harrus S, Day MJ, Waner T, et al. Presence of immune-complexes, and absence of antinuclear antibodies, in sera of dogs naturally and experimentally infected with Ehrlichia canis. Vet Microbiol 2001;83(4):343–9.
12. Margarito JM, Lucena R, Lopez R, et al. Levels of IgM and IgA circulating immune complexes in dogs with leishmaniasis. Zentralbl Veterinarmed B 1998; 45(5):263–7.
13. Matsumura K, Kazuta Y, Endo R, et al. Detection of circulating immune complexes in the sera of dogs infected with Dirofilaria immitis, by Clq-binding enzyme-linked immunosorbent assay. J Helminthol 1986;60(3):239–43.
14. Garden OA, Kidd L, Mexas AM, et al. ACVIM consensus statement on the diagnosis of immune-mediated hemolytic anemia in dogs and cats. J Vet Intern Med 2019;33(2):313–34.
15. Kidd L, Rasmussen R, Chaplow E, et al. Seasonality of immune-mediated hemolytic anemia in dogs from southern California. J Vet Emerg Crit Care (San Antonio) 2014;24(3):311–5.
16. Weinkle TK, Center SA, Randolph JF, et al. Evaluation of prognostic factors, survival rates, and treatment protocols for immune-mediated hemolytic anemia in dogs: 151 cases (1993–2002). J Am Vet Med Assoc 2005;226(11):1869–80.
17. Kidd L, Qurollo B, Lappin M, et al. Prevalence of vector-borne pathogens in Southern California dogs with clinical and laboratory abnormalities consistent with immune-mediated disease. J Vet Intern Med 2017;31(4):1081–90.
18. Little SE, Beall MJ, Bowman DD, et al. Canine infection with Dirofilaria immitis, Borrelia burgdorferi, Anaplasma spp., and Ehrlichia spp. in the United States, 2010-2012. Parasit Vectors 2014;7:257.
19. Qurollo BA, Chandrashekar R, Hegarty BC, et al. A serological survey of tick-borne pathogens in dogs in North America and the Caribbean as assessed by Anaplasma phagocytophilum, A. platys, Ehrlichia canis, E. chaffeensis, E. ewingii, and Borrelia burgdorferi species-specific peptides. Infect Ecol Epidemiol 2014;4.
20. Dantas-Torres F. Biology and ecology of the brown dog tick, Rhipicephalus sanguineus. Parasit Vectors 2010;3:26.
21. Parola P, Socolovschi C, Jeanjean L, et al. Warmer weather linked to tick attack and emergence of severe rickettsioses. PLoS Negl Trop Dis 2008;2(11):e338.
22. Aktas M, Ozubek S. Molecular evidence for trans-stadial transmission of Anaplasma platys by Rhipicephalus sanguineus sensu lato under field conditions. Med Vet Entomol 2018;32(1):78–83.
23. Bremer WG, Schaefer JJ, Wagner ER, et al. Transstadial and intrastadial experimental transmission of Ehrlichia canis by male Rhipicephalus sanguineus. Vet Parasitol 2005;131(1–2):95–105.

24. Di Cicco MF, Downey ME, Beeler E, et al. Re-emergence of Babesia conradae and effective treatment of infected dogs with atovaquone and azithromycin. Vet Parasitol 2012;187(1–2):23–7.

25. Drexler N, Miller M, Gerding J, et al. Community-based control of the brown dog tick in a region with high rates of Rocky Mountain spotted fever, 2012-2013. PLoS One 2014;9(12):e112368.

26. Beeler E, Abramowicz KF, Zambrano ML, et al. A focus of dogs and Rickettsia massiliae-infected Rhipicephalus sanguineus in California. Am J Trop Med Hyg 2011;84(2):244–9.

27. Nicholson WL, Gordon R, Demma LJ. Spotted fever group rickettsial infection in dogs from eastern Arizona: how long has it been there? Ann N Y Acad Sci 2006; 1078:519–22.

28. Demma LJ, Eremeeva M, Nicholson WL, et al. An outbreak of Rocky Mountain Spotted Fever associated with a novel tick vector, Rhipicephalus sanguineus, in Arizona, 2004: preliminary report. Ann N Y Acad Sci 2006;1078:342–3.

29. Wikswo ME, Hu R, Metzger ME, et al. Detection of Rickettsia rickettsii and Bartonella henselae in Rhipicephalus sanguineus ticks from California. J Med Entomol 2007;44(1):158–62.

30. Diniz PP, Beall MJ, Omark K, et al. High prevalence of tick-borne pathogens in dogs from an Indian reservation in northeastern Arizona. Vector Borne Zoonotic Dis 2010;10(2):117–23.

31. Kordick SK, Breitschwerdt EB, Hegarty BC, et al. Coinfection with multiple tick-borne pathogens in a Walker Hound kennel in North Carolina. J Clin Microbiol 1999;37(8):2631–8.

32. Drexler NA, Dahlgren FS, Heitman KN, et al. National Surveillance of Spotted Fever Group Rickettsioses in the United States, 2008-2012. Am J Trop Med Hyg 2016;94(1):26–34.

33. Telford SR. Status of the "East Side Hypothesis" (transovarial interference) 25 years later. Ann N Y Acad Sci 2009;1166:144–50.

34. Conrad P, Thomford J, Yamane I, et al. Hemolytic anemia caused by Babesia gibsoni infection in dogs. J Am Vet Med Assoc 1991;199(5):601–5.

35. Dear JD, Owens SD, Lindsay LL, et al. Babesia conradae infection in coyote hunting dogs infected with multiple blood-borne pathogens. J Vet Intern Med 2018; 32(5):1609–17.

36. Sykes JE. Canine and feline infectious diseases. St. Louis (MO): Elsevier; 2014.

37. Dambach DM, Smith CA, Lewis RM, et al. Morphologic, immunohistochemical, and ultrastructural characterization of a distinctive renal lesion in dogs putatively associated with Borrelia burgdorferi infection: 49 cases (1987-1992). Vet Pathol 1997;34(2):85–96.

38. Kelly DJ, Osterman JV, Stephenson EH. Rocky Mountain spotted fever in areas of high and low prevalence: survey for canine antibodies to spotted fever rickettsiae. Am J Vet Res 1982;43(8):1429–31.

39. Birkenheuer AJ, Correa MT, Levy MG, et al. Geographic distribution of babesiosis among dogs in the United States and association with dog bites: 150 cases (2000-2003). J Am Vet Med Assoc 2005;227(6):942–7.

40. Breitschwerdt EB, Malone JB, MacWilliams P, et al. Babesiosis in the Greyhound. J Am Vet Med Assoc 1983;182(9):978–82.

41. Taboada J, Harvey JW, Levy MG, et al. Seroprevalence of babesiosis in Greyhounds in Florida. J Am Vet Med Assoc 1992;200(1):47–50.

42. Fukumoto S, Suzuki H, Igarashi I, et al. Fatal experimental transplacental Babesia gibsoni infections in dogs. Int J Parasitol 2005;35(9):1031–5.

43. Levin ML, Killmaster LF, Zemtsova GE, et al. Clinical presentation, convalescence, and relapse of rocky mountain spotted fever in dogs experimentally infected via tick bite. PLoS One 2014;9(12):e115105.
44. Woods ME, Olano JP. Host defenses to Rickettsia rickettsii infection contribute to increased microvascular permeability in human cerebral endothelial cells. J Clin Immunol 2008;28(2):174–85.
45. Gasser AM, Birkenheuer AJ, Breitschwerdt EB. Canine Rocky Mountain Spotted fever: a retrospective study of 30 cases. J Am Anim Hosp Assoc 2001;37(1): 41–8.
46. Davidson MG, Breitschwerdt EB, Walker DH, et al. Vascular permeability and coagulation during Rickettsia rickettsii infection in dogs. Am J Vet Res 1990; 51(1):165–70.
47. Southern BL, Neupane P, Ericson ME, et al. Bartonella henselae in a dog with ear tip vasculitis. Vet Dermatol 2018;29(6). 537-e180.
48. Breitschwerdt EB, Maggi RG. A confusing case of canine vector-borne disease: clinical signs and progression in a dog co-infected with Ehrlichia canis and Bartonella vinsonii ssp. berkhoffii. Parasit Vectors 2009;2(Suppl 1):S3.
49. Maggi RG, Birkenheuer AJ, Hegarty BC, et al. Comparison of serological and molecular panels for diagnosis of vector-borne diseases in dogs. Parasit Vectors 2014;7:127.
50. Wardrop KJ, Birkenheuer A, Blais MC, et al. Update on canine and feline blood donor screening for blood-borne pathogens. J Vet Intern Med 2016;30(1):15–35.
51. Birkenheuer AJ, Levy MG, Breitschwerdt EB. Development and evaluation of a seminested PCR for detection and differentiation of Babesia gibsoni (Asian genotype) and B. canis DNA in canine blood samples. J Clin Microbiol 2003;41(9): 4172–7.
52. Carrade DD, Foley JE, Borjesson DL, et al. Canine granulocytic anaplasmosis: a review. J Vet Intern Med 2009;23(6):1129–41.
53. Starkey LA, Barrett AW, Chandrashekar R, et al. Development of antibodies to and PCR detection of Ehrlichia spp. in dogs following natural tick exposure. Vet Microbiol 2014;173(3–4):379–84.
54. Mylonakis ME, Koutinas AF, Billinis C, et al. Evaluation of cytology in the diagnosis of acute canine monocytic ehrlichiosis (Ehrlichia canis): a comparison between five methods. Vet Microbiol 2003;91(2–3):197–204.
55. Piccione J, Levine GJ, Duff CA, et al. Tick-borne relapsing fever in dogs. J Vet Intern Med 2016;30(4):1222–8.
56. Kidd L, Maggi R, Diniz PP, et al. Evaluation of conventional and real-time PCR assays for detection and differentiation of Spotted Fever Group Rickettsia in dog blood. Vet Microbiol 2008;129(3–4):294–303.
57. Nicholson WL, Allen KE, McQuiston JH, et al. The increasing recognition of rickettsial pathogens in dogs and people. Trends Parasitol 2010;26(4):205–12.
58. Jefferies R, Ryan UM, Jardine J, et al. Babesia gibsoni: detection during experimental infections and after combined atovaquone and azithromycin therapy. Exp Parasitol 2007;117(2):115–23.
59. Breitschwerdt EB, Davidson MG, Hegarty BC, et al. Prednisolone at anti-inflammatory or immunosuppressive dosages in conjunction with doxycycline does not potentiate the severity of Rickettsia rickettsii infection in dogs. Antimicrob Agents Chemother 1997;41(1):141–7.
60. Wang J, Zhang J, Kelly P, et al. First description of the pathogenicity of Babesia vogeli in experimentally infected dogs. Vet Parasitol 2018;253:1–7.

61. Baneth G, Harrus S, Ohnona FS, et al. Longitudinal quantification of Ehrlichia canis in experimental infection with comparison to natural infection. Vet Microbiol 2009;136(3–4):321–5.

62. Breitschwerdt EB, Maggi RG, Chomel BB, et al. Bartonellosis: an emerging infectious disease of zoonotic importance to animals and human beings. J Vet Emerg Crit Care (San Antonio) 2010;20(1):8–30.

63. Birkenheuer AJ, Levy MG, Savary KC, et al. Babesia gibsoni infections in dogs from North Carolina. J Am Anim Hosp Assoc 1999;35(2):125–8.

64. Parola P, Labruna MB, Raoult D. Tick-borne rickettsioses in America: unanswered questions and emerging diseases. Curr Infect Dis Rep 2009;11(1):40–50.

65. Breitschwerdt EB, Moncol DJ, Corbett WT, et al. Antibodies to spotted fever-group rickettsiae in dogs in North Carolina. Am J Vet Res 1987;48(10): 1436–40.

66. Harrus S, Waner T, Aizenberg I, et al. Amplification of ehrlichial DNA from dogs 34 months after infection with Ehrlichia canis. J Clin Microbiol 1998; 36(1):73–6.

67. Eddlestone SM, Diniz PP, Neer TM, et al. Doxycycline clearance of experimentally induced chronic Ehrlichia canis infection in dogs. J Vet Intern Med 2007;21(6): 1237–42.

68. Fukumoto S, Xuan X, Shigeno S, et al. Development of a polymerase chain reaction method for diagnosing Babesia gibsoni infection in dogs. J Vet Med Sci 2001;63(9):977–81.

69. Straubinger RK. PCR-Based quantification of Borrelia burgdorferi organisms in canine tissues over a 500-Day postinfection period. J Clin Microbiol 2000; 38(6):2191–9.

70. Farwell GE, LeGrand EK, Cobb CC. Clinical observations on Babesia gibsoni and Babesia canis infections in dogs. J Am Vet Med Assoc 1982;180(5): 507–11.

71. Anderson JF, Magnarelli LA, Sulzer AJ. Canine babesiosis: indirect fluorescent antibody test for a North American isolate of Babesia gibsoni. Am J Vet Res 1980;41(12):2102–5.

72. Yancey CB, Diniz P, Breitschwerdt EB, et al. Doxycycline treatment efficacy in dogs with naturally occurring Anaplasma phagocytophilum infection. J Small Anim Pract 2018;59(5):286–93.

73. Chandrashekar R, Mainville CA, Beall MJ, et al. Performance of a commercially available in-clinic ELISA for the detection of antibodies against Anaplasma phagocytophilum, Ehrlichia canis, and Borrelia burgdorferi and Dirofilaria immitis antigen in dogs. Am J Vet Res 2010;71(12):1443–50.

74. Breitschwerdt EB, Levy MG, Davidson MG, et al. Kinetics of IgM and IgG responses to experimental and naturally acquired Rickettsia rickettsii infection in dogs. Am J Vet Res 1990;51(8):1312–6.

75. Breitschwerdt EB, Walker DH, Levy MG, et al. Clinical, hematologic, and humoral immune response in female dogs inoculated with Rickettsia rickettsii and Rickettsia montana. Am J Vet Res 1988;49(1):70–6.

76. Grasperge BJ, Wolfson W, Macaluso KR. Rickettsia parkeri infection in domestic dogs, Southern Louisiana, USA, 2011. Emerg Infect Dis 2012;18(6):995–7.

77. Raoult D, Parola P. Rocky Mountain spotted fever in the USA: a benign disease or a common diagnostic error? Lancet Infect Dis 2008;8(10):587–9.

78. Solano-Gallego L, Bradley J, Hegarty B, et al. Bartonella henselae IgG antibodies are prevalent in dogs from southeastern USA. Vet Res 2004;35(5):585–95.

Diagnosis of Canine Leptospirosis

Krystle L. Reagan, DVM, PhD[a],*, Jane E. Sykes, BVSc(Hons), PhD[b]

KEYWORDS

- Leptospirosis • Diagnostics • Dog • Zoonotic disease

KEY POINTS

- Leptospirosis is an important zoonotic disease that can have a good prognosis provided it is identified early and treated appropriately.
- Several diagnostic tests are available to veterinarians, including serology and molecular diagnostics, each with its own benefits and limitations.
- A combination of diagnostic tests, including polymerase chain reaction, microscopic agglutination test, and/or point-of-care rapid diagnostics, may provide a practitioner with the most rapid and accurate overall diagnosis.

INTRODUCTION

Leptospirosis is an emerging zoonotic disease with a worldwide distribution caused by motile spirochete bacterium of the genus *Leptospira*. These aerobic bacteria are thin, spiraled organisms with hooked ends. Although there are more than 20 recognized species of *Leptospira*, the causative agents of disease in dogs are primarily of the species *L interrogans* and *L kirschneri*. These species are further classified into more than 250 serovars of pathogenic leptospires based on surface O antigen serology. Closely related serovars are grouped into serogroups, of which approximately 20 have been established. Leptospires also are increasingly differentiated into genotypes based on molecular methods, such as variable number tandem repeat analysis or genome sequencing.[1,2]

Individual *Leptospira* genotypes have adapted to have a reservoir host, most commonly rodents, which become infected and maintain a carrier state. Reservoir hosts harbor leptospires in the renal tubules and shed leptospires in their contaminating the environment. Incidental hosts become infected by contact with urine

Conflicts of Interest: Dr J.E. Sykes receives honoraria and research funding from Boehringer Ingelheim, Zoetis, and IDEXX Laboratories.
The authors have nothing to disclose.
[a] Veterinary Medical Teaching Hospital, University of California, 1 Shields Ave Davis, CA 95616, USA; [b] Department of Medicine and Epidemiology, University of California, 1 Shields Ave Davis, CA 95616, USA
* Corresponding author.
E-mail address: kreagan@ucdavis.edu

from a reservoir host or contaminated water or soil. Infections of incidental hosts, such as dogs or people, with pathogenic leptospires can lead to the clinical syndrome of leptospirosis. Dogs are known to be reservoir hosts for *L interrogans* sv Canicola; therefore, prolonged shedding of leptospires in the urine can be expected if no treatment is instituted.[3–6] It is increasingly recognized that dogs can shed other *Leptospira* serovars or species in the absence of clinical signs, raising concerns for zoonotic transmission.[3,7–10]

Although leptospires do not replicate outside of the host and are easily inactivated in harsh conditions, pathogenic serovars can remain viable in water or soil for weeks.[11] A wide variety of mammals can be infected with pathogenic *Leptospira* serovars when exposed to contaminated water or soil. Leptospirosis is described in both dogs and cats; however, cats seem more resistant to the disease.[12,13] Determining which serovars are the primary cause of disease is dogs is difficult because most studies report serology findings that may not represent the infecting serovar.[14] Antibodies to serovars Grippotyphosa, Bratislava, Canicola, Icterohaemorrhagiae, Autumnalis, and Pomona are frequently observed and serovars Canicola, Pomona, Bratislava, Icterohaemorrhagiae, and Grippotyphosa have been experimentally shown to induce disease in dogs.[14–20] Further epidemiologic studies are warranted to fully understand which serovars are predominantly responsible for disease in dogs.

Leptospires can penetrate intact mucosal surfaces or abrasions in the skin, leading to a bacteremic phase, which lasts for up to 10 days.[21] Bacteria then are able to invade the kidney and liver, among other organs, and leptospires are shed in the urine.[17] Antileptospiral IgM antibodies are detected in the first week of infection, increasing rapidly early during infection.[22] Antileptospiral IgG antibodies increase to detectable levels approximately 2 weeks after infection.[22] These principles can help guide the veterinarian on the appropriate diagnostic test and sample(s) to submit based on the timing of examination relative to the onset of illness.

Early diagnosis of leptospirosis in dogs is ideal due to both the zoonotic nature of the disease and need to initiate appropriate intervention in infected dogs. A significant hurdle to achieving a diagnosis is the often nonspecific clinical signs associated with leptospirosis, ranging in severity from no clinical signs to life limiting illness. Veterinarians should suspect leptospirosis in dogs with significant risk factors or consistent clinical signs and clinicopathologic abnormalities. Risk factors that have been associated with leptospirosis include exposure to water, male gender, and herding or working dogs in some studies[23,24] Other studies have found a similar seroprevalance in both large and small breed dogs from all age groups and genders, indicating that all breeds of dogs are at risk of exposure.[15,25] A machine learning boosted tree analysis based on location investigated the probability of dogs testing positive for leptospirosis based on MAT titers and identified areas of the United States at increased risk for exposure. Although there was wide geographic variation in predicted risk, there seemed to be associations with environmental factors, including residential area with houses on large lots, deciduous forested land, increased precipitation, and temperature.[26]

Leptospirosis in dogs can manifest with signs of vasculitis, acute kidney injury, and/or hepatic injury, which are variable based on infecting strain and host immune response. Other clinical presentations can include fever, pulmonary hemorrhage, uveitis, myositis, and reproductive failure. If any of these factors is identified, diagnostic tests for leptospirosis should be pursued and treatment initiated. When the disease is identified early and appropriate therapy is instituted, survival rates approach 80%.[27,28]

Several diagnostic tests are available for identification of leptospirosis in dogs and generally are categorized into 2 groups; those that detect the bacteria directly and those that detect antibodies directed at the bacteria. The first group includes direct visualization of the leptospires via culture, dark field microscopy, or detection of bacterial DNA using polymerase chain reaction (PCR). These diagnostic tests are most useful early in the course of disease and before the use of antimicrobial drugs when bacterial numbers are highest in the blood and urine. The second group are tests are designed to detect antibodies against *Leptospira*, traditionally using the microscopic agglutination test (MAT). Because MAT titers may be low or negative initially, acute and convalescent testing is recommended. In this review, the available diagnostic tests for leptospirosis in dogs are discussed, including recommendations for timing of specimen collection and the optimum specimens to be submitted to the laboratory.

CLINICOPATHOLOGIC ABNORMALITIES

Complete blood cell count (CBC), serum biochemistry, and urinalysis abnormalities have been described in dogs with leptospirosis, although none of these changes provides a definitive diagnosis. The most common serum biochemical findings are those consistent with kidney injury, including azotemia and hyperphosphatemia, and have been reported in 80% to 100% of cases.[27,29–31] Increased activity of serum liver enzymes is noted in approximately half of dogs with leptospirosis, but it is rarely noted in the apparent absence of kidney injury.[27,29,31–33] Other biochemical changes that have been reported include hypoalbuminemia in up to half of dogs and electrolyte abnormalities, including hyponatremia and hypochloremia.[33,34] In cases of oligoanuria, serum potassium values can paradoxically remain normal due to inhibition of sodium-potassium-ATPase by bacterial endotoxins.[35,36] Elevated creatinine kinase has been reported in 43% of cases of leptospirosis associated with myositis.[31] A CBC may reveal thrombocytopenia, which has been reported in 20% to 50% of dogs with leptospirosis.[27,29–31,34] Other reported abnormalities include a nonregenerative anemia, neutrophilia, and/or a lymphopenia.[34] Urinalysis findings that have been noted include hyposthenuria or isothenuria, proteinuria, and/or glucosuria.[29,30,32,33]

IMAGING

Pulmonary involvement has been reported in dogs with leptospirosis and abnormalities on thoracic radiography have been reported in up to 70% of cases.[33,37] Radiographic abnormalities can be noted with or without clinical signs of respiratory distress. Most commonly, a mild to moderate interstitial pattern is noted. Rarely, severe nodular interstitial to alveolar pattern is observed in association with leptospiral pulmonary hemorrhage syndrome.[29,31,37]

Abdominal ultrasound can reveal nonspecific changes associated with kidney injury in 85% to 100% of dogs, including 1 or more of the following: increased cortical echogenicity, renomegaly, mild pyelectasia, medullary rim sign, or perirenal effusion.[38,39] Other sonographic changes can include hepatic changes, including hypoechoic parenchyma, hepatomegaly, and evidence of biliary sludge.[39]

LABORATORY DIAGNOSIS BY DIRECT IDENTIFICATION OF LEPTOSPIRES
Darkfield Microscopy

Direct visualization of leptospires in blood and urine of infected dogs has been described using darkfield microscopy.[40,41] Because of the small size of the individual bacteria, conventional light microscopy does not permit organism visualization. Dark-field microscopy can be performed on blood or urine specimens. This technique requires special equipment and training to be reliable; however, with trained personnel, a positive result can lead to a rapid diagnosis. Sensitivity is low due to several factors, including short duration of leptospiremia or previous antimicrobial drug therapy.[42] False-positive results can occur when debris is mistaken for spirochetes.[42] Because of these limitations, this method is not used routinely in the clinical diagnosis of leptospirosis.

Bacterial Culture

Leptospira culture allows detection of leptospires, but it is technically difficult. Leptospires require special growth media that contain B vitamins and long-chain fatty acids, most commonly Ellinghausen-McCullough-Johnson-Harris medium. Cultures can be performed on fresh tissue, blood, or urine. It is recommended that blood is submitted in the first 10 days of signs and urine thereafter. Specimens must be transported on special growth medium to reference laboratories that offer this diagnostic test. Because the date of infection typically is not known, both specimens should be submitted to increase test sensitivity. Culture incubation times of up to several months are required to identify bacterial growth, making this test less helpful to obtain a clinical diagnosis. It is a useful tool, however, for identifying infecting serovars and can provide valuable epidemiologic information. Although culture of leptospires is highly specific, sensitivity is quite low, which may be related to low-level bacteremia, administration of antibiotics prior to specimen collection, or technical difficulties associated with the assay.[43–45]

Tissue Biopsy

Leptospires can be identified in tissue sections, such as kidney biopsies, when stained with Giemsa or silver stains.[42] For more definitive identification, immunohistochemistry and immunofluorescence protocols have been validated.[46] Fluorescent in situ hybridization assays for the detection of leptospiral DNA within tissue sections also are available.[47] These tests most commonly are performed on tissue samples obtained at necropsy rather than as an antemortem diagnostic test and can enhance understanding of the pathogenesis of leptospirosis.

Polymerase Chain Reaction

Molecular diagnostic tools, such as PCR, have become widely available through commercial diagnostic laboratories for the diagnosis of leptospirosis. These tests are able to detect leptospiral DNA before the development of a serologic response to infection, making them a valuable diagnostic tool early in the course of disease.[10,45] Multiple assays have been developed targeting different conserved genes within pathogenic *Leptospira* serovar genomes.[3,4,48] Real-time or quantitative PCR assays have improved assay sensitivity and are less prone to contamination compared with conventional (endpoint) PCR assays.[49–51]

Commercially available assays target conserved regions of pathogenic leptospires so cannot determine the infecting serovar when a positive result is obtained. Although this may not have an impact on individual case management, knowing the infecting serovar improves understanding of the epidemiology of leptospirosis in dogs and has implications for vaccine design. Some molecular assays used in research settings have shown some promise in differentiating among serovars and genotypes; however, these assays are not yet widely available.[7,52]

PCR in the clinical setting is performed most often on blood or urine specimens, but tissue specimens, such as kidney or lung tissue, also can be submitted for PCR. As with culture, it is recommended that whole blood is submitted for PCR within the first 10 days of illness and urine after the first week of illness, corresponding to the bacteremic and bacteriuric phases of disease. If the timeline of infection is unknown, both specimens can be submitted to increase sensitivity. False-negative results can be encountered if there are low bacterial loads as a result of disease phase, immune response, or administration of antimicrobial drugs. Positive results in a dog with consistent clinical signs and clinicopathologic changes suggest leptospirosis. Recent vaccination does interfere with real-time PCR detection of leptospires.[53]

In dogs that are clinically healthy, positive PCR results could indicate a chronic carrier state. Surveys of apparently healthy dogs have reported that leptospiral DNA can be detected at various rates, depending on geographic location. Some areas have low prevalence of positive urine PCR results, including no positives in 100 shelter dogs from Indiana; 1.5% of dogs in Bavaria, Germany; and 4.4% of dogs in New Caledonia.[6,8,51] Other areas have much higher prevalence reporting rates—11.3% in Egypt, 10.5% in Brazil, and 26.6% in Iran, in dogs without any clinical signs.[9,54,55] Positive PCR results should be interpreted in light of clinical signs, especially in hyperendemic areas.[3]

Commercially available tests through references laboratories vary and only few data are available on the performance of these assays. One PCR assay conducted on blood had a sensitivity of 86% in the first 6 days of infection, but this dropped significantly after 7 days of infection to 34%. The specificity of the same assay was 99%.[56] Further studies to determine the clinical sensitivity and specificity of these assays are warranted.

LABORATORY DIAGNOSTICS VIA SEROLOGIC ASSAYS
Microscopic Agglutination Test

Acute and convalescent phase serology using the MAT traditionally has been used as the reference method for the serologic diagnosis of leptospirosis.[17] This test, developed more than a century ago, uses serial dilutions of serum and reacts those with live cultures of leptospires.[42] The highest dilution for which 50% of the leptospires are agglutinated, as determined using darkfield microscopy, is reported. The MAT is conducted using a panel (typically 6–8) of serovars that are believed to represent the most common serogroups infecting dogs. The MAT has been well validated in canine patients; however, there can be considerable variation in results among different laboratories. In 1 study, convalescent samples from naturally infected dogs were submitted to 5 veterinary diagnostic laboratories. Results showed agreement among laboratories in only 3/11 samples.[57] It is recommended that veterinarians use a reference laboratory that participates in a quality assurance program overseen by the International Leptospirosis Society to ensure high-quality MAT results.[17]

Both acute and convalescent (collected 7–14 days later) specimens should be tested and a 4-fold rise in antibody titers for individual serovars is consistent with active infection. Negative MAT results are not uncommon during the first week of infection, and sensitivity of a single acute MAT is only 50%; however, this improves to 100% when paired samples are assessed, with specificity ranging between 70% and 100%.[58,59] The serologic response can be dampened by the administration of antimicrobial drugs, but the authors' clinical experiences suggest that usually a 4-fold rise in titer is still achieved.

Interpretation of positive titers must take into account previous exposure and vaccination status. Serologic surveillance shows variable positive rates in dogs, with up to half having positive MAT results ($\geq$1:100) in endemic regions.[55,60,61] Antibody titers of greater than or equal to 1:400 to nonvaccinal serogroups were present in 3.5% (7/200) of healthy dogs living in Germany.[8] Additionally, in a population of healthy unvaccinated dogs in the United States, MAT titers of greater than or equal to 1:400 were noted in 21% (61/291), and 2 dogs had titers greater than or equal to 1:6400.[14] Vaccination can induce a positive MATs to both vaccinal and nonvaccinal serogroups.[60] Antibody titers typically wane by 4 months after vaccination; however, they have been detected for up to 1 year postvaccination.[60,62] Although most dogs only develop a modest elevation in MAT titers postvaccination, titers of greater than or equal to 1:600 have been documented after vaccination.[62] These studies taken together indicate that although a single high MAT titer may be suggestive of leptospirosis when consistent clinical signs are present, the diagnosis cannot be confirmed without a convalescent sample.

MAT results are reported as titers against each serovar tested. The antibody response to each serovar does not predict the infecting serovar, because serologic cross-reactions occur among serovars. A paradoxic elevation in titers to a noninfecting serogroup often is seen due to broad cross-reactivity of antibodies in the acute stages of infection, which then becomes more serogroup specific as the infection progresses.[14] Most commercially available MAT panels contain only 6 to 8 serovars representing the most commonly encountered serogroups in a region; however, the World Health Organization recommends a panel containing 19 pathogenic serovars be used. Using limited panels decreases technical requirements but can reduce sensitivity if the infecting serovar is not on the panel.

Enzyme Linked Immunosorbent Assays

Several ELISAs have been developed to detect specific antibodies in dogs with leptospirosis, but until recently these tests were not widely available. Traditional ELISAs are rapid diagnostic tests that have the additional benefit of not requiring the live *Leptospira* cultures needed for the MAT. They do require, however, specialized training and equipment to perform and are run in commercial veterinary diagnostic laboratories.

Assays have been designed to detect IgM, IgG, or both antibody types in dogs.[63–68] IgG is produced in large quantities only after approximately 1 week to 3 weeks of infection. Assays that detect IgM may identify an antibody response during the first week of infection when the MAT has low sensitivity.[58,67]

ELISAs have been designed that detect antibodies against the whole bacterial cell and to single recombinant antigenic proteins from the bacterial surface to increase specificity. The LipL32 protein has been of particular interest because it is expressed only by pathogenic leptospires and is conserved across serogroups.[69,70]

Performance of traditional ELISAs has been variable and, due to lower overall sensitivity compared with the MAT, their use has not been previously recommended. Tests that can be performed rapidly with high sensitivity early in infection may be useful, however, before receiving results from MAT or PCR assays.

Point-of-Care Diagnostic Assays

Recently point-of-care (cageside), lateral-flow serologic assays have been made commercially available for the detection *Leptospira*-specific antibodies in dogs.[63,65] These diagnostic tests are designed to be performed in-clinic to provide rapid results to the practitioner.

SNAP Lepto (IDEXX Laboratories, Westbrook, ME, USA) is a point-of-care ELISA that detects antibodies against the LipL32, an abundant membrane protein of *Leptospira*. When the performance of this assay was compared with MAT in dogs that had serum submitted to a reference laboratory for diagnosis of leptospirosis, there was agreement between the 2 in 83.2% of clinical cases when the MAT titers were greater than or equal to 1:800.[65] When used to test for antibodies in dogs not suspected of having leptospirosis, the specificity was 96% when compared with MAT.[65] In a clinical setting, the SNAP Lepto was positive in 15/22 (68%) cases that were eventually confirmed to have leptospirosis and incorrectly identified 20/131 (15%) as positive when they were ultimately diagnosed with other causes of illness.[68] Antibodies resulting from *Leptospira* vaccination were detected with SNAP Lepto in 5/21 (24%) of dogs 52 weeks postvaccination and up to 1 year postvaccination.[65]

The Witness Lepto (Zoetis, Parsippany-Troy Hills, NJ, USA) is a lateral flow assay that detects IgM antibodies using whole-cell extracts from *L kirschneri* sv Grippotyphosa and *L interrogans* sv Bratislava.[63,64] When assessed in a group of dogs suspected of having leptospirosis in France, sensitivity was 98% and specificity 93.5% compared with the diagnosis via MAT.[63] An additional study of acute clinical cases in Germany found the Witness Lepto had a sensitivity of 75% whereas a single acute MAT had a sensitivity of 24% in dogs that were ultimately diagnosed with leptospirosis based on 4-fold or greater rise in MAT titer or positive PCR result.[64] Cross-reaction with antibodies produced in response to vaccination was reported in 6/25 (24%) vaccinated uninfected dogs at 12 weeks postvaccination.[64]

Two reports have compared the performance of the SNAP Lepto and the Witness Lepto point-of-care assays. In a study of 89 dogs suspected of having leptospirosis in Italy, the Witness Lepto, SNAP Lepto, and a single acute MAT were compared. A diagnosis of leptospirosis was based on a single MAT titer of greater than or equal to 1:800 or a 4-fold increase in titers between acute and convalescent MAT. Sensitivity for the Witness Lepto was 78.9% and for the SNAP Lepto was 86.5% whereas a single acute MAT was 70.3% compared with the final diagnosis. Specificity values were 100%, 97.6%, and 75% for the single acute MAT, Witness Lepto, and SNAP Lepto, respectively.[71] These results indicate that these 2 commercially point-of-care assays are sensitive early in the course of illness in this population. In another study of dogs that were experimentally infected with *Leptospira*, the Witness Lepto test detected antibodies in all dogs by day 10, the MAT detected antibodies in all dogs by day 14, and the SNAP Lepto detected antibodies in only 3/32 dogs at 2 weeks postinfection.[72] Differences in results between these 2 studies could be related to differences in sample timing after infection or differences in infecting serovars.

Other commercially available rapid ELISA tests have been developed for human medicine and been tested in canine populations with promising results.[66,67] Further validation of these tests should be pursued in a variety of geographic locations, because sensitivity could be affected by the circulating serovars present.

DIAGNOSTIC STRATEGY

No one diagnostic test described in this article is adequate in all clinical settings; each has its own advantages and limitations; therefore, using a combination of tests has been suggested. Practitioners should consider the suspected time of infection when collecting specimens, to optimize diagnostic test performance. In a clinical setting, the exact timing of infection not often is known, so the use of multiple tests in parallel or series may be warranted to ensure a rapid and accurate diagnosis. In 1 study, a combination of PCR and acute and convalescent MAT significantly improved sensitivity.[7] Consensus recommendations for the diagnosis of leptospirosis in dogs with appropriate clinical signs include PCR of both blood and urine before the administration of antibiotic therapy and paired MAT titers.[17,73] Cageside diagnostics tests can be used to provide valuable information while awaiting the results of PCR or MAT titers.

DIAGNOSTIC TESTS OF THE FUTURE

Many research efforts have been focused on the development of the next generation of diagnostic tools for leptospirosis that are rapid and accurate, are positive in the early stages of disease, differentiate between natural infection and vaccination, can identify to the serovar level, and do not pose a technical burden. Promising results have been obtained using isothermal PCR assays, which eliminate the special thermocyclers needed to conduct PCR. These methods can be completed within as little as 1 hour, making them valuable tools for point-of-care diagnostic tests.[74] One such test is commercially available for dogs, PCRun Canine Pathogenic Leptospira Molecular Detection Kit (Biogal – Galed Labs, Kibbutz Galed, Israel). Preliminary results show this assay correlates closely with real-time PCR assays at a diagnostic laboratory for both blood and urine samples.[75] Other assays that have been investigated in humans include microcapsule agglutination assays, which have similar sensitivity to the MAT for some serovars but cannot detect antibodies against a wider range of serovars.[76] Several latex card agglutination assays and lateral flow assays also are commercially available.[74] Diagnostics using urine as a substrate are attractive to small animal practitioners, because urine typically is easy to obtain from dogs. A dot-ELISA that detects *Leptospira* protein in urine from people with leptospirosis was found sensitive and reliable.[77] These assays have shown some promise in human medicine, but they are yet to be validated for use in dogs and cats.

SUMMARY

A diagnosis of leptospirosis can be challenging and depends on the stage of disease and factors, such as recent vaccination, the prevalence of subclinical exposure, and shedding within different geographic regions. The diagnostic tests reviewed in this article have characteristics that are advantageous in some situations but not others. Using a combination of diagnostic tests can increase the chances of gaining a rapid and accurate diagnosis. Research is needed to develop highly sensitive, rapid diagnostic assays that can identify infecting serovars accurately to help guide practitioners and provide valuable epidemiologic information that can be used to design vaccines, which are generally assumed to provide serovar-specific protection.

REFERENCES

1. Pailhoriès H, Buzelé R, Picardeau M, et al. Molecular characterization of Leptospira sp by multilocus variable number tandem repeat analysis (MLVA) from clinical samples: a case report. Int J Infect Dis 2015;37:119–21.
2. Hamond C, Pestana CP, Medeiros MA, et al. Genotyping of Leptospira directly in urine samples of cattle demonstrates a diversity of species and strains in Brazil. Epidemiol Infect 2016;144(01):72–5.
3. Rojas P, Monahan AM, Schuller S, et al. Detection and quantification of leptospires in urine of dogs: a maintenance host for the zoonotic disease leptospirosis. Eur J Clin Microbiol Infect Dis 2010;29(10):1305–9.

4. Harkin KR, Roshto YM, Sullivan JT. Clinical application of a polymerase chain reaction assay for diagnosis of leptospirosis in dogs. J Am Vet Med Assoc 2003; 222(9):1224–9.

5. Zakeri S, Khorami N, Ganji ZF, et al. Leptospira wolffii, a potential new pathogenic Leptospira species detected in human, sheep and dog. Infect Genet Evol 2010; 10(2):273–7.

6. Gay N, Soupé-Gilbert M-E, Goarant C. Though not reservoirs, dogs might transmit leptospira in New Caledonia. Int J Environ Res Public Health 2014;11(4): 4316–25.

7. Miotto BA, Tozzi BF, Penteado M de S, et al. Diagnosis of acute canine leptospirosis using multiple laboratory tests and characterization of the isolated strains. BMC Vet Res 2018;14(1):222.

8. Llewellyn J-R, Krupka-Dyachenko I, Rettinger AL, et al. Urinary shedding of leptospires and presence of leptospira antibodies in healthy dogs from Upper Bavaria. Berl Munch Tierarztl Wochenschr 2016;129(5–6):251–7.

9. Samir A, Soliman R, El-Hariri M, et al. Leptospirosis in animals and human contacts in Egypt: broad range surveillance. Rev Soc Bras Med Trop 2015;48(3): 272–7.

10. Harkin KR, Roshto YM, Sullivan JT, et al. Comparison of polymerase chain reaction assay, bacteriologic culture, and serologic testing in assessment of prevalence of urinary shedding of leptospires in dogs. J Am Vet Med Assoc 2003; 222(9):1230–3.

11. Zaĭtsev SV, Chernukha IG, Evdokimova OA, et al. Survival rate of Leptospira pomona in the soil at a natural leptospirosis focus. Zh Mikrobiol Epidemiol Immunobiol 1989;(2):64–8 [in Russian].

12. Bryson DG, Ellis WA. Leptospirosis in a British domestic cat. J Small Anim Pract 1976;17(7):459–65.

13. Rees H. Leptospirosis in a cat. N Z Vet J 1964;12(3):63–4.

14. Levett PN. Usefulness of serologic analysis as a predictor of the infecting serovar in patients with severe leptospirosis. Clin Infect Dis 2003;36(4):447–52.

15. Stokes JE, Kaneene JB, Schall WD, et al. Prevalence of serum antibodies against six Leptospira serovars in healthy dogs. J Am Vet Med Assoc 2007;230(11): 1657–64.

16. Davis MA, Evermann JF, Petersen CR, et al. Serological survey for antibodies to leptospira in dogs and raccoons in Washington State. Zoonoses Public Health 2008;55(8-10):436–42.

17. Sykes JE, Hartmann K, Lunn KF, et al. 2010 ACVIM Small animal consensus statement on leptospirosis: diagnosis, epidemiology, treatment, and prevention. J Vet Intern Med 2011;25(1):1–13.

18. Minke J, Bey R, Tronel J, et al. Onset and duration of protective immunity against clinical disease and renal carriage in dogs provided by a bi-valent inactivated leptospirosis vaccine. Veterinary microbiology 2009;137(1-2):137–45.

19. Greenlee J, Bolin C, Alt DP, et al. Clinical and pathologic comparison of acute leptospirosis in dogs caused by two strains of Leptospira kirschneri serovar grippotyphosa. Am J Vet Res 2004;65(8):1100–7.

20. Williams H, Murphy W, McCroan J, et al. An epidemic of Canicola fever in man with demonstration of Leptospira Canicola in dogs, swine and cattle. Am J Epidemiol 1956;64(1):46–58.

21. Greenlee JJ, Alt DP, Bolin CA, et al. Experimental canine leptospirosis caused by Leptospira interrogans serovars pomona and bratislava. Am J Vet Res 2005; 66(10):1816–22.

22. Frik JF, Hartman EG, van Houten M, et al. Determination of specific anti-leptospiral immunoglobulins M and G in sera of experimentally infected dogs by solid-phase enzyme-linked immunosorbent assay. Vet Immunol Immunopathol 1984;7(1):43–51.

23. Ward MP, Glickman LT, Guptill LF. Prevalence of and risk factors for leptospirosis among dogs in the United States and Canada: 677 cases (1970-1998). J Am Vet Med Assoc 2002;220(1):53–8.

24. Ward MP, Guptill LF, Prahl A, et al. Serovar-specific prevalence and risk factors for leptospirosis among dogs: 90 cases (1997–2002). J Am Vet Med Assoc 2004; 224(12):1958–63.

25. Gautam R, Wu C-C, Guptill LF, et al. Detection of antibodies against Leptospira serovars via microscopic agglutination tests in dogs in the United States, 2000-2007. J Am Vet Med Assoc 2010;237(3):293–8.

26. White AM, Zambrana-Torrelio C, Allen T, et al. Hotspots of canine leptospirosis in the United States of America. Vet J 2017;222:29–35.

27. Goldstein RE, Lin RC, Langston CE, et al. Influence of infecting serogroup on clinical features of Leptospirosis in dogs. J Vet Intern Med 2006;20(3): 489–94.

28. Brown CA, Roberts AW, Miller MA, et al. Leptospira interrogans serovar grippo-typhosa infection in dogs. J Am Vet Med Assoc 1996;209(7):1265–7.

29. Birnbaum N, Barr SC, Center SA, et al. Naturally acquired leptospirosis in 36 dogs: serological and clinicopathological features. J Small Anim Pract 1998; 39(5):231–6.

30. Tangeman LE, Littman MP. Clinicopathologic and atypical features of naturally occurring leptospirosis in dogs: 51 cases (2000–2010). J Am Vet Med Assoc 2013;243(9):1316–22.

31. Mastrorilli C, Dondi F, Agnoli C, et al. Clinicopathologic features and outcome predictors of Leptospira interrogans australis serogroup infection in dogs: a retrospective study of 20 cases (2001-2004). J Vet Intern Med 2007;21(1):3–10.

32. Geisen V, Stengel C, Brem S, et al. Canine leptospirosis infections - clinical signs and outcome with different suspected Leptospira serogroups (42 cases). J Small Anim Pract 2007;48(6):324–8.

33. Knöpfler S, Mayer-Scholl A, Luge E, et al. Evaluation of clinical, laboratory, imaging findings and outcome in 99 dogs with leptospirosis. J Small Anim Pract 2017; 58(10):582–8.

34. Sykes JE. Canine and feline infectious diseases. St. Louis (MO): Elsevier Health Sciences; 2013.

35. Lacroix-Lamandé S, d'Andon MF, Michel E, et al. Downregulation of the Na/K-ATPase pump by leptospiral glycolipoprotein activates the NLRP3 inflammasome. J Immunol 2012;188(6):2805–14.

36. Younes-Ibrahim M, Burth P, Faria MV, et al. Inhibition of Na,K-ATPase by an endotoxin extracted from Leptospira interrogans: a possible mechanism for the physiopathology of leptospirosis. C R Acad Sci III 1995;318(5):619–25.

37. Kohn B, Steinicke K, Arndt G, et al. Pulmonary abnormalities in dogs with Leptospirosis. J Vet Intern Med 2010;24(6):1277–82.

38. Forrest LJ, O'Brien RT, Tremeling MS, et al. Sonographic renal findings in 20 dogs with leptospirosis. Vet Radiol Ultrasound 1998;39(4):337–40.

39. Sonet J, Barthélemy A, Goy-Thollot I, et al. Prospective evaluation of abdominal ultrasonographic findings in 35 dogs with leptospirosis. Vet Radiol Ultrasound 2018;59(1):98–106.

40. Goldstein RE. Canine leptospirosis. Vet Clin North Am Small Anim Pract 2010; 40(6):1091–101.
41. Chandrasekaran S, Pankajalakshmi VV. Usefulness of dark field microscopy after differential centrifugation in the early diagnosis of leptospirosis in dog and its human contacts. Indian J Med Sci 1997;51(1):1–4.
42. Levett PN. Leptospirosis. Clin Microbiol Rev 2001;14(2):296–326.
43. Merien F, Baranton G, Perolat P. Comparison of polymerase chain reaction with microagglutination test and culture for diagnosis of Leptospirosis. J Infect Dis 1995;172(1):281–5.
44. Bolin CA, Zuerner RL, Trueba G. Comparison of three techniques to detect Leptospira interrogans serovar hardjo type hardjo-bovis in bovine urine. Am J Vet Res 1989;50(7):1001–3.
45. Brown PD, Gravekamp C, Carrington DG, et al. Evaluation of the polymerase chain reaction for early diagnosis of leptospirosis. J Med Microbiol 1995;43(2): 110–4.
46. Ellis WA, Neill SD, O'Brien JJ, et al. Bovine leptospirosis: microbiological and serological findings in normal fetuses removed from the uteri after slaughter. Vet Rec 1982;110(9):192–4.
47. De Brito T, Menezes LF, Lima DMC, et al. Immunohistochemical and in situ hybridization studies of the liver and kidney in human leptospirosis. Virchows Arch 2006;448(5):576–83.
48. Xu C, Loftis A, Ahluwalia SK, et al. Diagnosis of canine leptospirosis by a highly sensitive FRET-PCR targeting the lig genes. In: Dellagostin OA, editor. PLoS One 2014;9(2):e89507.
49. Smythe LD, Smith IL, Smith GA, et al. A quantitative PCR (TaqMan) assay for pathogenic Leptospira spp. BMC Infect Dis 2002;2(1):13.
50. Levett PN, Morey RE, Galloway RL, et al. Detection of pathogenic leptospires by real-time quantitative PCR. J Med Microbiol 2005;54(1):45–9.
51. Fink JM, Moore GE, Landau R, et al. Evaluation of three 5′ exonuclease–based real-time polymerase chain reaction assays for detection of pathogenic Leptospira species in canine urine. J Vet Diagn Invest 2015;27(2):159–66.
52. Cai C-S, Zhu Y-Z, Zhong Y, et al. Development of O-antigen gene cluster-specific PCRs for rapid typing six epidemic serogroups of Leptospira in China. BMC Microbiol 2010;10(1):67.
53. Midence JN, Leutenegger CM, Chandler AM, et al. Effects of recent Leptospira vaccination on whole blood real-time PCR testing in healthy client-owned dogs. J Vet Intern Med 2012;26(1):149–52.
54. Khorami N, Malmasi A, Zakeri S, et al. Screening urinalysis in dogs with urinary shedding of leptospires. Comp Clin Path 2010;19(3):271–4.
55. Miotto BA, Guilloux AGA, Tozzi BF, et al. Prospective study of canine leptospirosis in shelter and stray dog populations: identification of chronic carriers and different Leptospira species infecting dogs. PloS one 2018;13(7):e0200384.
56. Riediger IN, Stoddard RA, Ribeiro GS, et al. Rapid, actionable diagnosis of urban epidemic leptospirosis using a pathogenic Leptospira lipL32-based real-time PCR assay. In: Lin T, editor. PLoS Negl Trop Dis 2017;11(9): e0005940.
57. Miller MD, Annis KM, Lappin MR, et al. Variability in results of the microscopic agglutination test in dogs with clinical Leptospirosis and dogs vaccinated against Leptospirosis. J Vet Intern Med 2011;25(3):426–32.
58. Fraune CK, Schweighauser A, Francey T. Evaluation of the diagnostic value of serologic microagglutination testing and a polymerase chain reaction assay for

diagnosis of acute leptospirosis in dogs in a referral center. J Am Vet Med Assoc 2013;242(10):1373–80.

59. Miller M, Annis K, Lappin M, et al. Sensitivity and specificity of the microscopic agglutination test for the diagnosis of leptospirosis in dogs. abstract# 287. Available at: insights.ovid.com. Accessed September 1, 2018.

60. Barr SC, McDonough PL, Scipioni-Ball RL, et al. Serologic responses of dogs given a commercial vaccine against Leptospira interrogans serovar pomona and Leptospira kirschneri serovar grippotyphosa. Am J Vet Res 2005;66(10):1780–4.

61. Meeyam T, Tablerk P, Petchanok B, et al. Seroprevalence and risk factors associated with leptospirosis in dogs. Southeast Asian J Trop Med Public Health 2006;37(1):148–53.

62. Martin LER, Wiggans KT, Wennogle SA, et al. Vaccine-associated *leptospira* antibodies in client-owned dogs. J Vet Intern Med 2014;28(3):789–92.

63. Kodjo A, Calleja C, Loenser M, et al. A rapid in-clinic test detects acute Leptospirosis in dogs with high sensitivity and specificity. Biomed Res Int 2016;1–3.

64. Lizer J, Grahlmann M, Hapke H, et al. Evaluation of a rapid IgM detection test for diagnosis of acute leptospirosis in dogs. Vet Rec 2017;180(21):517.

65. Curtis K, Foster P, Simth P, et al. Performance of a recombinant LipL32 based rapid in-clinic ELISA (SNAP ® Lepto) for the detection of antibodies against Leptospira in dogs. Intern J Appl Res Vet Med 2015;13(3):182–9.

66. Dey S, Mohan CM, Ramadass P, et al. Recombinant antigen-based dipstick ELISA for the diagnosis of leptospirosis in dogs. Vet Rec 2007;160(6):186–8.

67. Abdoel TH, Houwers DJ, van Dongen AM, et al. Rapid test for the serodiagnosis of acute canine leptospirosis. Vet Microbiol 2011;150(1–2):211–3.

68. Winzelberg S, Tasse SM, Goldstein RE, et al. Evaluation of SNAP® Lepto in the diagnosis of leptospirosis infections in dogs: twenty two clinical cases. Intern J Appl Res Vet Med 2015;13(3):193–8.

69. Haake DA, Chao G, Zuerner RL, et al. The leptospiral major outer membrane protein LipL32 Is a lipoprotein expressed during mammalian infection. Infect Immun 2000;68(4):2276–85.

70. Dey S, Mohan CM, Kumar TMAS, et al. Recombinant LipL32 antigen-based single serum dilution ELISA for detection of canine leptospirosis. Vet Microbiol 2004;103(1–2):99–106.

71. Troìa R, Balboni A, Zamagni S, et al. Prospective evaluation of rapid point-of-care tests for the diagnosis of acute leptospirosis in dogs. Vet J 2018;237:37–42.

72. Lizer J, Velineni S, Weber A, et al. Evaluation of 3 serological tests for early detection of *leptospira* -specific antibodies in experimentally infected dogs. J Vet Intern Med 2018;32(1):201–7.

73. Schuller S, Francey T, Hartmann K, et al. European consensus statement on leptospirosis in dogs and cats. J Small Anim Pract 2015;56(3):159–79.

74. Picardeau M, Bertherat E, Jancloes M, et al. Rapid tests for diagnosis of Leptospirosis: current tools and emerging technologies. Diagn Microbiol Infect Dis 2014;78(1):1–8.

75. Thiel BE, Larson LJ, Okwumabua O SR, Comparison of a novel point-of-care diagnostic, PCRun, with real time Leptospira PCR for detection of Leptospira antigen in canine samples. In: Conference of research workers in animal diseases. Chicago, December 7-9, 2014.

76. Sehgal SC, Vijayachari P, Subramaniam V. Evaluation of leptospira micro capsule agglutination test (MCAT) for serodiagnosis of leptospirosis. Indian J Med Res 1997;106:504–7.
77. Saengjaruk P, Chaicumpa W, Watt G, et al. Diagnosis of human Leptospirosis by monoclonal antibody-based antigen detection in urine. J Clin Microbiol 2002; 40(2):480–9.

Update on Feline Hemoplasmosis

Emi N. Barker, BSc, BVSc, PhD, MRCVS

KEYWORDS

- Mycoplasma haemofelis • Clearance • Haemoplasma • Fluoroquinolone
- Doxycycline

KEY POINTS

- Hemoplasmosis due to *Mycoplasma haemofelis* infection is an uncommon cause of potentially fatal, moderate-severe hemolytic anemia in cats.
- "*Candidatus* Mycoplasma haemominutum" infection, detected in approximately 20% of cats, can result in mild anemia; however, a subclinical carrier state is common.
- Decision to treat should be based on accurate diagnosis of hemoplasma infection, including speciation, using molecular diagnostic techniques (ie, polymerase chain reaction).
- Tetracyclines (eg, doxycycline) and fluoroquinolones (eg, marbofloxacin; pradofloxacin) are considered appropriate choices of antibiotics for hemoplasmosis.
- Monotherapy rarely results in persistent clearance of infection; however, the chronic carrier state is uncommonly of clinical concern.

INTRODUCTION

Hemotropic mycoplasmas (hemoplasmas) are wall-less bacteria that parasitize red blood cells. They can induce potentially life-threatening hemolytic anemia in a wide variety of mammals, including the domestic cat, in which they are the agent of feline infectious anemia.

WHAT IS IN A NAME?

Hemoplasmas were first described in laboratory rodents in the 1920s, appearing in association with anemia following splenectomy.[1–3] Originally thought to be members of the *Bartonella* genus due to their hemotropic properties, small size (<1 μm), and suspected role of arthropods in their transmission, their reclassification within the order

Disclosure Statement: Employed by Langford Vets, a wholly owned subsidiary of University of Bristol, who offers a quantitative polymerase chain reaction assay for the detection of canine and feline hemoplasmas. Author's PhD on the molecular characterization of companion animal hemoplasmas was partly funded by Zoetis (previously Pfizer Animal Health).
Langford Vets, University of Bristol, Bristol BS40 5DU, UK
E-mail address: emi.barker@bristol.ac.uk

Rickettsiales in the family Anaplasmataceae was suggested a decade later due to their uncultivatable status and lack of cutaneous lesions.[4] However, questions still remained as to the correct positioning of these organisms within the family Anaplasmataceae because of their lack of a cell wall, lack of flagellae, inability to invade erythrocytes, and apparent antibiotic sensitivities (resistant to penicillin; sensitive to tetracyclines). Following the advent of DNA sequencing and phylogenetic analysis based on ribosome gene sequence comparisons, many of the hemoplasmas became officially reclassified as mycoplasmas.[5–7] Reclassification remains incomplete, as the first description of the rodent hemoplasma *Eperythrozoon coccoides* predates that of the type species for the *Mycoplasma* genus *Mycoplasma mycoides*.[8]

In 1942, the first description of such bacteria in association with anemia in a cat appeared, with the name *Eperythrozoon felis*.[9] Further descriptions, using the name *Haemobartonella felis*, appeared shortly afterward.[10–12] Outside the United States, this feline hemoplasma continued to be referred to as *E felis* into the 1970s before it became universally known as *H felis*, with subsequent reclassification as *Mycoplasma haemofelis* at the turn of the twenty-first century.[7,13] Of note, by contrast with rodents and dogs, clinical disease was reported in cats that had not been splenectomized.

Before gene-based phylogenetic analysis, it had been recognized that *"H felis"* existed in different forms of differing pathogenicities, with the "large" form (a.k.a. Illinois, Florida, Ohio, and Oklahoma strains) most frequently associated with disease compared with the "small" form (a.k.a. California and Birmingham strains).[14] Ribosomal gene analysis (16S ribosomal RNA [rRNA] gene and *rnpB*) confirmed the presence of 2 distinct organisms: *Mycoplasma haemofelis* and "*Candidatus* Mycoplasma haemominutum."[7,13,14] More recently, a further feline hemoplasma "*Candidatus* Mycoplasma turicensis" was described in association with hemolytic anemia.[15] All 3 of these organisms have since been described worldwide, sometimes in combination, with variable prevalences.[16] These prevalence studies, mostly based on convenience samples, have also described the detection of "*Candidatus* Mycoplasma haematoparvum" and "*Candidatus* Mycoplasma haematoparvum"-like organisms in cats[17,18]; however, their role in disease is unknown.

CLINICAL RELEVANCE

Many of the clinical signs reported with hemoplasmosis (lethargy, weakness, depression, collapse, pallor, tachycardia, dyspnea/tachypnea, cardiac "hemic" murmur, hepatosplenomegaly, lymphadenopathy, dehydration, fever, weight loss, pica, icterus) result from anemia or the underlying immune-mediated process, which can be fatal in severe cases.

The presence of a chronic carrier state has limited the ability of epidemiologic studies to associate hemoplasma infection with disease. In experimental feline studies, acute infection with *M haemofelis* often results in severe hemolytic anemia in previously immunocompetent cats.[19–21] However, at other times, only mild anemia is seen and it has been suggested that age may play a role in outcome, with younger cats more likely to develop more severe anemia. Although experimental infection with *"Ca* M haemominutum" and "*Ca* M turicensis" can result in a decreased hematocrit, they are infrequently associated with clinical signs in the absence of concurrent disease or immunosuppression. It should be noted that these studies comprise only handful of hemoplasma isolates, and that it is unclear whether strains of differing pathogenicity exist within an individual species. Experimental studies have also demonstrated protective immunity against rechallenge with the same hemoplasma species for both *M haemofelis* and "*Ca* M turicensis".[22,23]

Consistent with an immune-mediated hemolytic anemia, auto-agglutination or positive Coombs testing may be detectable during acute *M haemofelis* infection.[21] However, hemoplasmosis remains an infrequent cause of immune-mediated hemolytic anemia, positive auto-agglutination results, or a positive Coombs test.[24]

DIAGNOSIS

Blood should be collected for analysis before the administration of any treatments, particularly antibiotics with known activity against mycoplasmas (ie, tetracyclines and fluoroquinolones).

Although cytologic detection of organisms during acute hemoplasmosis could be considered as a point-of-care test, this is limited by the experience of the slide reviewer, as misdiagnosis can potentially arise from artifact (stain precipitate, poor slide preparation), Howell-Jolly bodies, and other infecting species. One study demonstrated that cytology has a sensitivity of 11.1%, with a specificity of 84%,[25] whereas another reported a detection rate of 37.5% based on blood smear examination, compared with 100% for polymerase chain reaction (PCR) in cats experimentally infected with *M haemofelis* and "*Ca* M haemominutum."[26] In addition, the presence of the anticoagulants EDTA and heparin have been suggested to result in the disassociation of hemoplasmas from erythrocytes over time, necessitating the preparation of fresh blood smears if assessment for their presence is desired.[27,28] Cytologic visualization of organisms may not be possible for some hemoplasma species; for example, in cats experimentally infected with "*Ca* M turicensis" blood copy numbers remain very low, even during acute infection.[15,29]

Accurate diagnosis is currently reliant on the detection of bacterial DNA using PCR assays, which have been repeatedly demonstrated to be both more sensitive and specific than cytology.[14,19–21,26,30] Newer quantitative PCRs determine hemoplasma numbers within samples collected.[18,31] In common with most PCRs, due to small volumes of reagents used in these assays, the limit of detection for a typical assay is 200 organisms per mL blood. This is based on the detection of a single copy of a target gene within the 5 µL purified DNA added to the PCR reaction, where DNA is purified from blood and eluted in an equivalent volume, and where the gene is present in a single copy within the organism.

In a US study of cats with signs consistent with hemoplasmosis, 4.8% were found to be infected with *M haemofelis*, 23.2% to be infected with "*Ca* M haemominutum," and 6.5% to be infected with "*Ca* M turicensis," of which 6.5% represented coinfections.[32] A similar UK study found lower prevalences of hemoplasma infection, with 2.8% infected with *M haemofelis*, 11.2% infected with "*Ca* M haemominutum," and 1.7% infected with "*Ca* M turicensis," of which 1.6% represented coinfections.[31] A higher prevalence of *M haemofelis* (7.6%) was reported in a convenience sample population of cats, in which 21.7% were also infected with "*Ca* M haemominutum," although hematological parameters were not determined for these cats.[33] However, where hemoplasma prevalence has been compared between anemic and nonanemic cats, some investigators have found no detectable difference,[24,34] whereas another study reported that "*Ca* M haemominutum"–infected cats were less likely to be anemic.[18]

Due to the presence of a chronic carrier state, detection of lower pathogenicity hemoplasmas "*Ca* M haemominutum" and "*Ca* M turicensis" in an anemic cat should prompt continued investigation of concurrent contributory factors to the etiopathogenesis of the anemia. However, knowledge of their presence is of use when considering treatment options, particularly if these would involve immune suppression, for example, in the treatment of idiopathic immune-mediated hemolytic anemia or lymphoma, or where no additional factors are identified.

It should be noted that the design of highly species-specific PCR assays can limit the detection of novel or incompletely described hemoplasmas. In the rare event that clinical suspicion persists, further advice from the laboratory performing the assay should be sought.

TREATMENT
When to Treat

Cats with severe anemia resulting in cardiovascular compromise, including those with anemia caused by hemoplasmosis, are fragile and require careful management pending confirmation of underlying etiology. However, confirmation of diagnosis by PCR is often subject to a time delay, as samples are submitted to external commercial laboratories. Clinical hemoplasmosis, when confirmed, can often be successfully managed with a course of an appropriate antibiotic (see later in this article), in conjunction with basic supportive care.[19,35–37]

Despite clinical resolution of hemoplasmosis, infection will be eliminated in only a minority of cases, and some cats can spontaneously clear the infection without antibiotic treatment. It should be noted that most cats found to be infected with hemoplasmas in prevalence studies, particularly those infected with "*Ca* M haemominutum" or "*Ca* M turicensis," were likely asymptomatic chronic carriers and that, for *M haemofelis* and "*Ca* M turicensis" at least, rechallenge with the original infecting species does not appear to result in clinical disease.[22,23]

In some situations, clearance of infection may be desirable in addition to clinical cure. For example, when the cat is immunocompromised by concurrent infection (particularly by retroviruses feline immunodeficiency virus [FIV] and feline leukemia virus [FeLV]), as a result of treatments administered such as chemotherapy, or following splenectomy. Clearance of infection may also be considered when the cat represents a risk to either other cats by both horizontal or vertical transmission, or to an immunocompromised owner.[38] Although horizontal spread remains the most likely route of infection, a possible case of vertical spread from queen to litter of kittens resulting in clinical anemia has been described[39]; unfortunately, this study predated molecular confirmation of infection and hemoplasma speciation. Molecular techniques have more recently strongly supported vertical transmission in ruminant species.[40,41] Zoonotic *M haemofelis* infection has been described in a man positive for human immunodeficiency virus with concurrent *Bartonella henselae* infection.[38] The source of infection was suspected to have been one of the *M haemofelis*–infected cats in the household. Human infections with swine and ovine hemoplasmas have also been reported.[42,43] Finally, as was the case in the experimentally hemoplasma-infected cats included in a recent study,[44] clearance of infection may be a requirement of rehoming.

The consequences of the chronic hemoplasma infection ("carrier state") are poorly understood. Anemic-stress has been shown to be a trigger for myelogenous leukemia in susceptible rodents (eg, irradiated rats and leukemia-prone RF strain of mice).[45,46] One early experimental study suggested that cats infected simultaneously with FeLV and *M haemofelis* were more likely to develop FeLV viremia and aplastic anemia than those not infected with *M haemofelis*.[47] In another, preexisting retrovirus infection (FeLV or FeLV/FIV) in apparently healthy cats potentiated the severity of anemia following "*Ca* M haemominutum" infection.[48] The latter study also reported a high incidence of myeloproliferative disease (eg, leukemia, myelodysplastic syndrome, lymphoma); however, the absence of a control population of hemoplasma uninfected cats limited conclusions. Further studies are required to determine the long-term impact of chronic hemoplasma infection on the risk of bone marrow disorders, particularly in association with retrovirus infection.

SUPPORTIVE MANAGEMENT

When cats are dehydrated, which is very common in hemoplasmosis, fluid deficits and electrolyte imbalances should be addressed with isotonic crystalloids. Conversely, chronically anemic cats are at risk of fluid overload due to increased circulating volume that, particularly in the presence of occult cardiac disease, may precipitate congestive heart failure. Care should be taken when history, physical examination findings, and clinicopathological results do not indicate the degree of chronicity. Following rehydration, red cell parameters should be reassessed, as the severity of anemia may have been exacerbated.

In cats in which the anemia has rapidly developed or when the anemia is severe (≤12%), cardiovascular compromise may be evident, despite correction of fluid deficits. In such cases, administration of either whole blood, or preferably packed red blood cells, should be considered. AB system blood-typing should be performed before the administration of the first unit, and a unit of the same type administered. Cross-matching has been recommended from 4 days after administration of the initial unit, although in some cats antibodies can be detected, by way of a positive cross-match result, as early as 2 days posttransfusion.[49] Due to the presence of non-AB system feline erythrocyte antigens,[50] some experts have advocated cross-matching the initial blood product, in addition to all subsequent ones; however, a recent study did not find that cross-matching the initial blood product altered outcome or posttransfusion red blood cell parameters.[51]

The role of corticosteroids in the management of hemoplasmosis is unclear. In *M haemofelis*–infected cats, clinical signs have resolved without their administration,[19,21] suggesting that they are not necessary. Moreover, immunosuppression induced by corticosteroid administration has been used in experimental studies with the aim of enhancing infection or inducing recrudescence of bacteremia.[15,44,52] Further studies are required to determine whether corticosteroids at any dose rate are detrimental or beneficial; however, it is generally accepted that they may be indicated pending confirmation of diagnosis.

SPECIFIC MANAGEMENT: HEMOPLASMOSIS

Like their relatives the mucosal mycoplasmas, hemoplasmas lack a cell wall, and as such are inherently resistant to antibiotics that are cell wall active, such as the β-lactams (eg, penicillin-derivatives and cephalosporins) and glycopeptides (eg, vancomycin). In addition, due to the parasitic nature of the hemoplasmas, they are predicted to be inherently resistant to anti-metabolite antibiotics (eg, trimethoprim sulfonamide), as are the mucosal mycoplasmas. In contrast, both tetracyclines and fluoroquinolones have been shown to have efficacy for the treatment of clinical hemoplasmosis in cats.[19,30,35–37,53–57]

Antibiotics of the tetracycline group (eg, oxytetracycline, doxycycline) inhibit protein synthesis by blocking access of transfer RNA molecules to the 30S ribosomal subunit and are considered bacteriostatic. In contrast, antibiotics of the fluoroquinolone group (eg, enrofloxacin, marbofloxacin, pradofloxacin) interfere with DNA replication by inhibiting the bacterial gyrase and/or the topoisomerase IV enzyme and are considered bactericidal. Experimentally, there is a well-characterized antagonism between fluoroquinolone ciprofloxacin and tetracycline in the killing of the model bacterium

Escherichia coli.[58,59] However, one report documents unpublished studies of *Mycoplasma genitalium* that provide evidence of a synergistic effect between moxifloxacin and doxycycline in moxifloxacin-susceptible strains.[60] To date, there are no data to support concurrent administration of fluoroquinolones and tetracyclines for feline hemoplasmas other than a single case report of the successful management of hemoplasmosis in a human.[61]

In cats experimentally infected with *M haemofelis*, rapid resolution of the clinical signs of hemoplasmosis occurred during the administration of both tetracycline (doxycycline 5 mg/kg orally twice daily for 14 days) and fluoroquinolones (enrofloxacin 5 mg/kg or 10 mg/kg orally once daily for 14 days; marbofloxacin 2 mg/kg orally once daily for 28 days; marbofloxacin 2.75 mg/kg orally once daily for 14 days; pradofloxacin 5 mg/kg or 10 mg/kg orally once daily for 14 days).[19,35,36,52] Where different antibiotics, and doses, were compared, none were found to be clinically superior,[35,36] potentially due to low numbers in each treatment group. Simultaneous administration of tetracyclines and fluoroquinolones was also associated with a significant and marked decrease in *M haemofelis* load. It should be noted that these studies included untreated control cats, all of which recovered without antibiotic administration, with some being administered fluid therapy if dehydrated, inappetent, or severely anemic. Clearance of *M haemofelis* infection was not achieved in most cases treated with doxycycline, enrofloxacin, or marbofloxacin. Of the cats treated with pradofloxacin, although 50% (n = 6) were initially negative by PCR, subsequently repeated testing found 3 of these to have very low hemoplasma copy numbers present, with a further 2 becoming intermittently PCR positive following immunosuppression.[36]

In cats experimentally infected with "*Ca* M haemominutum," administration of marbofloxacin (2 mg/kg orally once daily for 28 days) resulted in a significant decrease in hemoplasma load, compared with the nontreatment control group, although this response was less dramatic, delayed, and was nonsustained compared with the response of *M haemofelis*–infected cats to marbofloxacin.[19,57]

One experimental study assessed the response of "*Ca* M turicensis" infection to antibiosis, in a limited number of cats (n = 3). After doxycycline treatment (10 mg/kg once daily for 14 days), one cat showed a sustained decline in hemoplasma load following treatment. The other 2 cats were initially administered marbofloxacin (2 mg/kg once daily for 10 days), with negative "*Ca* M turicensis" PCRs obtained 4 days later; however, detectable hemoplasma loads were obtained on the 10th day of treatment. Treatment was switched to doxycycline (10 mg/kg once daily for 14 days), and negative "*Ca* M turicensis" PCR results were obtained 14 days later. Neither of these 2 cats was monitored further. A single case study describes the clearance of "*Ca* M turicensis" from a naturally infected cat following a course of doxycycline (10 mg/kg once daily for 14 days), with no subsequent recrudescence.[34]

The European Advisory Board on Cat Diseases currently recommends doxycycline (10 mg/kg orally once daily or 5 mg/kg orally twice daily) as a first-line therapy for clinical hemoplasmosis, typically for 2 to 4 weeks.[62] Due to the risk of esophagitis and stricture formation,[63] particularly with the hyclate form of doxycycline, tablets or capsules should be administered followed by water or a small amount of food. Fewer adverse effects are reported when doxycycline is administered in divided doses or in the monohydrate form, such as those found in some liquid or paste formulations.[62] Fluoroquinolones could be considered as an alternative, although enrofloxacin should be avoided where possible due to risks of retinal toxicity and acute blindness,[64] particularly when alternative fluoroquinolones are available.

SPECIFIC MANAGEMENT: CHRONIC CARRIER STATUS

A recent study described a treatment protocol that consistently cleared *M haemofelis* infection in a small number (n = 15) of chronically infected cats.[44] Furthermore, following immunosuppression, recrudescence was not detected. The protocol comprised a course of doxycycline (5 mg/kg orally twice daily for 28 days) followed, if organisms were still detectable in the blood, by a course of marbofloxacin (2 mg/kg orally once daily for 14 days). Delays of up to 4 weeks' duration between the administration of doxycycline and marbofloxacin were not detrimental to outcome. It should be noted that to determine clearance of infection, the *M haemofelis* quantitative PCR was performed in quadruplicate/triplicate to increase assay sensitivity (from ≥200 copies per mL to ≥50–66 copies per mL) on a weekly basis. However, neither drug is labeled for the treatment of hemoplasmosis in the cat and the suggested course durations for both doxycycline and marbofloxacin were relatively long. These findings should not be extrapolated to other feline hemoplasmas.

In case reports of canine and human hemoplasmosis with clinical remission and apparent clearance of infection, as demonstrated by serial PCR testing, treatments have comprised extended administration of either tetracycline alone[65] or combinations of tetracycline and fluoroquinolone.[61] A dog infected with *Mycoplasma haemocanis* was administered doxycycline for nearly 3 months.[65] A second canine case infected with *M haemocanis,* clinically responded to extended courses of antibiotics (2 months oxytetracycline followed by 8 months enrofloxacin), although persistent clearance of infection was not achieved.[66] Both canine cases involved dogs that had been splenectomized for non-neoplastic disease. In a human infected with "*Candidatus* Mycoplasma haemohominis" there was a marked clinical improvement (resolution of hemolytic anemia) and achievement of nondetectable hemoplasma levels in blood in response to doxycycline alone; however, relapse occurred following discontinuation.[61] Clinical cure followed 6-months' worth of both doxycycline and moxifloxacin, with a 1-year follow-up.

GROUP CONSIDERATIONS

Arthropods, particularly the cat flea *Ctenocephalides felis*, have been implicated in the transmission of feline hemoplasmas; however, confirmation of transmission by fleas by experimental demonstration has been limited.[67,68] Currently, regular administration of anti-ectoparasitic treatment seems prudent in cats. Aggressive interactions leading to the subcutaneous inoculation of infected blood have also been implicated in transmission of hemoplasma infection[69]; therefore, indoor housing and separation of cats between which aggressive interactions are known to have occurred also seems sensible. Spread of infection has also been reported between cats housed together in the absence of arthropods and without reports of aggressive interactions.[68] Therefore, when the aim is to maintain hemoplasma-free status, uninfected cats should not be housed with hemoplasma-infected cats.

SUMMARY

Hemoplasmosis due to *M haemofelis* infection is an uncommon cause of moderate-severe anemia in cats. In contrast, "*Ca* M haemominutum" is detected in approximately 1 in every 5 cats, and can result in mild anemia during acute infection; however, as a carrier state is common, concurrent disease should be investigated in clinically anemic cats. Infection may be exacerbated by immunosuppression; therefore, prompt identification of the infecting hemoplasma species and appropriate antibiotic administration (eg, tetracycline; fluoroquinolone) is necessary. Although cats with hemoplasmosis respond rapidly to antibiosis and supportive care, initial monotherapy courses rarely result in clearance of infection. A protocol now exists for the clearance of the most pathogenic feline hemoplasma *M haemofelis*.

REFERENCES

1. Mayer M. Über einige Bakterienähnliche Parasiten der Erythrozyten bei Menschen und Tieren. Arch Schiffs Trop Hyg 1921;25:150–2.
2. Ford WW, Eliot CP. The transfer of rat anemia to normal animals. J Exp Med 1928; 48(4):475–92.
3. Schilling V. *Eperythrozoon coccoides*, eine neue durch splenektomie aktivierbare dauerinfektion der weissen maus. Klin Wochenschr 1928;7:1853–5.
4. Tyzzer EE, Weinman D, Haemobartonella NG. (*Bartonella* olim pro parte), *H. microti*, N.Sp., of the field vole *Microtus pennsylvanicus*. Am J Hyg 1939; 30(3):141–57.
5. Messick JB, Walker PG, Raphael W, et al. "*Candidatus* Mycoplasma haemodidelphidis" sp. nov., "*Candidatus* Mycoplasma haemolamae" sp. nov. and *Mycoplasma haemocanis* comb. nov., haemotrophic parasites from a naturally infected opossum (*Didelphis virginiana*), alpaca (*Lama pacos*) and dog (*Canis familiaris*): phylogenetic and secondary structural relatedness of their 16S rRNA genes to other mycoplasmas. Int J Syst Evol Microbiol 2002;52(Pt 3):693–8.
6. Neimark H, Hoff B, Ganter M. *Mycoplasma ovis* comb. nov. (formerly *Eperythrozoon ovis*), an epierythrocytic agent of haemolytic anaemia in sheep and goats. Int J Syst Evol Microbiol 2004;54(Pt 2):365–71.
7. Neimark H, Johansson KE, Rikihisa Y, et al. Proposal to transfer some members of the genera *Haemobartonella* and *Eperythrozoon* to the genus *Mycoplasma* with descriptions of "*Candidatus* Mycoplasma haemofelis", "*Candidatus* Mycoplasma haemomuris", "*Candidatus* Mycoplasma haemosuis" and "*Candidatus* Mycoplasma wenyonii". Int J Syst Evol Microbiol 2001;51(Pt 3):891–9.
8. Tindall BJ. The request for an opinion that the current use of the genus name *Mycoplasma* be maintained and *Mycoplasma coccoides* be considered a legitimate name is denied. Opinion 92. Judicial Commission of the International Committee on Systematics of Prokaryotes. Int J Syst Evol Microbiol 2014;64(Pt 10):3586–7.
9. Clark R. *Eperythrozoon felis* (sp. Nov) in a cat. J S Afr Vet Med Assoc 1942;13(1): 15–6.
10. Flint JC, McKelvie DH. Feline infectious anaemia - Diagnosis and treatment. 92nd Annual Meeting of the American Veterinary Medical Association. Minneapolis, August 15-18, 1955.
11. Flint JC, Moss LC. Infectious anaemia in cats. J Am Vet Med Assoc 1953; 122(910):45–8.
12. Flint JC, Roepke MH, Jensen R. Feline infectious anaemia. II. Experimental cases. Am J Vet Res 1959;20:33–40.
13. Neimark H, Johansson KE, Rikihisa Y, et al. Revision of haemotrophic *Mycoplasma* species names. Int J Syst Evol Microbiol 2002;52:683.
14. Foley JE, Pedersen NC. "*Candidatus* Mycoplasma haemominutum", a low-virulence epierythrocytic parasite of cats. Int J Syst Evol Microbiol 2001; 51(Pt 3):815–7.
15. Willi B, Boretti FS, Cattori V, et al. Identification, molecular characterization, and experimental transmission of a new hemoplasma isolate from a cat with hemolytic anemia in Switzerland. J Clin Microbiol 2005;43(6):2581–5.

16. Barker EN, Tasker S. Haemoplasmas: lessons learnt from cats. N Z Vet J 2013; 61(4):184–92.
17. Martinez-Diaz VL, Silvestre-Ferreira AC, Vilhena H, et al. Prevalence and co-infection of haemotropic mycoplasmas in Portuguese cats by real-time polymerase chain reaction. J Feline Med Surg 2013;15(10):879–85.
18. Sykes JE, Drazenovich NL, Ball LM, et al. Use of conventional and real-time polymerase chain reaction to determine the epidemiology of hemoplasma infections in anemic and nonanemic cats. J Vet Intern Med 2007;21(4):685–93.
19. Tasker S, Caney SM, Day MJ, et al. Effect of chronic FIV infection, and efficacy of marbofloxacin treatment, on *Mycoplasma haemofelis* infection. Vet Microbiol 2006;117(2–4):169–79.
20. Tasker S, Helps CR, Day MJ, et al. Use of real-time PCR to detect and quantify *Mycoplasma haemofelis* and *"Candidatus* Mycoplasma haemominutum" DNA. J Clin Microbiol 2003;41(1):439–41.
21. Tasker S, Peters IR, Papasoulotis K, et al. Description of outcomes of experimental infection with feline haemoplasmas: haematology, Coombs" testing and blood glucose concentrations. Vet Microbiol 2009;139(3–4):323–32.
22. Hicks CAE, Willi B, Riond B, et al. Protective immunity against infection with *Mycoplasma haemofelis*. Clin Vaccine Immunol 2015;22(1):108–18.
23. Novacco M, Boretti FS, Franchini M, et al. Protection from reinfection in "Candidatus Mycoplasma turicensis"-infected cats and characterization of the immune response. Vet Res 2012;43(1):82.
24. Tasker S, Murray JK, Knowles TG, et al. Coombs", haemoplasma and retrovirus testing in feline anaemia. J Small Anim Pract 2010;51(4):192–9.
25. Tasker S, Binns SH, Day MJ, et al. Use of a PCR assay to assess the prevalence and risk factors for *Mycoplasma haemofelis* and *"Candidatus* Mycoplasma haemominutum" in cats in the United Kingdom. Vet Rec 2003;152(7):193–8.
26. Westfall DS, Jensen WA, Reagan WJ, et al. Inoculation of two genotypes of *Hemobartonella felis* (California and Ohio variants) to induce infection in cats and the response to treatment with azithromycin. Am J Vet Res 2001;62(5):687–91.
27. Hall SM, Cipriano JA, Schoneweis DA, et al. Isolation of infective and non-infective *Eperythrozoon suis* bodies from the whole blood of infected swine. Vet Rec 1988;123(25):651.
28. Tasker S. Haemotropic mycoplasmas: what's their real significance in cats? J Feline Med Surg 2010;12(5):369–81.
29. Willi B, Museux K, Novacco M, et al. First morphological characterization of *"Candidatus* Mycoplasma turicensis" using electron microscopy. Vet Microbiol 2011; 149(3–4):367–73.
30. Berent LM, Messick JB, Cooper SK. Detection of *Haemobartonella felis* in cats with experimentally induced acute and chronic infections, using a polymerase chain reaction assay. Am J Vet Res 1998;59(10):1215–20.
31. Peters IR, Helps CR, Willi B, et al. The prevalence of three species of feline haemoplasmas in samples submitted to a diagnostics service as determined by three novel real-time duplex PCR assays. Vet Microbiol 2008;126:142–50.
32. Sykes JE, Terry JC, Lindsay LL, et al. Prevalences of various hemoplasma species among cats in the United States with possible hemoplasmosis. J Am Vet Med Assoc 2008;232(3):372–9.
33. Lappin MR, Griffin B, Brunt J, et al. Prevalence of *Bartonella* species, haemoplasma species, *Ehrlichia* species, *Anaplasma phagocytophilum*, and *Neorickettsia risticii* DNA in the blood of cats and their fleas in the United States. J Feline Med Surg 2006;8(2):85–90.

34. Willi B, Boretti FS, Baumgartner C, et al. Prevalence, risk factor analysis, and follow-up of infections caused by three feline hemoplasma species in cats in Switzerland. J Clin Microbiol 2006;44(3):961–9.

35. Dowers KL, Olver CS, Radecki SV, et al. Use of enrofloxacin for treatment of large-form *Haemobartonella felis* in experimentally infected cats. J Am Vet Med Assoc 2002;221(2):250–3.

36. Dowers KL, Tasker S, Radecki SV, et al. Use of pradofloxacin to treat experimentally induced *Mycoplasma hemofelis* infection in cats. Am J Vet Res 2009;70(1): 105–11.

37. Tasker S, Helps CR, Day MJ, et al. Use of a Taqman PCR to determine the response of *Mycoplasma haemofelis* infection to antibiotic treatment. J Microbiol Methods 2004;56(1):63–71.

38. dos Santos AP, dos Santos RP, Biondo AW, et al. Hemoplasma infection in HIV-positive patient, Brazil. Emerg Infect Dis 2008;14(12):1922–4.

39. Fisher EW, Toth S, Collier WO. Anaemia in a litter of Siamese kittens. J Small Anim Pract 1983;24(4):215–9.

40. Pentecosta RL, Marsha AE, Niehausa AJ, et al. Vertical transmission of *Mycoplasma haemolamae* in alpacas (*Vicugna pacos*). Small Rumin Res 2012; 106(2–3):181–8.

41. Hornok S, Micsutka A, Meli ML, et al. Molecular investigation of transplacental and vector-borne transmission of bovine haemoplasmas. Vet Microbiol 2011; 152(3–4):411–4.

42. Sykes JE, Lindsay LL, Maggi RG, et al. Human co-infection with *Bartonella henselae* and two hemotropic mycoplasma variants resembling *Mycoplasma ovis*. J Clin Microbiol 2010;48(10):3782–5.

43. Yuan CL, Liang AB, Yao CB, et al. Prevalence of *Mycoplasma suis (Eperythrozoon suis)* infection in swine and swine-farm workers in Shanghai, China. Am J Vet Res 2009;70(7):890–4.

44. Novacco M, Sugiarto S, Willi B, et al. Consecutive antibiotic treatment with doxycycline and marbofloxacin clears bacteremia in *Mycoplasma haemofelis*-infected cats. Vet Microbiol 2018;217:112–20.

45. Gong JK. Anemic stress as a trigger of myelogenous leukemia in rats rendered leukemia-prone by X-ray. Science 1971;174(4011):833–5.

46. Gong JK, Glomski CA, Braunsch PG. Anemic stress as a trigger of myelogenous leukemia in unirradiated RF mouse. Science 1972;177(4045):274–6.

47. Kociba GJ, Weiser MG, Olsen RG. Enhanced susceptibility to feline leukaemia virus in cats with *Haemobartonella felis* infection. Leuk Rev Int 1983;1:88–9.

48. George JW, Rideout BA, Griffey SM, et al. Effect of preexisting FeLV infection or FeLV and feline immunodeficiency virus coinfection on pathogenicity of the small variant of *Haemobartonella felis* in cats. Am J Vet Res 2002;63(8):1172–8.

49. Hourani L, Weingart C, Kohn B. Alloimmunisation in transfused patients: serial cross-matching in a population of hospitalised cats. J Feline Med Surg 2017; 19(12):1231–7.

50. Weinstein NM, Blais MC, Harris K, et al. A newly recognized blood group in domestic shorthair cats: the Mik red cell antigen. J Vet Intern Med 2007;21(2): 287–92.

51. Sylvane B, Prittie J, Hohenhaus AE, et al. Effect of cross-match on packed cell volume after transfusion of packed red blood cells in transfusion-naive anemic cats. J Vet Intern Med 2018;32(3):1077–83.

52. Ishak AM, Dowers KL, Cavanaugh MT, et al. Marbofloxacin for the treatment of experimentally-induced *Mycoplasma haemofelis* infection in cats. J Vet Intern Med 2008;22(2):288–92.

53. Foley JE, Harrus S, Poland A, et al. Molecular, clinical, and pathologic comparison of two distinct strains of *Haemobartonella felis* in domestic cats. Am J Vet Res 1998;59(12):1581–8.

54. Harvey JW, Gaskin JM. Experimental feline hemobartonellosis. J Am Anim Hosp Assoc 1977;13(1):28–38.

55. Harvey JW, Gaskin JM. Feline haemobartonellosis - Attempts to induce relapses of clinical disease in chronically infected cats. J Am Anim Hosp Assoc 1978; 14(4):453–6.

56. Rikihisa Y, Kawahara M, Wen B, et al. Western immunoblot analysis of *Haemobartonella muris* and comparison of 16S rRNA gene sequences of *H. muris*, *H. felis*, and *Eperythrozoon suis*. J Clin Microbiol 1997;35(4):823–9.

57. Tasker S, Caney SM, Day MJ, et al. Effect of chronic feline immunodeficiency infection, and efficacy of marbofloxacin treatment, on "*Candidatus* Mycoplasma haemominutum" infection. Microbes Infect 2006;8(3):653–61.

58. Ocampo PS, Lazar V, Papp B, et al. Antagonism between bacteriostatic and bactericidal antibiotics is prevalent. Antimicrob Agents Chemother 2014;58(8): 4573–82.

59. Bollenbach T, Quan S, Chait R, et al. Nonoptimal microbial response to antibiotics underlies suppressive drug interactions. Cell 2009;139(4):707–18.

60. Bradshaw CS, Jensen JS, Waites KB. New horizons in mycoplasma genitalium treatment. J Infect Dis 2017;216(suppl_2):S412–9.

61. Steer J, Tasker S, Barker EN, et al. A novel hemotropic mycoplasma (hemoplasma) in a patient with hemolytic anemia and pyrexia. Clin Infect Dis 2011; 53(11):e147–51.

62. Tasker S, Hofmann-Lehmann R, Belak S, et al. Haemoplasmosis in cats: European guidelines from the ABCD on prevention and management. J Feline Med Surg 2018;20(3):256–61.

63. McGrotty YL, Knottenbelt CM. Oesophageal stricture in a cat due to oral administration of tetracyclines. J Small Anim Pract 2002;43(5):221–3.

64. Gelatt KN, van der Woerdt A, Ketring KL, et al. Enrofloxacin-associated retinal degeneration in cats. Vet Ophthalmol 2001;4(2):99–106.

65. Pitorri F, Dell"Orco M, Carmichael N, et al. Use of real-time quantitative PCR to document the successful treatment of *Mycoplasma haemocanis* infection with doxycycline in a dog. Vet Clin Pathol 2012;41(4):493–6.

66. Hulme-Moir KL, Barker EN, Stonelake A, et al. Use of real-time polymerase chain reaction to monitor antibiotic therapy in a dog with naturally acquired *Mycoplasma haemocanis* infection. J Vet Diagn Invest 2010;22(4):582–7.

67. Woods JE, Wisnewski N, Lappin MR. Attempted transmission of "*Candidatus* Mycoplasma haemominutum" and *Mycoplasma haemofelis* by feeding cats infected *Ctenocephalides felis*. Am J Vet Res 2006;67(3):494–7.

68. Lappin MR. Feline haemoplasmas are not transmitted by Ctenocephalides felis. Symposium of the CVBD World Forum. Barcelona, 20th March 2014.

69. Museux K, Boretti FS, Willi B, et al. In vivo transmission studies of "*Candidatus* Mycoplasma turicensis" in the domestic cat. Vet Res 2009;40(5):45.

Cutaneous and Renal Glomerular Vasculopathy

What Do We Know so Far?

Rosanne E. Jepson, BVSc, MVetMed, PhD, FHEA, MRCVS[a],[*],
Jacqueline M. Cardwell, MA, VetMB, MScVetEd, PhD, FHEA, MRCVS[b],
Stefano Cortellini, DMV, MVetMed, FHEA, MRCVS[a],
Laura Holm, BVM&S, CertSAM, MRCVS[c],
Kim Stevens, PhD, MScAgric, PGCAP[b], David Walker, MRCVS[c]

KEYWORDS

- CRGV • Thrombotic microangiopathy • Alabama rot • Acute kidney injury
- Skin lesion

KEY POINTS

- Cutaneous renal glomerular vasculopathy is a condition resulting in thrombotic microangiopathy recognized with apparently increasing prevalence in the United Kingdom since 2012.
- An infectious cause has not been identified to date.
- Clinical progression of cases usually involves identification of ulcerated skin lesions, typically affecting the distal limb and progression to oligoanuric acute kidney injury. However, subclinical manifestations of this condition with less severely affected individuals are thought to occur.
- Mortalities for dogs that develop oligoanuric acute renal failure are very high, although a limited number of dogs have been reported to survive with intensive supportive care.

INTRODUCTION

Cutaneous renal glomerular vasculopathy (CRGV) or the condition that has colloquially been termed "Alabama rot" has been recognized with apparently increasing frequency in the United Kingdom since 2012. The etiopathogenesis of this condition remains

Disclosure Statement: The authors have nothing to disclose.
[a] Department of Clinical Science and Services, Royal Veterinary College, Queen Mother Hospital for Animals, Hawkshead Lane, North Mymms, Herts, London AL9 7TA, UK; [b] Department of Pathobiology and Population Sciences, Royal Veterinary College, Hawkshead Lane, North Mymms, Herts, London AL9 7TA, UK; [c] Anderson Moores Veterinary Specialists, The Granary, Bunstead Barns, Poles Lane, Hursley, Winchester SO21 2LL, UK
* Corresponding author.
E-mail address: rjepson@rvc.ac.uk

Vet Clin Small Anim 49 (2019) 745–762
https://doi.org/10.1016/j.cvsm.2019.02.010
0195-5616/19/© 2019 Elsevier Inc. All rights reserved.

incompletely understood. Despite speculation and preliminary infectious disease testing of confirmed cases, an infectious cause has not been identified. However, the chronology of presentation, diagnostic testing, and small sample size are limiting factors. The condition has gained much attention because of the high mortality reported in dogs that develop oligoanuric acute renal failure associated with CRGV. Lack of a definitive antemortem diagnostic test and reliance on renal histopathology for confirmation of this condition mean that the true prevalence and incidence of CRGV within the canine population remains unknown. Continued work is required to better understand the epidemiology of CRGV and to explore individual, genetic, environmental, or infectious associations that underpin the risk of dogs developing CRGV. Ultimately it is likely that only through a better understanding of the pathogenesis of CRGV, that diagnostic tests can be developed that may facilitate early diagnosis and intervention that improves survival.

HISTORY OF CUTANEOUS RENAL GLOMERULAR VASCULOPATHY AND "ALABAMA ROT"

Conditions compatible with CRGV were first reported in the veterinary literature in greyhounds from the United States in the late 1980s.[1–3] These cases were variably associated with both skin lesions and acute kidney injury (AKI), and an underlying cause was not identified. Since 2012, a form of CRGV has been recognized in the United Kingdom. It is unclear whether the cause for these UK cases is the same as historical cases, but the clinical progression of cases and histopathologic manifestations are similar. Dogs that develop CRGV commonly present with ulcerated skin lesions, with development of AKI a median of 4 days after skin lesions are noted.[4] The presence of skin lesions is rarely reported in dogs, with other causes of AKI making the clinical presentation of dogs with CRGV unique. The common feature of all dogs with CRGV is the histopathologic finding of thrombotic microangiopathy (TMA) in renal tissue. Differential diagnoses for TMA in dogs include CRGV but also hemolytic uremic syndrome (HUS). HUS has previously been reported in 5 dogs, including several different breeds, such as the Yorkshire terrier, miniature poodle, Labrador retriever, and German shepherd dog.[5,6] Of the HUS cases reported in the literature, skin lesions were not reported.

THROMBOTIC MICROANGIOPATHIES IN HUMANS

TMA is a term used to describe a pathologic process that includes endothelial damage and thrombosis within the microvasculature, with high stress leading to platelet aggregation, a consumptive thrombocytopenia, and red cell shearing, resulting in a microangiopathic hemolytic anemia.[7] These features lead to ischemia and infarction, which particularly affect the kidney. TMA is a histopathologic diagnosis, and features of this are identified in several specific clinical conditions, including HUS, atypical hemolytic uremic syndrome (a-HUS), and thrombotic thrombocytopenic purpura (TTP).[7] TMA may be associated with underlying conditions, such as malignancy, administration of chemotherapy and other drugs, transplantation, sepsis, and disseminated intravascular coagulation.[8,9]

Hemolytic Uremic Syndrome

HUS in humans is triggered by infectious organisms and/or their toxins, for example, shiga toxin–producing bacteria (eg, *Escherichia coli* [STEC] and *Shigella dysenteriae* type 1) or infection with *Streptococcus pneumoniae* (pneumococcal HUS). However, in some individuals, HUS is not infection or toxin triggered and is therefore referred to as "atypical" (a-HUS). In human patients with STEC-HUS, renal failure is commonly associated with prodromal hemorrhagic diarrhea and is most commonly recognized in children.[8] In this condition, shiga toxin binds with high affinity to globotriaosylceramide 3 receptors expressed on glomerular endothelial cells.[10] Injury to the glomerular endothelium precipitates a prothrombotic cascade leading to microthrombi formation.[7] Diagnostic investigations in these patients typically include fecal culture and evaluation for E coli endotoxin antibodies (immunoglobulin M).[11]

Noninfection-associated triggers, including genetic or acquired risk factors for defective regulation of the alternative complement pathway (AP), play a role in the pathogenesis of a-HUS. Clinical features of a-HUS can be indistinguishable from other causes of TMA, with renal involvement predominating. Prodromal diarrhea is reported in up to 25% of patients ultimately considered to have a-HUS.[12,13] AP complement dysregulation involves uncontrolled complement activation as a result of deficient or functionally impaired regulatory proteins or hyperactive C3 convertase components. It is hypothesized that the glomerular endothelium may be particularly susceptible to complement dysregulation, although the exact mechanism by which microthrombi formation ensues is not fully elucidated.[13] Identification of familial associations leads to the recognition of genetic predispositions, which are identified in approximately 50% to 60% of individuals with a-HUS.[9] These genetic variants have been identified in complement regulators (factor H, factor I, CD46, and thrombomodulin) and complement activators (C3 and factor B). Acquired autoantibody production against factor H may also give a similar a-HUS phenotype, both with and without predisposing genetic variability in factor H. Low plasma concentrations of C3 are consistent with a diagnosis of a-HUS but are neither specific nor sensitive, given the most common variants in complement factor H result in normal circulating C3 and factor H concentrations.[7] Diagnosis of a-HUS in humans is therefore usually based on a combination of immunologic and genetic testing. When a human patient presents with clinical signs compatible with a-HUS, initial investigations will include assessment of complement concentrations (C3, C4, factor H, and factor I), mutation screening (CFH, CF1, CD46, C3, CFB, THBD, and DGKE), and detection of factor H autoantibodies.[11]

Thrombotic Thrombocytopenic Purpura

TTP is an uncommon TMA, which has been most commonly associated with acquired deficiency or genetic mutations in ADAMTS13.[7] ADAMTS13 is the cleaving protein of von Willebrand factor (vWF). vWF is required for primary hemostasis, facilitating platelet aggregation, and thrombus formation at sites of endothelial injury. In health, vWF is gradually degraded into progressively smaller circulating forms by ADAMTS13 with the influence of shear stress. Since the 1980s, it has been known that there is an association between TTP and highly thrombogenic "ultralarge" multimers of vWF, which was only later recognized to be due to deficiency or lack of functionality of ADAMTS13. Although genetic mutations in ADAMTS13 have been reported, these account for the minority of TTP cases, and it is more common for ADAMTS13 deficiency to be the result of an acquired inhibitory autoantibody.[7] Very low ADAMTS13 activities are required for TTP, typically less than 5% to 10% of normal protease activity. However, in individuals where TTP is present in conjunction with coexisting TMA risk factors, for example, sepsis, malignancy, or transplantation, then ADAMTS13 activity may not be markedly suppressed, so that quantification of ADAMTS13 is not a perfect diagnostic test.[11]

Interestingly, all 3 conditions have variable penetrance. For example, it is reported that some patients with hereditary forms of TTP do not manifest the disease until greater than 20 years of age; not all patients infected with STEC will develop STEC-HUS, and only 40% to 50% of carriers of the recognized CFH, membrane cofactor protein, and CFI mutations will manifest disease.[9] The pathogenesis of TMA is therefore complex and multifactorial, with interplay between genetic predispositions, environmental factors, and other disease conditions determining whether an individual clinically manifests a disease phenotype. In humans, extensive exploration of clinical history, combined with advanced immunologic and genetic diagnostic testing, is usually required in order to differentiate between causes of TMA.

CLINICAL PRESENTATION OF UNITED KINGDOM CASES OF CUTANEOUS RENAL GLOMERULAR VASCULOPATHY

Many different breeds of dog (>25, data courtesy of Anderson Moores Veterinary Specialists Ltd) have been identified with CRGV, which is in contrast to American data, where the disease appeared to affect only racing greyhounds.[1,14,15]

Dogs diagnosed with CRGV are initially presented to veterinarians for assessment of skin lesions, affecting the limbs (77%), body (20%), face/muzzle (7%), and tongue (4%). Systemic signs are also sometimes present (**Table 1**), but rarely noted before the development of skin lesions (1% of cases; n = 102, data courtesy of Anderson Moores Veterinary Specialists Ltd).

Skin lesion appearance is variable, ranging from small, superficial abrasions (0.5 cm), to large areas of full-thickness ulceration and necrosis (>30 cm), with surrounding bruising and edema. Lesions are commonly circular and erythematous. Central necrosis and ulceration develop subsequently. Lesions affecting digits frequently appear similar to pododermatitis or paronychia. Oral cavity lesions generally affect the tongue as circular erosions/ulcers, whereas lesions affecting the muzzle can be erosive/ulcerative or vesicular in appearance. Facial lesions commonly appear similar to acute moist dermatitis (**Fig. 1**).

CRGV may cause skin lesions without systemic illness,[2] whereas some dogs develop AKI that may or may not lead to azotemia.[16] Currently, in the United Kingdom, the relative proportion of azotemic versus nonazotemic CRGV remains unknown, because of the voluntary nature of case reporting and the difficulties in achieving a definitive antemortem diagnosis. One case series (n = 160 dogs) reported that 74% were nonazotemic[1]; however, diagnosis in these canine patients relied solely on

Table 1 Clinical signs at initial presentation	
Clinical Signs at Initial Presentation	Percentage of Dogs Affected (n = 102)
Skin lesions	99
Lameness	33
Anorexia	28
Vomiting	21
Lethargy	18
Pyrexia	17
Signs of bleeding	4
Diarrhea	3
Neurologic signs	2
Jaundice	1
Hypothermia	1

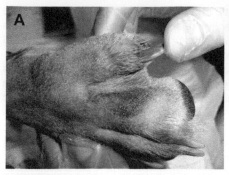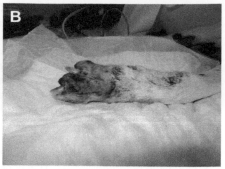

Fig. 1. Typical skin lesions identified in dogs with CRGV. (*A*) Interdigital skin lesion identified in dog with CRGV. (*B*) Progressive ulcerated skin lesions identified in dog with CRGV.

clinical signs and expert opinion. In a further case series (n = 12), renal histopathology was performed in both azotemic and nonazotemic cases, via light and electron microscopy, and confirmed the presence of glomerular TMA in all dogs. The changes observed in the nonazotemic group were less severe and widespread than in the azotemic group.[14] In another report (n = 18), 56% developed azotemia, whereas 44% remained nonazotemic, but diagnosis for all cases was reached by expert opinion based on clinical signs, blood and urine test results, without dermal or renal histopathology.[16]

Classification of CRGV into either nonazotemic or azotemic groups may be overly simplistic. The largest case series from the United States (n = 160)[1] reported the following 4 possible clinical manifestations:

1. Skin lesions with no systemic signs, remaining nonazotemic (a population potentially seen in the United Kingdom)
2. Pyrexia and skin lesions, followed rapidly by azotemic AKI (this presentation appears to account for a low number of confirmed UK cases [19% of 102 cases; unpublished data, 2018, courtesy of Anderson Moores Veterinary Specialists Ltd])
3. Skin lesions with development of azotemic AKI within 10 days (60% of 102 cases; unpublished data, 2018, courtesy of Anderson Moores Veterinary Specialists Ltd)
4. Azotemia before development of skin lesions (which appears rare in the United Kingdom; 1% of 102 cases; unpublished data, 2018, courtesy of Anderson Moores Veterinary Specialists Ltd)

In the United Kingdom, in 3% of dogs, azotemic AKI was detected more than 10 days after development of skin lesions (11, 20, and 21 days later). This finding could suggest that another, delayed, clinical manifestation of azotemic CRGV exists; however, it is also possible that these cases developed AKI before biochemistry and urinalysis was performed.

Approach to Suspected Cases and Clinicopathologic Findings

Antemortem diagnosis of CRGV can be challenging. There is no single, noninvasive diagnostic test available with high sensitivity and specificity.

- Renal histopathology: Demonstration of TMA on renal histopathology is considered the reference standard for diagnosis. Fibrinoid necrosis and thrombosis, affecting the glomerular arterioles, are the most commonly reported findings with congestion of the glomerular tufts, and tubular degeneration and necrosis also reported.[1,4,14] Unfortunately, given the relative contraindication for renal biopsy in dogs at risk of, or diagnosed with, AKI and sometimes thrombocytopenia, this is usually obtained postmortem with retrospective confirmation of CRGV.

- When presented with a dog for evaluation of skin lesions, which could be compatible with CRGV, baseline complete blood cell count, biochemistry, and urinalysis should be performed to assess for abnormalities, which may further suggest CRGV. This also provides a baseline for ongoing monitoring. The frequency and duration of monitoring for development of AKI will depend on many factors, including the level of clinical concern, owner preferences, dog temperament, and any financial considerations.

- Complete blood cell count: This is normally unremarkable in dogs suspected to have nonazotemic CRGV, whereas most cases that develop AKI (95%) have some combination of neutrophilia, nonregenerative anemia or preregenerative anemia, or thrombocytopenia (**Table 2**). In these cases, blood smear examination may identify evidence of microangiopathic hemolysis (Burr cells, acanthocytes, or schistocytes: 38% of 13 cases, Holm and colleagues[4]; 29% of 7 cases, Carpenter and colleagues[1]; 78% of 9 cases, Cowan and colleagues[16]).

- Biochemistry: Serum biochemical analysis is generally unremarkable in suspected nonazotemic CRGV cases; however, mildly elevated serum liver enzyme activity has been identified (51/102 cases, median alanine aminotransferase [ALT] activity 50 μ/L, range 35–117; reference range <25 μ/L).[17] Of the dogs developing AKI, 87% to 96% have abnormal serum urea and/or creatinine concentrations at the time of initial biochemistry. Azotemia has most frequently been documented 3 days after the development of skin lesions (n = 102, range: 3 days before to 21 days later). Other biochemical abnormalities include hyperphosphatemia, hyperbilirubinemia, elevated serum liver enzyme activity, mildly elevated serum muscle enzyme activity, and mild hypoalbuminemia (**Table 3**). Abnormal canine pancreatic lipase results have also been identified (79% of 14 cases, unpublished data, 2018, courtesy of Anderson Moores Veterinary Specialists Ltd).

- International Renal Interest Society (IRIS) AKI grading: IRIS grading can be helpful to document severity of AKI but has not yet been shown to be prognostically significant for CRGV cases. Median IRIS AKI grade for UK CRGV cases (n = 102) was III, range I--V.[17]

- Urinalysis: This is generally unremarkable in nonazotemic cases, although mild proteinuria has been reported (2 of 6 nonazotemic cases had Urine protein to creatinine ratio (UP:Cr) >1.0, Cowan and colleagues[16]; 14% of 13 cases had elevated UP:Cr, median value 0.85, range 0.56–1.14, reference range <0.5, Holm and Walker[17]). Commonly identified abnormalities in azotemic cases are similar to those seen in dogs with AKI of any cause and include proteinuria (n = 5, UP:Cr 1.19–7.0, Cowan and colleagues[16]; n = 102, median UP:Cr 3.42, range 1.81–7.64, reference <0.5)[17], hematuria/hemoglobinuria (95%), glycosuria (32%), and granular or hyaline casts (n = 102).

- Oligoanuria: Reduced or absent urine production is common in dogs with CRGV that developed AKI (urine output data available for 61 of 102 cases revealed 70% were oliguric or anuric (30/61 oliguric and 13/61 anuric; unpublished data, 2018, courtesy of Anderson Moores Veterinary Specialists Ltd; 8 of 10 azotemic cases were oliguric or anuric; Cowan and colleagues[16]). The authors are aware of 9 cases suspected to have had CRGV, which developed severe AKI (median IRIS grade III; range II–V), but recovered with intensive management. Urine output data were available for 7 of these cases: 3 had normal urine output,

Table 2
Selected hematology results for cutaneous renal glomerular vasculopathy cases

Publication	Abnormality	Number of Dogs in Report	% of Dogs Affected	Median Value	Range	Normal Reference Range
Carpenter et al,[1] 1988 (US)	Thrombocytopenia	7	86	103×10^9/L	$45{-}241 \times 10^9$/L	—
	Anemia	7	71	41%	37%–51%	>55%
Hertzke et al,[14] 1995 (US)	Thrombocytopenia	12	100	43×10^9/L	$<10{-}173 \times 10^9$/L	$>200 \times 10^9$/L
Cowan et al,[16] 1997 (US)	Thrombocytopenia	18: 10 azotemic, 8 nonazotemic	100	Mean values: azotemic 43.9×10^9/L Nonazotemic 114.6×10^9/L	Azotemic cases: $6{-}97 \times 10^9$/L Nonazotemic: $6{-}>120 \times 10^9$/L	$>180 \times 10^9$/L
	Anemia	18: 10 azotemic, 8 nonazotemic	100% of azotemic cases 75% of nonazotemic cases	Mean values: azotemic 29% Nonazotemic 47%	—	—
	Neutrophilia	18: 10 azotemic, 8 nonazotemic	—	Mean values: azotemic 17.053×10^9/L Nonazotemic 8.881×10^9/L 47%	—	—
Holm et al,[4] 2015 (UK)	Thrombocytopenia	30	50	78×10^9/L	$1{-}401 \times 10^9$/L	$175{-}500 \times 10^9$/L
	Anemia	30	23	43.9%	26%–65.3%	37%–55%
Holm & Walker,[17] in press (UK)	Thrombocytopenia	102	78% (n = 76 cases)	40×10^9/L	$0{-}60 \times 10^9$/L	$175{-}500 \times 10^9$/L
	Anemia	102	22 (n = 22 cases)	30.6%	24%–36%	37%–55%
	Neutrophilia	102	52 (n = 53 cases)	13.7×10^9/L	$10.6{-}37.9 \times 10^9$/L	$2.8{-}10.5 \times 10^9$/L

Table 3
Selected biochemistry results for cutaneous renal glomerular vasculopathy cases

Publication	Abnormality	Number of Dogs in Report	Dogs Affected (%)	Median Value	Range	Normal Reference Range
Carpenter et al,[1] 1988 (US)	Elevated urea/serum urea nitrogen (BUN)	7, data available for 5	44 of 168 (26)	105 mg/dL (37.5 mmol/L)	24–453 mg/dL (15–161.8 mmol/L)	—
	Elevated creatinine	7, data available for 5	44 of 168 (26)	7.2 mg/dL (636.5 µmol/L)	2.2–23.3 mg/dL (194.5–2059.7 µmol/L)	—
	Increased ALT activity	7	5 of 7 (71)	—	74–510 µ/L	—
Hertzke et al,[14] 1995 (US)	Elevated urea/BUN	12	7 of 12 (58)	240 mg/dL (85.7 mmol/L)	80–450 mg/dL (28.6–160 mmol/L)	<40 mg/dL
	Elevated creatinine	12	7 of 12 (58)	5.6 mg/dL (495 µmol/L)	2.5–19.6 mg/dL (221–1732.7 µmol/L)	<2.0 mg/dL
Cowan et al,[16] 1997 (US)	Elevated creatinine	18	10 of 18 (56)	—	—	>1.8 mg/dL
	Increased ALT activity	18	11 of 18 (61)	—	—	—
	Increased CK activity	18, data available for 15	3/8 nonazotemic (38) 6/7 azotemic (86)	Mean in nonazotemic cases 556 µ/L Mean in azotemic cases 4136 µ/L	—	—
	Hypoalbuminemia	18	2/8 nonazotemic (25) 9/10 azotemic (90)	Mean in nonazotemic cases 2.33 g/dL Mean in azotemic cases 1.66 g/dL	—	—

Source	Parameter	n (data available)	Count (%)	Value	Reference range
Holm et al,[4] 2015 (UK)	Elevated urea/BUN	30	100%	46.4 mmol/L	3.6–85.1 mmol/L	2.0–9.0 mmol/L
	Elevated creatinine	30	30/30 (100)	406.5 µmol/L	71–900 µmol/L	40–159 µmol/L
	Increased ALT activity	30, data available for 25	21/25 (84)	119 µ/L	48–950 µ/L	<100 µ/L
	Increased ALKP activity	30, data available for 28	11/28 (39)	91.5 µ/L	16–650 µ/L	<212 µ/L
	Hyperbilirubinemia	30, data available for 27	9/27 (33)	12 µmol/L	0–338 µmol/L	0–15 µmol/L
	Hyperphosphatemia	30, data available for 26	21/26 (81)	3.12 mmol/L	1.28–6.2 mmol/L	0.8–2.20 mmol/L
	Increased CK activity	30, data available for 8	4/8 (50)	206 µ/L	112–881 µ/L	<190 µ/L
	Increased aspartate aminotransferase (AST) activity	30, data available for 6	6/6 (100)	76.5 µ/L	51–473 µ/L	<49 µ/L
	Hypoalbuminemia	30, data available for 27	10/27 (37)	27 g/L	14–36 g/L	26–40 g/L
Holm & Walker, in press (UK); and some unpublished data, 2018, courtesy of Anderson Moores Veterinary Specialists Ltd	Elevated urea/BUN	102	98/102 (96)	41.9 mmol/L (n = 102)	4.7–92.6 mmol/L (n = 102)	2.0–9.0 mmol/L
	Elevated creatinine	102	96/102 (94)	304 µmol/L (n = 102)	68–1606 µmol/L (n = 102)	40–106 µmol/L
	Increased ALT activity	102, data available for 83	79/83 (95)	199 µ/L (n = 79)	34–950 µ/L (n = 79)	<25 µ/L (n = 24) <100 µ/L (n = 59)
	Increased ALKP activity	102, data available for 86	37/86 (43)	335 µ/L (n = 37)	76–2920 µ/L (n = 37)	<50 µ/L (n = 24) <212 µ/L (n = 62)
	Hyperbilirubinemia	102, data available for 76	51/76 (67)	27 µmol/L (n = 51)	16–603 µmol/L (n = 51)	<15 µmol/L
	Hyperphosphatemia	102, data available for 83	65/83 (78)	3.42 mmol/L (n = 65)	1.81–7.64 mmol/L (n = 65)	0.8–1.6 mmol/L (n = 30) 0.81–2.2 mmol/L (n = 53)
	Increased CK activity	102, data available for 17	12/17 (71)	295 µ/L (n = 12)	217–881 µ/L (n = 12)	<190 µ/L
	Increased AST activity	102, data available for 10	10/10 (100)	86 µ/L (n = 10)	51–473 µ/L (n = 10)	<49 µ/L
	Hypoalbuminemia	102, data available for 85	24/85 (20)	23 g/L (n = 24)	14–25 g/L (n = 24)	26–40 g/L (n = 53)

4 were oliguric, and none were anuric (unpublished data, 2018, courtesy of Anderson Moores Veterinary Specialists Ltd).

- Abdominal ultrasonography: In azotemic dogs, abdominal ultrasonography is useful to further assess renal architecture and exclude other postrenal causes of azotemia. Findings tend to be largely unremarkable in CRGV cases. Hyperechoic renal cortices are sometimes identified (approximately one-third of cases; unpublished data, 2018, courtesy of Anderson Moores Veterinary Specialists Ltd), and some dogs have small-volume abdominal effusions (because of hemorrhage or volume overloading).
- Dermal histopathology: Skin biopsy, with dermal histopathology, *may* help to confirm the diagnosis and can be considered for suspected cases. However, it commonly reveals nonspecific, ischemic changes, including ulceration of the epidermis with coagulative necrosis of the subjacent dermis. In just more than one-third of cases with dermal histopathology performed as part of a postmortem examination (39% of 89 cases, unpublished data, 2018, courtesy of Anderson Moores Veterinary Specialists Ltd), fibrinoid necrosis and thrombosis were identified in the small dermal arterioles, demonstrating a TMA process, supporting the diagnosis of CRGV.

ETIOPATHOGENESIS EXPLORED TO DATE

At this time, the cause of CRGV remains unknown. When CRGV was first recognized in greyhounds in the 1980s and 1990s, it was postulated that it was associated with the ingestion of uncooked ground beef,[16] and STEC strains have been isolated more frequently from the feces of greyhounds with CRGV than from healthy greyhounds. However, STEC strains were not isolated from all greyhounds diagnosed with CRGV.[18]

In the largest case series of dogs with CRGV to date, fecal culture was performed in 7 dogs and yielded *E coli*.[4] However, multiplex polymerase chain reactions (PCRs) for *E coli* virulence genes (eaeA, stx 1 and 2, LT1, and ST1 and 2) were negative in all of these dogs. Although shiga toxin has been identified in various species,[3,19] it has not been identified in dogs with HUS,[5,20] and both fluorescent in situ hybridization (FISH; n = 6) and PCR (n = 4) for shiga toxin on renal tissue in the UK CRGV dogs were negative.[4] Reasons for failing to identify toxin, or causative bacteria, may have included previous antibiotic administration, inappropriate sample handling, or late collection of samples. In humans, recovery of toxin producing *E coli* is highly dependent on fecal culture being performed within 6 days of the onset of diarrhea.[21]

Other gram-negative bacteria, including *Rickettsia rickettsii* and the leptospirae, were postulated as causative agents in greyhounds; however, serology did not yield a definitive diagnosis.[1] Leptospirosis was considered possible and has been explored further, although renal histopathology in dogs with leptospirosis would not be compatible with CRGV.[22] Leptospirosis microscopic agglutination testing was performed in 15 cases.[4] Ten dogs had negative titers, obtained a median of 3 days (1–8 days) after the development of systemic signs but without available convalescent titers. Five dogs had positive titers, albeit at a low concentration (1:100–1:800), and all of these dogs had been vaccinated less than 1 year before testing. Although vaccinal titers often decline by 4 months after vaccination, they can sometimes persist for longer, leading to false positive results.[23] In addition, only single titers greater than 1:1600 are considered significant for indicating infection in vaccinated dogs.[24] FISH and *Leptospira* PCR have been performed in low numbers of dogs confirmed to have CRGV, but have yielded discordant results.[25]

In the UK case series, viral metagenomics was performed on fresh kidney tissue (n = 2), liver (n = 1), and lymph node (n = 1), by random nucleic acid amplification. All results were negative, and histopathologically there was no evidence of viral cytopathic effect (cytoplasmic inclusion bodies) in any of the tissues examined.[4] PCR for canine circovirus was also performed on splenic tissue (n = 4) and blood (n = 3), and FISH was performed on renal tissue (n = 6); all results were negative.[26] Negative results for viral metagenomics do not completely exclude a viral cause. These results could indicate that virus was present in low copy numbers, or that the virus was too remotely related to known viruses used for sequence alignment, or that the sample used was too autolyzed to preserve the virus.

Renal tissue from 2 dogs was submitted to 2 separate laboratories, with both laboratories receiving identical samples for evaluation with a broad spectrum set of 16S ribosomal RNA–directed probes. One laboratory identified a clear 16S band in the tissue of 1 dog and a faint band in the other, and Staphylococcaceae were identified in both samples; however, this was thought to be the result of contamination with commensal skin bacteria. Urine and renal tissue culture results were negative in both dogs.[4] The second laboratory only identified leptospires in both samples.

Several other causes were considered in the UK case series; Borrelia PCR (n = 5) and serology (n = 2) were negative, and renal heavy metal concentrations (n = 3; lead, arsenic and cadmium) were below reported reference intervals in all 3.[4] A botanist from the Natural History Museum, London visited one of the sites that an affected dog had walked over the weeks before developing disease, and no plant species observed were considered likely to be either causal or a cofactor in the development of CRGV (David Walker, 2018, personal communication). The only fungi identified have a long history in the United Kingdom and were considered unlikely to be the cause of this emerging disease. Urine toxicology was negative in 5 of 6 dogs tested. Pentaethylene glycol (trace) was detected in 1 dog.[4] A brown recluse spider bite was considered a possible cause with a bite eliciting a pattern of necrotizing dermatitis with subsequent vasculitis and necrosis in the kidney, but this spider is not endemic in the United Kingdom and arachnid envenomation would not correlate with the seasonality of the disease in the United Kingdom.[27,28] No evidence of ricinine was found in the urine of 7 histopathologically confirmed cases (unpublished data, 2018, courtesy of Anderson Moores Veterinary Specialists Ltd).

EPIDEMIOLOGY OF CUTANEOUS RENAL GLOMERULAR VASCULOPATHY

The first known cases of CRGV in UK dogs were reported in 2012, and although initial numbers were very low (n = 3), the annual frequency of reported cases showed a steady increase, albeit exhibiting occasional year-on-year variation. The outbreak pattern of CRGV in the United Kingdom is in accord with the definition of a newly emerging disease.[29] However, that does not mean that the disease was completely unknown in the United Kingdom, because it may simply not have been recognized, owing to a very low incidence in the population before 2012.

Breed Risk Factors

Previous non-UK studies have suggested that CRGV is associated primarily with greyhounds,[1,2,14,16] with a single case reported in a great Dane in Germany.[3] However, a comparison of 101 dogs diagnosed with CRGV between November 2012 and May 2017, with a denominator population of 446,453 UK dogs from the

VetCompass database (VetCompass 2014),[15] reported that greyhounds did not have a significantly higher odds of CRGV diagnosis (odds ratio [OR] 1.65, P = .629) and that the disease was instead associated with multiple breeds. In general, hounds (OR 10.68, P<.001), gundogs (OR 9.69, P<.001), and pastoral dogs (OR 3.50, P = .046) had the highest risk of being diagnosed with CRGV, whereas toy dogs were absent from the case population. Compared with crossbreds, specific breeds with increased odds of being a CRGV case included the flat-coated retriever (OR 84.48), Hungarian Vizsla (OR 40.98), Manchester terrier (OR 41.41), Saluki (OR 27.46), Whippet (OR 22.43), English springer spaniel (OR 11.41), and bearded collie (OR 10.85).[15] Breeds with decreased odds of being a case were the Staffordshire bull terrier (OR 0.50), German shepherd dog (OR 0.45), and Jack Russell terrier (OR 0.37). Female dogs were more likely to be diagnosed with CRGV (OR 1.51), as were neutered dogs (OR 3.36).[15]

Spatiotemporal Distribution in the United Kingdom

CRGV in the United Kingdom has been characterized by annual outbreaks, which display a distinct seasonal pattern. More than 90% of cases between 2012 and 2017 occurred between November and May,[30] and Kuldorff's seasonal scan statistics identified a significant temporal cluster from December to April (P = .001; Kim Stevens, 2018, unpublished work, 2018). In general, negligible numbers of cases are reported during the summer months.[30]

The number of cases has increased incrementally from 3 in 2012 to greater than 60 in the 2017/2018 "season." The New Forest region on England's southern coast was the initial focus of the disease, although cases have subsequently been identified across most of southern and western England.[30] The eastern half of England, however, has remained relatively free of the disease and is consequently predicted to be a low-risk region.[30] Small, localized spatiotemporal clusters exhibiting significantly higher proportions of cases than the rest of the United Kingdom were identified between February and March 2013 in the New Forest area (P = .004) and between January and April 2014 in Manchester (P = .087), although these clusters appeared to be transient, because they were not apparent every year.[30] In fact, no cases were reported from the New Forest area in either 2016 or the 2017/2018 "season." Interestingly, between April 2015 and May 2017, the area immediately to the east of the New Forest reported a significantly lower proportion of CRGV cases (P = .002) than the rest of the United Kingdom.[30]

Agroecological Risk Factors

A boosted regression tree model[30] identified habitat, specifically, woodlands and lowland dry heath communities, as the variable with the highest relative contribution to CRGV occurrence (20.3%). However, UK woodlands are highly diverse, each characterized by different types of trees, and largely influenced by geology, soils, climate, and history, making it difficult to identify a potential source of the disease. Pastures were the habitat least associated with CRGV occurrence, suggesting it is unlikely CRGV is the result of a livestock-related pathogen to which dogs are exposed while walking across pastures. In addition to associations with specific habitat types, increasing relative probability of CRGV presence was associated with increasing mean maximum temperatures in winter, spring, and autumn, increasing mean rainfall in winter and spring, and increasing mean temperature in spring.[30] Stevens and colleagues[30] suggest that appropriate climatic conditions on their own appear to be insufficient for CRGV occurrence; the concomitant presence of suitable habitats appears to be essential, citing the fact that Wales and most of southwest England, where the disease has yet to gain any noticeable foothold, are dominated by pastures.

MANAGEMENT OF CUTANEOUS RENAL GLOMERULAR VASCULOPATHY CASES

On the basis of the current understanding of CRGV, management is as for many dogs with AKI. Treatment goals are aimed at limiting further renal damage and enhancing cellular recovery.[31] Correction of fluid, electrolyte, and acid-base disorders, achieving and maintaining normotension, and establishing/maintaining urine flow are the most important aspects of therapy.[32,33] Readers are directed to review articles for more specific information on the optimal medical management of AKI.

Hypertension is a common complication of AKI.[34] The median blood pressure in dogs with CRGV was 176 mm Hg (range 102–280 mm Hg) at the time of onset of AKI.[4] Treatment is indicated if systolic blood pressure is greater than 180 mm Hg or if there is evidence of "end-organ" damage.[32,35]

Immunomodulatory and Antiplatelet Therapy

Management of human TMAs is dependent on the underlying cause. Plasma therapy, antibiotic administration, monoclonal shiga toxin antibodies, and renal transplantation have been used in STEC-HUS. A recombinant, anti-C5 antibody (eculizumab) is the treatment of choice for human a-HUS.[36–38] One dog with CRGV was reportedly ineffectively managed with immunosuppressive therapy.[3] The efficacy of monoclonal antibody therapy has yet to be evaluated in CRGV.

Antiplatelet therapy seems like a potential therapeutic consideration, given the etiopathogenesis of CRGV. Aspirin was part of the standard treatment protocol in the 2 largest studies of plasma exchange in TTP,[39,40] and there have been reports of sudden deterioration and death among patients with TTP during recovery, when not taking platelet inhibitors.[41] Antiplatelet agents are usually not recommended for patients with TTP when bleeding is observed or when they also have severe thrombocytopenia. Low-dose aspirin is recommended by the British Committee for Standards in Hematology for patients with TTP with platelet counts greater than 50,000 per cubic millimeter.[42] Clopidogrel has been associated with the development of TTP.[43] Therefore, although there is no reported association with TTP in dogs, aspirin therapy may be preferred to clopidogrel.

Wound Management

Skin lesions in CRGV should be appropriately managed once the dog is clinically stable; sedation or anesthesia should be avoided for wound management unless deemed absolutely necessary, but analgesia should be provided, taking into account potentially compromised renal function.[44–47] Debridement is rarely needed for lesions that develop in CRGV.[48,49] Samples for cytology and bacteriology should be collected, ideally before topical or systemic antimicrobial therapy is initiated.[50] Even if microorganisms are isolated from a lesion, the initiation of systemic antimicrobial treatment is contraindicated if there are no clinical signs that indicate infection.[51–53] If antimicrobial use is deemed appropriate, drug selection should initially be based on the most likely pathogen and their prevailing susceptibility patterns. Once the results of bacterial culture and sensitivity testing are available, the antimicrobial should be switched to the narrowest spectrum possible.[51] A sterile dressing should be applied to provide a physical barrier to prevent contamination and infection and to maintain a wound environment that accelerates wound healing.[50,54]

UTILITY OF ADVANCED THERAPIES FOR CUTANEOUS RENAL GLOMERULAR VASCULOPATHY CASES

In many subtypes of TMA in people, the severity of the disease and underlying cause are not easily treatable.[55] Renal replacement therapy (RRT) offers ongoing support to reduce azotemia and maintain an appropriate fluid status and acid-base and electrolyte imbalance in patients with severely reduced kidney function, while awaiting either resolution of the AKI or renal transplantation.[55]

RRT has been used in dogs with CRGV with severe AKI resulting in oligoanuria and has allowed for treatment to be extended for a few weeks. However, this therapy alone, in the absence of specific treatments, has not been shown to be effective in improving survival in cases with severe renal damage (Rosanne Jepson, 2019, personal communication). To date, there are no reports of the use of RRT beyond a few weeks in dogs; it is currently unknown whether providing RRT over a longer period may allow full recovery of the renal lesions induced by CRGV.

Given the high mortality associated with certain types of TMA in people, research efforts have been focused on mediating the dysregulation of the immune system associated with these conditions. Implementation of alternative treatments has been necessary to target the activation of the complement system occurring in a-HUS or the presence of anti-ADAMTS13 autoantibodies in TTP, as previously described in this review.

A novel immune modulator, Eculizumab, a monoclonal antibody that binds to C5, impeding its hydrolysis and the subsequent activation of the complement pathway, has proven successful in treating a-HUS compared with traditional immunosuppressive treatment.[55] This therapy, which is currently highly recommended in people with a-HUS, is cost-prohibitive for veterinary patients, and there is no evidence for its efficacy in dogs with CRGV.

In people with anti-ADAMTS13 autoantibodies, therapeutic plasma exchange (TPE, also known as plasmapheresis) has been successful in improving survival rates.[55] This therapy consists of diverting blood in an extracorporeal circuit and removing plasma, either by filtration or by centrifugation of the blood, and then replacing it with allogenic plasma from healthy donors. This therapy removes autoantibodies, replaces ADAMTS-13, and reduces further activation of the coagulation system, thus limiting the progression of clinical signs. Current human guidelines advise the exchange of 1.5 times the plasma volume for each cycle, repeated every day until platelet numbers normalize.[56] Because this therapy has been proven effective in people with TTP, leading to a substantial increase in survival if performed in an early phase of the disease,[55] a recent case series study described the use of TPE in 6 dogs with severe CRGV.[57] Although 2 dogs with severe AKI in the report survived, it still remains unknown if this therapy is superior to conservative management because of the uncontrolled study design. In addition, this therapy is usually effective in people with TTP if performed early and for extended periods, but dogs described in this study were already in an advanced stage of the disease and only received 1 or 2 treatments in total; hence, it remains unclear if this therapy could be useful if applied earlier in the disease.

OUTCOME AND PROGNOSIS

Previous reports suggest that the prognosis for dogs with nonazotemic CRGV is excellent.[1,17] In the United States, dogs presenting with lethargy, pyrexia, and skin lesions, with rapid development of AKI, also appeared to have a fair prognosis with intensive management (25/30 survived). Dogs that developed azotemia before skin lesions were also reported to recover fully (7/7 survived).[1] This finding is in contrast with the 100% mortality observed when dogs developed AKI within 10 days of the appearance of skin lesions,[1] which is similar to the experience in the United Kingdom, and also to later experiences in the United States, where most dogs that developed significant azotemia were euthanized (100% of azotemic cases, Cowan and colleagues[16]; 83% of azotemic cases, Holm and colleagues[4]; 92% of azotemic cases, Holm and Walker[17]).

For UK cases, the median time from the development of skin lesions to euthanasia was 5 days (n = 102; range 1–31 days, unpublished data, 2018, courtesy of Anderson Moores Veterinary Specialists Ltd). Reasons for euthanasia included oligoanuria refractory to medical management (n = 29), progressive azotemia (n = 25), perceived poor prognosis (n = 15), development of seizures (n = 4), development of suspected acute lung injury/acute respiratory distress syndrome (n = 4), financial constraints (n = 4), progressive anemia (n = 2), suspected DIC (n = 2), and suspected sepsis (n = 2). A further 2 dogs died, and the reason for euthanasia was not stated for 13 cases. It is possible that prognosis for some cases could have been more favorable if more intensive management had been pursued, but this is unknown.

The authors are aware of a small number of suspected cases (n = 3) that developed IRIS grade I AKI, which responded well to intravenous fluid therapy ± furosemide and recovered uneventfully. These cases either developed an increase in serum creatinine concentration (>26.4 μmol/L above baseline, while remaining within the reference range) or oliguria (urine output <1 mL/kg/h). Again, the difficulty of confirming the diagnosis without renal histopathology has hampered efforts to better understand the true prognosis for CRGV in dogs in the United Kingdom. The small number of suspected cases with severe azotemia that survived could suggest that CRGV with AKI is not invariably fatal with appropriate intensive management.

SUMMARY

CRGV is an emerging disease in the United Kingdom, but the cause and any association with an infectious agent remains uncertain at this time. A population of nonazotemic dogs with CRGV exists, and for such cases, prognosis may be good. For the population of dogs that develop azotemia, and particularly oligoanuric AKI, the prognosis can be guarded, but intensive medical therapy is indicated in these cases because successful outcomes have been achieved. At this stage, further work must focus on the underlying infectious triggers and immune dysregulation, which have been associated with similar TMA conditions in humans, in order to determine whether risk factors can be identified for the canine population.

REFERENCES

1. Carpenter JL, Andelman NC, Moore FM, et al. Idiopathic cutaneous and renal glomerular vasculopathy of greyhounds. Vet Pathol 1988;25(6):401–7.
2. Hendricks A. Akute ulzerative dermatitis bei einem Greyhound. Proceedings of the 46th Annual Congress of the Small Animal division of the German Veterinary Association, Dusseldorf, Germany, November 9-12, 2000. p. 62–3.
3. Rotermund A, Peters M, Hewicker-Trautwein M, et al. Cutaneous and renal glomerular vasculopathy in a great dane resembling 'Alabama rot' of greyhounds. Vet Rec 2002;151(17):510–2. Available at: http://veterinaryrecord.bmj.com/content/151/17/510.abstract.
4. Holm LP, Hawkins I, Robin C, et al. Cutaneous and renal glomerular vasculopathy as a cause of acute kidney injury in dogs in the UK. Vet Rec 2015;176(15):384. Available at: http://veterinaryrecord.bmj.com/content/176/15/384.abstract.

5. Holloway S, Senior D, Roth L, et al. Hemolytic uremic syndrome in dogs. J Vet Intern Med 1993;7(4):220–7.
6. Marta D, Walter B, Luigi P, et al. Hemolytic-uremic syndrome in a dog. Vet Clin Pathol 2008;34(3):264–9.
7. Barbour T, Johnson S, Cohney S, et al. Thrombotic microangiopathy and associated renal disorders. Nephrol Dial Transplant 2012;27(7):2673–85.
8. Shenkman B, Einav Y. Thrombotic thrombocytopenic purpura and other thrombotic microangiopathic hemolytic anemias: diagnosis and classification. Autoimmun Rev 2014;13(4–5):584–6.
9. Franchini M. Atypical hemolytic uremic syndrome: from diagnosis to treatment. Clin Chem Lab Med 2015;53:1679.
10. Karpman D, Sartz L, Johnson S. Pathophysiology of typical hemolytic uremic syndrome. Semin Thromb Hemost 2010;36(6):575–85.
11. Scully M, Goodship T. How I treat thrombotic thrombocytopenic purpura and atypical haemolytic uraemic syndrome. Br J Haematol 2014;164(6):759–66.
12. Sellier-Leclerc A-L, Fremeaux-Bacchi V, Dragon-Durey M-A, et al. Differential impact of complement mutations on clinical characteristics in atypical hemolytic uremic syndrome. J Am Soc Nephrol 2007;18(8):2392–400.
13. Edey MM, Mead PA, Saunders RE, et al. Association of a factor H mutation with hemolytic uremic syndrome following a diarrheal illness. Am J Kidney Dis 2008; 51(3):487–90.
14. Hertzke DM, Cowan LA, Schoning P, et al. Glomerular ultrastructural lesions of idiopathic cutaneous and renal glomerular vasculopathy of greyhounds. Vet Pathol 1995;32(5):451–9.
15. Stevens K, O'Neill D, Jepson RE, et al. Signalment risk factors for cutaneous and renal glomerular vasculopathy (Alabama Rot) in dogs in the UK. Vet Rec 2018; 183(14):448.
16. Cowan LA, Hertzke DM, Fenwick BW, et al. Clinical and clinicopathologic abnormalities in Greyhounds with cutaneous and renal glomerular vasculopathy: 18 cases (1992-1994). J Am Vet Med Assoc 1997;210(6):789–93.
17. Holm LP, Walker DJ. Dealing with cutaneous and renal glomerular vasculopathy in dogs. In Practice 2018;40(10):426–38.
18. Fenwick BW, Cowan LA. Canine Model of hemolytic-uremic syndrome. In: Kaper JB, O'Brien DA, editors. Escherichia Coli 0157:H7 and other shiga toxin producing E.coli strains. Chapter 26. Washington DC: ASM Press; 1998. p. 268–77.
19. Dickinson CE, Gould DH, Davidson AH, et al. Hemolytic-uremic syndrome in a postpartum mare concurrent with encephalopathy in the neonatal foal. J Vet Diagn Invest 2008;20(2):239–42.
20. Chantey J, Chapman PS, Patterson-Kane JC. Haemolytic uraemic syndrome in a dog. J Vet Med A Physiol Pathol Clin Med 2002;49:470–2.
21. Tarr PI, Gordon CA, Chandler WL. Shiga-toxin-producing Escherichia coli and haemolytic uraemic syndrome. Lancet 2005;365(9464):1073–86.
22. Van Den Ingh TS, Van Winkle T, Cullen JM, et al. Morphological classification of parenchymal disorders of the canine and feline liver. In: WSAVA Standards for Clinical and Histological Diagnosis of Canine and Feline Liver Diseases. 1st Edition. Philadelphia: Elsevier; 2006. p. 93–5.
23. Sykes J, Hartmann K, Lunn KF, et al. 2010 ACVIM small animal consensus statement on leptospirosis: diagnosis, epidemiology, treatment, and prevention. J Vet Intern Med 2010;25(1):1–13.

24. Tangeman LE, Littman MP. Clinicopathologic and atypical features of naturally occurring leptospirosis in dogs: 51 cases (2000–2010). J Am Vet Med Assoc 2013;243(9):1316–22.

25. Monahan AM, Callanan JJ, Nally JE. Review paper: host-pathogen interactions in the kidney during chronic leptospirosis. Vet Pathol 2009;46(5):792–9.

26. Li L, McGraw S, Zhu K, et al. Circovirus in tissues of dogs with vasculitis and hemorrhage. Emerg Infect Dis 2013;19(4):534–41. https://doi.org/10.3201/eid1904.121390.

27. Elston DM, Eggers JS, Schmidt WE, et al. Histological Findings After Brown Recluse Spider Envenomation. Am J Dermatopathol 2000;22(3):242–6. Available at: https://journals.lww.com/amjdermatopathology/Fulltext/2000/06000/Histological_Findings_After_Brown_Recluse_Spider.6.aspx.

28. Anwar S, Torosyan R, Ginsberg C, et al. Clinicopathological course of acute kidney injury following brown recluse (Loxoscles reclusa) envenomation. Clin Kidney J 2013;6(6):609–12.

29. Morens DM, Folkers GK, Fauci AS. The challenge of emerging and re-emerging infectious diseases. Nature 2004;430:242.

30. Stevens K, Jepson RE, Holm LP, et al. Spatio-temporal patterns and agroecological risk factors for cutaneous and renal glomerular vasculopathy (Alabama Rot) in dogs in the UK. Vet Rec 2018;183:502–12.

31. Pruchnicki MC, Dasta JF. Acute renal failure in hospitalized patients: part I. Ann Pharmacother 2002;36(7–8):1261–7.

32. Langston CE. Acute kidney injury. In: Ettinger S, Feldman E, editors. Textbook of veterinary internal medicine. 8th edition; 2017. p. 1926–9.

33. Labato MA. Strategies for management of acute renal failure. Vet Clin North Am Small Anim Pract 2001;31(6):1265–87.

34. Geigy A, Schweighauser A, Doherr M, et al. Occurrence of systemic hypertension in dogs with acute kidney injury and treatment with amlodipine besylate. J Small Anim Pract 2011;52(7):340–6.

35. Acierno M, Brown S, Coleman A, et al. Guidelines for the identification, evaluation and management of systemic hypertension in dogs and cats. J Vet Intern Med 2018;32(6):1803–22.

36. Kavanagh D, Goodship TH, Richards A. Atypical hemolytic uremic syndrome. Semin Nephrol 2013;33(6):508–30.

37. Salvadori M. Update on hemolytic uremic syndrome: diagnostic and therapeutic recommendations. World J Nephrol 2013;2(3):56–76.

38. Blombery P, Scully M. Management of thrombotic thrombocytopenic purpura: current perspectives. J Blood Med 2014;5:15–23.

39. Bell WR, Braine HG, Ness PM, et al. Improved survival in thrombotic thrombocytopenic purpura–hemolytic uremic syndrome. N Engl J Med 1991;325(6):398–403.

40. Rock GA, Shumak KH, Buskard NA, et al. Comparison of plasma exchange with plasma infusion in the treatment of thrombotic thrombocytopenic purpura. N Engl J Med 1991;325(6):393–7.

41. Gordon LI, Kwaan HC, Rossi EC. Deleterious effects of platelet transfusions and recovery thrombocytosis in patients with thrombotic microangiopathy. Semin Hematol 1987;24:194–201.

42. Allford SL, Hunt BJ, Rose P, et al, Haemostasis and Thrombosis Task Force, British Committee for Standards in Haematology. Guidelines on the diagnosis and management of the thrombotic microangiopathic haemolytic anaemias. Br J Haematol 2003;120(4):556–73.

43. Bennett CL, Connors JM, Carwile JM, et al. Thrombotic thrombocytopenic purpura associated with clopidogrel. N Engl J Med 2000;342(24):1773–7.
44. Edlich RF, Rodeheaver GT, Morgan RF, et al. Principles of emergency wound management. Ann Emerg Med 1988;17(12):1284–302.
45. Cockbill S, Turner T. Management of veterinary wounds. Vet Rec 1995;136(14): 362–5.
46. Strohal R, Dissemond J, Jordan O'Brien J, et al. EWMA Document: Debridement: An updated overview and clarification of the principle role of debridement. J Wound Care 2013;22(Sup1):S1–49.
47. Shetty R, Paul MK, Barreto E, et al. Syringe-based wound irrigating device. Indian J Plast Surg 2012;45(3):590–1.
48. Edlich RF, Madden JE, Prusak M, et al. Studies in the management of the contaminated wound: VI. The therapeutic value of gentle scrubbing in prolonging the limited period of effectiveness of antibiotics in contaminated wounds. Am J Surg 1971;121(6):668–72.
49. Devriendt N, de Rooster H. Initial management of traumatic wounds. Vet Clin North Am Small Anim Pract 2017;47(6):1123–34.
50. Dernell WS. Initial wound management. Vet Clin North Am Small Anim Pract 2006; 36(4):713–38.
51. Bowler PG, Duerden BI, Armstrong DG. Wound microbiology and associated approaches to wound management. Clin Microbiol Rev 2001;14(2):244–69.
52. Mouro S, Vilela CL, Niza MMRE. Clinical and bacteriological assessment of dog-to-dog bite wounds. Vet Microbiol 2010;144(1–2):127–32.
53. Davies J, Davies D. Origins and evolution of antibiotic resistance. Microbiol Mol Biol Rev 2010;74(3):417–33.
54. Percival NJ. Classification of wounds and their management. Surgery 2001;20(5): 114–7.
55. Bommer M, Wölfle-Guter M, Bohl S, et al. The differential diagnosis and treatment of thrombotic microangiopathies. Dtsch Arztebl Int 2018;115(19):327–34.
56. Joseph S, Anand P, Nicole A, et al. Guidelines on the use of therapeutic apheresis in clinical practice–evidence-based approach from the writing committee of the American Society for Apheresis: the seventh special issue. J Clin Apher 2016; 31(3):149–338.
57. Skulberg R, Cortellini S, Chan DL, et al. Description of the use of plasma exchange in dogs with cutaneous and renal glomerular vasculopathy. Front Vet Sci 2018;5:161. Available at: https://www.frontiersin.org/article/10.3389/fvets. 2018.00161.

Canine Brucellosis
Old Foe and Reemerging Scourge

Lin K. Kauffman, DVM[a], Christine A. Petersen, DVM, PhD[b,c],*

KEYWORDS

- *Brucella* • Zoonosis • Reproduction • Abortion • Control • Prevention

KEY POINTS

- *Brucella canis* causes canine brucellosis, an emerging zoonosis.
- Dogs at highest risk of *B canis* infection are used for breeding programs or come from the Southeastern United States or countries where this disease is enzootic.
- Antimicrobial treatment of *B canis* does not lead to sterile cure; recrudescence of infection often occurs.
- Control of *B canis* is through testing all animals and removing animals that are infected, through either spay/neuter or euthanasia.
- Testing for *B canis* should be mandated before import or interstate travel.

HISTORY OF *BRUCELLA* INFECTION

Brucella spp, in the class alpha-Proteobacteria, were first described on the island of Malta in 1860[1] and were isolated from pure culture in 1887. The genus was originally thought to contain only 3 species: *Brucella abortus*, *Brucella melitensis*, and *Brucella suis*.[2] Several new species were added to the genus and more species are under consideration. Newer species include *Brucella canis*, *Brucella ovis*, *Brucella ceti*, *Brucella microti*, *Brucella neotomae*, *Brucella pinnipedialis*, and *Brucella inopinata*.[3–5] Genetic sequencing studies indicate that there is much homology across the *Brucella* genus, although small sequence differences between species exist. Some investigators propose a "One species" theory that states all *Brucella* spp are the same.[2,6] Although each species has a preferred reservoir host, most *Brucella* species infect numerous mammalian hosts; hence, its propensity as a zoonotic infection.[7–9] *B canis*, like other *Brucella* spp, has strong tropism for the reproductive and

Disclosure Statement: The authors have nothing to disclose.
^a Prairie View Animal Hospital, Grimes, IA 50111, USA; ^b Department of Epidemiology, College of Public Health, University of Iowa, 145 North Riverside Drive, Iowa City, IA 52242, USA; ^c Center for Emerging Infectious Diseases, University of Iowa Research Park, Coralville, IA 52241, USA
* Corresponding author. Department of Epidemiology, College of Public Health, University of Iowa, 145 North Riverside Drive, Iowa City, IA 52242.
E-mail address: christine-petersen@uiowa.edu

Vet Clin Small Anim 49 (2019) 763–779
https://doi.org/10.1016/j.cvsm.2019.02.013
0195-5616/19/© 2019 Elsevier Inc. All rights reserved.

lymphoendoreticular systems.[10] Colonization of reproductive tissue, mammary glands, and the spleen, as defined by positivity on culture, is common.

BRUCELLA CANIS PATHOGENESIS

Brucellae enter the host by penetrating mucosal epithelium, usually of the reproductive tract, after sexual or reproductive transmission, or through oral transmission, and are transported as free bacteria, or within phagocytic cells, to regional lymph nodes.[11] Colonization of regional lymph nodes causes lymph node hypertrophy, lymphatic and reticuloendothelial hyperplasia, leading to inflammation. If bacteria are not phagocytosed and killed within phagocytic cells, they replicate and spread via blood and particularly lymph, collecting within reproductive organs. Continued proliferation of B canis within the uterine wall, testis, and mammary tissue, as well as lymph nodes and spleen, leads to reproductive failure and nonspecific, cyclical, febrile disease.[12]

BRUCELLA INTRACELLULAR LIFE

Bacteremia is short-lived, because B canis is rapidly engulfed into host phagocytic cells. Smooth strains of Brucella spp rely on the actin cytoskeleton of host cells for internalization. B canis is usually a rough strain[13] but is similarly phagocytosed into monocytes and macrophages. Low intracellular pH (<4.5) is required for intracellular replication of wild-type Brucella spp. Low pH induces expression of the VirB operon that controls expression of genes associated with a type IV secretion system,[14] associated with strain virulence.[2] Brucella spp lipopolysaccharide (LPS) O-polysaccharide seems to be a key molecule for the interaction with lipid rafts and internalization.[15,16] LPS O-polysaccharide prevents complement-mediated bacterial lysis and stops host cell apoptosis, allowing the bacteria to survive.[11] Multiple mechanisms are used by Brucella spp for intracellular survival and to avoid the host immune system.

BRUCELLA CANIS VIRULENCE: DIFFERENCES FROM OTHER BRUCELLA SPP

B canis was first recognized and isolated in the United States from beagles in 1966[2,17,18] and was shown to cause human disease shortly thereafter.[19] The bacteria were described as small, gram-negative, aerobic, coccobacillary organisms with rough, colonial morphology.[20] Most Brucella spp bacteria have smooth colonial morphology associated with the LPS of the outer capsular membrane. B canis lacks expression of the mucoid "O" polysaccharide side chain of LPS, which causes the roughness observed in culture. B canis has other virulence factors that aid host cell entry and cause disease,[21,22] such as ligands normally hidden by the "O" side chain, which when exposed, facilitate adherence to macrophages. B canis is internalized through LPS interaction with Toll-like receptors4, or mannose receptor recognition of the bacterial surface.[23–25] A crucial component of Brucella immunity that leads to maintenance of chronic infection is production of interferon-γ secondary to the recognition of bacterial cell wall components. These components interact with Toll-like receptors, which lead to intracellular signaling, and the production of interleukin-12 and tumor necrosis factor-α by monocytes and macrophages.[26] Acquired antibodies from recovered dogs have a limited role in protecting naïve dogs from disease, based on several passive transfer studies.[26]

ROUTES OF TRANSMISSION OF BRUCELLA CANIS INFECTION

B canis causes similar disease to the other Brucella spp: abortion, infertility, and reproductive loss. Susceptible hosts are infected by bacteria penetrating mucosal membranes of the conjunctiva, oral cavity, and vagina. The minimum canine infectious oral dose is around 10^6 colony-forming units (CFU), whereas the conjunctival infectious dose is around 10^4 to 10^5 CFU.[27] Transmission of bacteria most commonly occurs by oronasal contact with aborted fetal material, which can contain up to 10^{10} bacteria per milliliter,[10,27] but can also occur venereally, which is important in breeding kennels.[18,28–32] Bacteria are shed in viscous, serosanguinous vaginal discharge for up to 6 weeks after infection[18] and are also found in milk, seminal fluid, and urine. Fomite transmission of *B canis* is possible, commonly by contaminated syringes, vaginoscopy equipment, and artificial insemination.[18] *Brucella* bacteria are easily inactivated by common disinfectants and are short lived outside the host.

GLOBAL EPIDEMIOLOGY OF BRUCELLOSIS

Brucellosis remains one of the most important zoonotic diseases in the world with the highest prevalence of human disease currently found in the Middle East, Africa, Asia, and Latin America.[2] An estimated 500,000 new human infections occur annually worldwide, usually due to *B abortus*, *B suis*, or *B mellitensis*.[11] Most human cases report "flulike" symptoms and lymphadenopathy. Diagnosis of human cases is difficult, with blood culture being the most common method. Most cases respond to antimicrobial therapy, but reemergence of disease is common. No approved human vaccine is available.

BRUCELLA GENUS RESERVOIR HOSTS AND SPECIES/STRAINS

- *B abortus*, *B suis*, *B melitensis*, *B ovis* (ruminant, swine)
- *B ceti* and *B pinnipedialis* (marine)
- *B neotomae* and *B microti* (rat and vole)
- *B canis* (dog, wild and domestic)
- *B inopinata* (isolated from human breast implant infection)[5]

EPIDEMIOLOGY OF CANINE BRUCELLOSIS

Canine brucellosis has been detected worldwide (**Fig. 1**). There is a higher seroprevalence of disease in the rural southeastern United States[18] and urban slums, due to populations of free-ranging, intact dogs in these areas, which serve as reservoirs for *B canis*.

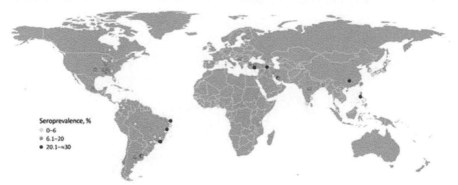

Fig. 1. Global map of locations of *B canis* surveillance in dogs and detected seroprevalence. Yellow = 0%–6%; orange = 6.1%–20%; red = 21% or greater. (*From* Hensel ME, Negron M, Arenas-Gamboa AM. Brucellosis in dogs and public health risk. Emerg Infect Dis 2018;24(8):1401–6; with permission. Available at: https://dx.doi.org/10.3201/eid2408.171171.)

HIGH-RISK POPULATIONS FOR CANINE BRUCELLOSIS

The highest prevalence of canine brucellosis is in purebred dogs, especially from large commercial breeding kennels. In these locations, dogs are housed in close contact, and there is constant movement of dogs for breeding or sale. Recent outbreaks in Sweden, Hungary, Columbia, and the United States highlighted links between the international movement of breeding dogs and outbreaks of *B canis*.[17] Unrestricted movement of reproductively intact dogs or puppies is a known risk factor for the spread of *B canis*, leading to human infections.[28,29]

Any sexually mature, reproductively active, dog is susceptible to *B canis*. Even dogs not reproductively active can contract the disease if exposed to infected bodily fluid or aborted materials.[33] Puppies can be infected in utero, while nursing, or while being housed with an infected bitch. Early embryonic death and resorption, normally diagnosed as conception failure, occurs if the bitch is exposed to *B canis* up to 20 days after conception.[34] If infection occurs later in gestation, abortion normally occurs around day 45 to 59 of gestation. The aborted fetus is normally partially autolyzed with subcutaneous edema, hemorrhage, and congestion (**Fig. 2**). Fetal lesions caused by *B canis* infection can include the following: bronchopneumonia, lymphadenitis, hepatitis, multifocal renal hemorrhage, and myocarditis.[2] Puppies not aborted and born to an infected bitch may die shortly after birth and have similar lesions to aborted fetuses. Infected puppies may seem healthy at birth but shed bacteria into their environment, risking transmission to in-contact dogs and humans. Bacteria are shed for at least several months,[18] and these puppies develop clinical disease after puberty[35] (**Box 1**).

Feral and stray dogs are the predominant reservoirs for *B canis*; these dogs are more likely to be intact than pet dogs.[36–40] Testing of feral dogs has documented a higher prevalence of *B canis*, raising concerns that the disease could easily spill over to the human population.[17] In the United States, many of these dogs are placed into animal shelters and foster care systems with the intent of adopting them into "forever homes." Approximately 30% of US pet dogs are adopted from shelters, and this number is growing.[41] However, testing for *B canis* is not a standard procedure before adoption, thereby risking zoonotic transmission in adoptive homes (**Box 2**).

ZOONOTIC RISK FACTORS FOR CANINE BRUCELLOSIS

Human infections are uncommon, although actual case numbers are not known due to underreporting and misdiagnosis, both within and outside the United States.[27]

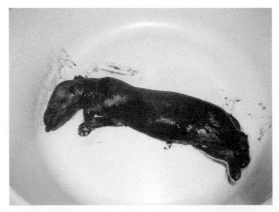

Fig. 2. Image of aborted canine fetus, partially autolyzed, secondary to *B canis* infection at day 48 of gestation. (*Courtesy of* Dr L. Kauffman, DVM, Grimes, IA.)

Box 1
Puppies

Keep in mind that your clinic may be presented with
- Pups born to infected female dogs
- Pups born in infected facilities
  - Pups may die shortly after birth due to disease
  - Pups may seem healthy but they are infected
- Infected dogs shed *B canis* bacteria for several months
  - Infected dogs can infect other dogs and humans
  - Infected pups become clinically affected after puberty
  - Pups should be tested for *B canis*; discuss culling any pups that test positive

---

Multiple surveillance studies have been performed globally to estimate the incidence of *B canis*. Results vary greatly, from 4.6% to 13.3% in healthy adults,[42,43] to greater than 80% seropositivity rates in people with fever of unknown origin.[44] Differences in human seroprevalence are due to differences in the relative diagnostic accuracy of tests used to identify *B canis* infection in each population.[17] Risk factors include pregnancy, childhood, and immunosuppression. Veterinarians, laboratory workers, and animal caretakers have increased risks for exposure to *B canis*,[17] which occurs either by direct contact with infected dogs or by infected samples. Human infections due to *B canis* are an emerging problem in people of lower socioeconomic status, especially in urban slums,[2] associated with poor hygiene in dog handling and increasing numbers of local free-roaming dogs.[29]

VETERINARIANS, ANIMAL CARETAKERS, DOG BREEDERS, PET OWNERS

Veterinarians, dog breeders, and animal caretakers have an increased risk of exposure to *B canis* because of their increased interactions with sick dogs.[17] Exposure occurs by direct contact with infected dogs or by exposure to infected animal by-products (aborted material, seminal fluid, vaginal discharge, urine, and so forth). Newly acquired brood stock may have unknown medical histories, so have the potential to bring *Brucella* into the kennel. Many kennels and dog breeders invoke a minimalist approach to the quarantine of new breeding stock. The highest bacterial load is found in fetal material and the vaginal discharge of the bitch after abortion. Contact with or

---

Box 2
***Brucella canis* routine screening and monitoring**

Breeding stock
- Test female and male dogs serologically before breeding
  - Any dogs with positive results should receive additional testing using AGID or PCR
- Test all dogs using serology in problem kennels every 3 months as a surveillance strategy
  - Any confirmed positives should be removed from kennel, and the remainder of the kennel placed under quarantine
  - Quarantine is lifted once all dogs test negative by serology every 90 days for a total of 3 consecutive tests
  - One positive test result takes the entire kennel back to the beginning of testing
- New additions to the kennel must be placed in isolation until *B canis* testing is complete
  - Test using serology every 30 days for a total of 3 tests
  - If all 3 tests are negative, new dogs can be added to the general population
  - If any of the 3 tests are positive, additional testing is warranted
  - Confirmed positives must be removed from kennel facility

accidental consumption of this material facilitates the spread of disease, especially in high-risk groups such as breeders and veterinarians.

Pet owners also have an increased risk of exposure to B canis by potentially adopting an infected dog. Even though the dog may be spayed or neutered, it still can shed bacteria in secretions and urine.[17] Pregnant women, children, and immunosuppressed individuals are at heightened risk of zoonotic infection due to decreased immune protection, so should avoid contact with dogs considered "high risk" or suspect for B canis infection. Good hygiene, including frequent hand washing, is paramount, especially after handling household pets.

REGULATIONS AND GUIDELINES FOR CANINE *BRUCELLA CANIS* INFECTION

There are no federal guidelines or regulations for mandatory B canis testing before interstate or international movement of dogs. Infected dogs can be shipped across the country and internationally, transmitting disease to dogs and humans, as in recent outbreaks of disease in Sweden, Hungary, Colombia, and the United States.[17] B canis is a reportable disease at the state level in the United States, like any other Brucella species, and several states have protocols in place for reporting positive cases. These protocols require that a mandatory quarantine is placed on the kennel or breeding facility when a positive case is reported to the state veterinarian office; no dog can enter or exit the facility until quarantine is lifted. Because of the limitations of some currently available serologic screening tests, some dogs with false positive results could be euthanized if additional confirmation testing is not performed. Mandatory quarantine remains in place until follow-up B canis testing is completed for the entire kennel. All dogs in the kennel must be screened for B canis infection every 30 days for a total of 2 or 3 negative tests, depending on state requirements.[18] If 1 dog tests positive, it is removed from the kennel, and testing for the kennel starts over again. This regimen of testing can take months and can be financially devastating for the kennel owner.

Human cases of disease caused by B canis must be reported to the National Notifiable Disease Surveillance System in the United States.[17] Infrequent reporting is thought to be due to unreliable diagnostic tools to confirm human cases and the nonspecific nature of the typical presentation (flulike symptoms). Blood cultures are the routine diagnostic test for human infection, but bacteremia with B canis infection is sporadic at best, making culture less sensitive than molecular methods. Commercially available serologic tests screen for antibodies against smooth Brucella species and do not detect antibodies against B canis.[17] Serologic surveys to determine the true incidence of brucellosis from B canis infection are rare.

CANINE CLINICAL SIGNS

Nonspecific general signs of B canis infection can include lethargy, poor hair coat, fatigue, weight loss, exercise intolerance, and lymphadenopathy early in the disease process.[12,18,34,35] As B canis infection progresses, splenomegaly and recurrent uveitis can occur. In addition, orthopedic issues, such as lameness, muscle weakness, spinal pain, and neurologic dysfunction, can be associated with spinal compression.[12,17,35] These clinical signs are related to vertebral osteomyelitis and diskospondylitis. Veterinarians should always have B canis on their differential list when dealing with cases of uveitis and any lameness or spinal pain, especially if the dog is intact. Spinal disease is more prevalent in male dogs, because the prostate acts as a reservoir for B canis, promoting intermittent bacteremia.[17] Radiographic lesions can include unaffected vertebral architecture with either focal or multifocal inflammatory lesions involving the intervertebral disk. Even though these nonspecific signs are less common presentations, *B canis* should always be on the differential list for any intact dog.

MALE-SPECIFIC CLINICAL SIGNS

Clinical signs seen in stud dogs are mainly testicular. Acute epididymitis and prostatitis are more common, whereas orchitis is less frequent[2,12,17,34] (**Fig. 3**). Initially, there is a moist scrotal dermatitis secondary to licking, which can progress to permanent testicular atrophy. Any testicular disease can lead to spermatic changes: sperm agglutination, sperm abnormalities, and inflammatory cells.[18,34,35] Experimentally, abnormal sperm have been noted as soon as 2 weeks after infection, and by 20 weeks after infection, 90% sperm were affected.[2]

Infertility is another *B canis* presentation, and there may be a history of infertility documented as a series of missed matings with different proven female dogs. Alternatively, the stud may present with testicular or scrotal abnormalities that are noted on physical or ultrasound examination. Semen analysis can provide crucial clues, such as sperm agglutination, bent tails, double tails, swollen mid pieces, retained protoplasmic droplets, and deformed acrosomes[16,18,35] (**Fig. 4**). The ejaculate might contain abnormally high numbers of white blood cells. Obtaining accurate case histories and performing a thorough diagnostic workup can be challenging in infertility cases. It should be borne in mind that infected male dogs can spread the disease to other dogs and humans, so care must be taken to minimize exposure to the stud until the cause of the infertility can be confirmed. *B canis* testing must be part of any infertility workup, even if the risk of infection is considered low.

FEMALE-SPECIFIC CLINICAL SIGNS

The most common presentation of *B canis* in the bitch is late-term abortion, after day 45 to 59 gestation.[12,17,18,34] Any breeding bitch that presents for late-term abortion should be evaluated for bacterial, viral, fungal, genetic, traumatic causes, but if the abortion occurs within the day 45 to 59 timeframe, canine brucellosis must be ruled out. Aborted fetuses from these cases are usually partially autolyzed with subcutaneous edema, hemorrhage, and congestion. Aborting bitches have a vaginal discharge that is dark and fetid and can last for 1 to 6 weeks after abortion.[17,18] Bacterial loads in

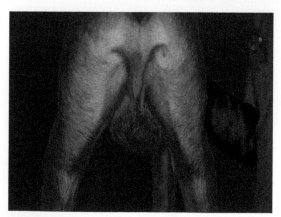

Fig. 3. Scrotum from a dog with orchitis involving right testicle secondary to *B canis* infection. (*Courtesy of* Dr L. Evans, Ames, IA.)

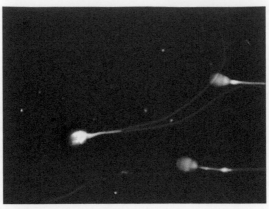

Fig. 4. Abnormal sperm secondary to *B canis* infection: note double tails, retained protoplasmic droplets, and swollen midpiece (100× magnification, stained with Eosin and Nigrosin). (*Courtesy of* Dr L. Kauffman, DVM, Grimes, IA.)

this discharge are substantial; therefore, infection risk is high if appropriate biosecurity measures are not taken when working with these dogs.[18] Gross pathology of the uterus after abortion commonly reveals endometritis and placentitis with the typical discharge[2] (**Fig. 5**).

Bitches may have a history of chronic infertility or abortion, followed by several successful litters, only to have issues with infertility or abortion again.[35] Keep in mind that the female dog can spread the disease to other dogs and people, so care must be taken to minimize exposure until the cause of the infertility can be confirmed. As with stud dogs, *B canis* testing is mandatory for any infertility workup, even in low-risk situations.

HUMAN CLINICAL SIGNS, SYMPTOMS, AND IDENTIFICATION

Symptoms of *B canis* infection can be much more difficult for physicians to recognize, because this is a low-prevalence disease in healthy people in the United States. Signs are nonspecific and "flulike," such as headache, back pain, chills/night sweats, recurrent/undulant fever, and overall weakness or malaise,[12,17,34] which

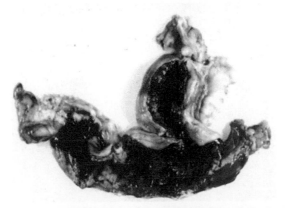

Fig. 5. Uterus from *B canis*–infected bitch after abortion: Note dark, fetid material within uterine lumen and endometritis. (*Courtesy of* Dr L. Carmichael, Ithaca, NY.)

are easily misdiagnosed as other illnesses. In more severe cases, additional signs, such as polyarthritis, meningitis, endocarditis, hepatomegaly, and splenomegaly, can be observed. Peripheral lymphadenomegaly is regularly diagnosed in association with B canis infection.[12,17,34] The most important element is the history of exposure to a dog, possibly with reproductive disease, but often such questions are not asked during a routine physical examination. As previously mentioned, infected dogs are typically clinically healthy[34] but can transmit B canis to humans through secretions, making the possibility of zoonotic disease less apparent to health care workers. Immunosuppressed individuals, including young children, pregnant women, cancer and transplant patients, and those living with HIV, are at higher risk of zoonotic infection.[18]

Low physician awareness of brucellosis also poses challenges for the recognition of B canis infection in human patients. In addition, B canis antigen testing, such as blood culture, may be required to diagnose some human cases, because there is no cross-reactivity between antibodies against B canis and the standard B abortus serology used in human medicine.[45] The Centers for Disease Control and Prevention Web site is an excellent place to start for information on human brucellosis and zoonotic transmission.[46]

DIAGNOSIS OF DISEASE
Case History

Diagnosing canine brucellosis based on case history alone is unlikely; additional diagnostics are required to confirm the suspicion of infection. Not all B canis clinical signs are present in every case, and infertility may be the only presenting clinical sign in bitches or stud dogs. Veterinarians providing services to reproductively active dogs may suspect or identify this disease on prebreeding examinations and testing of bitches and stud dogs. B canis testing is recommended every 3 months ("semester") for active breeding dogs[35] (see **Box 2**).

Physical Examination and Laboratory Screening

A thorough physical examination is essential for all cases presenting for prebreeding examinations or any type of reproductive problem. In most cases, physical examination findings are unremarkable, but occasionally abnormalities associated with B canis infection, such as lymphadenopathy, uveitis, back pain, vaginal discharge, scrotal dermatitis, or testicular changes, are identified and warrant further investigation. Complete blood count, serum biochemistry, and urinalysis should be performed to screen organ function and help assess overall health. There are no routine abnormalities noted on blood work or urinalysis that directly associate with, or specifically predict, B canis infection.

Blood Culture

Blood culture is considered the "best method" for diagnosis of early infection of B canis in dogs that have not yet received antimicrobial therapy.[35] More than 50% of dogs are bacteremic for at least 1 year following infection, and bacteremia usually commences by 2 weeks after infection.[18] If left untreated, bacteremia can last at least 1 to 2 years.[27]

A series of 3 blood culture samples should be collected consecutively, at least 24 hours apart.[18] Culture requires up to 9 days for growth to occur, which increases the risk of pathogen exposure for laboratory personnel.[17] Negative culture does not rule out B canis infection because bacteria may not be present in blood.[35]

Culture of Other Fluids

Various fluids and tissues can be submitted for *B canis* culture. Urine collected by cystocentesis (to avoid urethral contaminants[18]) can be a useful diagnostic sample, especially from stud dogs, because urine from intact male dogs might also contain seminal fluids[47]; male urine may contain 10^3 to 10^6 bacteria per milliliter.[2] Postabortion vaginal discharge, aborted placenta, and aborted fetal tissue also contain high *B canis* loads and are excellent samples for culture. Semen and seminal fluid (prostatic portion of the ejaculate) are good fluid samples to culture, especially during the first 3 months of infection.[27]

The best male reproductive tissues to collect at necropsy and submit for culture are prostatic, testicular, and epididymal tissue. Semen and seminal fluid may be collected from the epididymis, which can contain high numbers of *B canis* organisms. Female reproductive samples for culture include vaginal and uterine swabs as well as any fluid found in the vaginal tract or uterus. Lochia can contain as many as 10^{10} bacteria per milliliter.[2] Lymph nodes, spleen, liver, and bone marrow collected at necropsy should also be submitted for culture on any suspected *B canis* case.[35] In addition, any aborted canine fetal material and placentas submitted for necropsy analysis should be sampled for *B canis* culture, if only to rule out brucellosis as a possible cause. It is important to remember that negative culture results cannot be used to rule out this disease, because *B canis* bacteria may not always be present in the tissues or fluids cultured.[35]

Serology

Serologic testing for *B canis* uses an agglutination reaction between canine *B canis* antibodies and bacterial cytoplasmic protein antigens.[18] It usually takes 3 to 4 weeks (sometimes as long as 8–12+ weeks) after exposure for anti–*B canis* antibodies to become detectable, producing a positive test result. Although serology can be positive as early as 2 weeks after infection, negative serologic results are not reliable before 12 weeks after infection.[35] Antibody titers can fluctuate even if bacteremia is persistent, and the magnitude of the titer does not reflect the stage of disease.[18] *Infected dogs may initially test negative on serology.* Chronically infected dogs can also test seronegative due to low circulating antibody titers.[12] Although serologic tests detect agglutinating antibodies from infected dogs, those antibodies do not protect the dog from clinical disease.[18] Serologic tests designed to detect infections with smooth *Brucella* spp will *not* detect infection with *B canis*.[17]

Rapid Slide Agglutination Test

Rapid slide agglutination test (RSAT or card test) was first developed in 1974 and is still commercially available as D-Tec CB (Zoetis). The test uses rose bengal–stained, heat-killed *B ovis* cell wall antigen instead of *B canis* for ease of manufacturing.[5,18,34,35] Positive test results may occur from 2 to 4 weeks after infection, although it may take up to 8 to 12+ weeks for positive test results in some cases.[12] The RSAT test is a cheap and easy screening test that produces results within 2 minutes. It is a highly sensitive test but not overly specific.[18] This test has decreased sensitivity in chronically infected dogs due to intermittent bacteremia, which affects antibody levels.[17] False negative results are rare with this test, but false positives can occur in around 60% of dogs whose sera agglutinate to RSAT antigen,[34] because of cross-reactions between test antigen and large capsule organisms, such as *Staphylococcus* spp, *Streptococcus* spp, and *Moraxella*-type organisms, and some gram-negative bacteria, such as *Bordetella bronchiseptica*, *Pseudomonas* spp, and *Actinobacillus equuli*.[7,17,18] If a dog tests negative on the RSAT test, then the dog is likely negative. If a dog tests positive with the RSAT test, then more testing is required for *B canis* infection to be confirmed.

MODIFIED RAPID SLIDE AGGLUTINATION TEST

The modified rapid slide agglutination test (ME-RSAT) test incorporates 2-mercapto-ethanol (2ME) into the traditional RSAT test to inactivate immunoglobulin M (IgM) on the surface of *B ovis* bacteria, which prevents misidentification of positive sera because of the presence of other large capsule bacteria or certain gram-negative bacteria.[18] If a positive RSAT sample is treated with the 2ME, the IgM pentamers that can interfere with evaluation of IgG in the sample are destroyed, preventing cross-reactions. If the sample becomes negative after 2ME treatment, the dog should be retested at least 15 days later.[17,35] Another modification of the RSAT test uses a less mucoid variant of *B canis* (the M-antigen) instead of the original *B ovis*, to increase test specificity and enable confirmation of any screening test.[18,27]

Agar Gel Immunodiffusion Test

Agar gel immunodiffusion test (AGID) is a confirmation test for suspected *B canis* cases detected initially by RSAT or ME-RSAT. Positive test results usually occur 8 to 12 weeks after infection and become negative 3 to 4 years later.[18] AGID cytoplasmic protein assay (AGIDcpa) uses cytoplasmic protein antigens extracted from *B canis* cytoplasm, but is only performed by a few laboratories. This test is highly specific for *Brucella* and is useful to distinguish between infected and noninfected dogs.[34] This test should not be used as a screening test because other tests such as RSAT and culture are more sensitive for early *B canis* infections.[18] AGID cell wall antigen (AGIDcwa) is less specific than the AGIDcpa test.[18,35] AGID testing is usually negative early in the course of disease. Cornell University, University of Florida, and the Tifton Veterinary Diagnostic and Investigatory Laboratory in Georgia[48] currently offer AGID testing for *B canis*.

Tube Agglutination Test

The tube agglutination test (TAT) was historically the most widely used serodiagnostic procedure done to confirm infection in ME-RSAT–positive dogs.[27] The antigen solution for this test is made by the US Department of Agriculture (USDA). The solution contains heat-killed and washed *B canis* bacteria.[18] Availability of this solution for testing purposes is erratic. There is still an issue with cross-reactions between other infections agents, as with the RSAT test, so 2ME clarification is still needed with this test,[27] but false positive test results are still possible.[12,18] Test results are semiquantitative with a 1:200 titer considered evidence of an active infection.[18] When titers are low, those dogs should be considered suspect positive and need to be retested 2 weeks later, when *B canis* diagnosis will likely be confirmed.[35] Positive test results often correlate with positive blood cultures. Because of a lack of standardized reagents or testing methods, it is difficult to compare ME-TAT titers from 1 case to another for diagnostic purposes. No commercial tests for TAT are available on the market.[35]

MOLECULAR DETECTION OF *BRUCELLA CANIS*

Polymerase chain reaction (PCR) primers have been designed to detect *B canis* DNA in whole blood, vaginal secretions, urine, and semen.[49–51] PCR detection of *B canis* DNA from urine, semen, or vaginal fluids is more sensitive and specific than blood cultures or serology.[12] PCR can be used as a confirmatory test for seropositive dogs and has the potential to rapidly screen kennel populations for the presence of infection[17] and also allows for species and biovar identification. Minimal biological containment is required for PCR testing, and turnaround time for results is relatively short. It can open opportunities for genetic fingerprinting, which can facilitate disease tracing and determining sources of infection.[12] However, B canis PCR testing is not available at most diagnostic laboratories and is cost prohibitive for most kennels (see **Box 2**).

MEDICAL TREATMENT VERSUS DISEASE CONTROL

Management of canine brucellosis by medical treatment alone *is not recommended*. B canis bacteria hide from the host immune system inside cells for extended periods, and bacteremia can be episodic, making effective treatment problematic.[27,35,52] No single antimicrobial regimen has been 100% successful to achieve B canis sterile cure; therefore, antimicrobials cannot be the sole answer to management of this disease. Multiple courses of antimicrobials have been tried, but recrudescence of infection is common. It is widely thought that antimicrobial therapy, either single or multiple courses, cannot eliminate persistent infection in dogs.[12] B canis–infected dogs that have been spayed or neutered can still shed bacteria in the urine, allowing for transmission of infection to dogs and humans. Even after antimicrobial treatment, indefinite testing of affected dogs is recommended because of concern that the dog could shed organisms into the environment via the urine.[12,18,34] Disease prevention rather than treatment should be the focus of disease management. Identification of the source of infection is ideal, but breeders are sometimes reluctant to cooperate with disease tracking because poor animal husbandry practices might be uncovered. Some states have mandated that all B canis–infected dogs be euthanized, in an attempt to eliminate or at least slow its spread.

PREVENTION AND OWNER EDUCATION

Currently, prevention is focused on limiting kennel exposure to infection, coupled with identification and elimination of B canis–infected dogs from the kennel. Limiting dog exposure to infection requires yearly testing of all breeding stock. All dogs introduced into the kennel should be tested before entry into the kennel. Two consecutive negative tests, performed 4 to 6 weeks apart, should be a prerequisite for entry and contact with kenneled dogs.[18,34,53] Only dogs with no known history of B canis exposure and no clinical signs of brucellosis at time of entry into the kennel should be considered for purchase. All dogs used for breeding should be seronegative for B canis. Biosecurity is of the upmost importance once negative B canis status has been obtained for the kennel.[12] The USDA and Georgia Department of Agriculture Web sites[48,54,55] contain information on management strategies for breeding facilities to help prevent disease caused by B canis.[6]

In the United States, there are published recommendations to follow for case detection in the kennel if a B canis–seropositive dog is identified in a breeding kennel.[17] Veterinary diagnostic laboratories that obtain positive results on any confirmatory test must notify state health authorities. Owner education by the veterinarian is also critical for B canis control and prevention; suitable materials designed to educate about all aspects of biosecurity should be provided to dog owners, especially if they own B canis–positive dogs.[17] These materials should detail optimal hygiene when handling canine urine and reproductive secretions, and options for managing B canis–positive dogs, including spay/neuter, antimicrobial drug treatment, and euthanasia if owners cannot or do not want to treat (**Box 3**). Appropriate biosecurity measures must also be used by all in-contact personnel during and after any suspect cases of brucellosis are presented to veterinary hospitals, especially bitches with frank vaginal

---

Box 3
Spay/neuter as part of *B canis* treatment

- Remember that dogs can still be a reservoir for disease after antimicrobial treatment has been completed
  - Bacteria persist in the prostate and lymphoid tissues and sequester intracellularly for long periods
  - Dogs can shed bacteria in saliva, nasal secretions, and urine
  - Male urine contains higher loads of *B canis* than female urine because male urine can be contaminated with seminal fluid
  - There is possible legal liability due to potential human zoonotic infection

---

discharge.[56] Such dogs should be placed directly into an examination room, bypassing the waiting area to reduce potential exposure events.

DRUG RESISTANCE

Because *B canis* is an intracellular pathogen with a tropism for reproductive and lymphoid tissues, antimicrobial penetration at the site of infection can challenge efficacy. Therefore, if antimicrobial therapy is under consideration, long course lengths, often several months, are required. However, even with prolonged courses, antimicrobial therapy does not guarantee bacterial clearance and relapse or reinfection is common. Prolonged courses can also predispose to the development of antimicrobial resistance, and as such, combination antimicrobial therapy may be warranted.[18,27] Several studies have indicated that treatment with doxycycline, enrofloxacin, and streptomycin can lead to loss of seropositivity, suggesting the possibility of cure, but this is yet to be determined.[57]

FUTURE POSSIBILITIES
Nanotechnology or Other Drug Formulation Changes

There are ongoing research efforts to develop antimicrobial agents with improved tissue penetration to treat *B canis* infection. Among these are liposomal formulations and drugs that release microparticles or nanoparticles that target monocytes and macrophages, which are frequent immunologic target cells in *B canis* infections.[52,58,59] To date, although liposomal formulations are available for some antifungal drugs and parasiticides, the development of these formulations for antimicrobials with activity against *B canis* has lagged behind, perhaps because of market forces.

Vaccine

A vaccine against *B canis* is not currently available, but could drastically decrease the incidence of infection in a population of dogs and therefore reduce the risk of transmission of disease to humans. There is some concern that a vaccine for *B canis* would invoke an antibody response that could interfere with serologic testing; however, some other licensed vaccines, such as *B abortus* (RB51), use vaccine modifications to allow the differentiation of vaccinated and infected animals.[34,53]

Legislative and Bureaucratic Challenges

Many countries do not have regulations for *B canis* testing or control, probably because of a lack of awareness of the potential disease morbidity and associated economic losses. Few surveillance studies have been performed, especially in humans, facilitating international spread over years.[17] Testing of breeding dogs and their offspring, at national and international levels, should be mandatory before interstate and international movement. Only with such regulations worldwide can we hope to decrease the risk of zoonotic and reverse zoonotic (zooanthroponotic) transmission of B canis.[17]

SUMMARY

B canis is enzootic in dogs in many parts of the world and is an important zoonotic disease that is (re)emerging in dogs. General practitioners need a clear understanding of all clinical aspects of canine brucellosis, including risk factors, clinical signs, diagnostic modalities, biosecurity, and management strategies for household pets and breeding kennels. Science-based advice to dog owners on proper screening, treatment, and kennel management is paramount. On a larger scale, brucellosis will remain an underrecognized threat to animal welfare and human health until there are international guidelines for infection control and management.[17] A good first step in this process would be for testing of any dog before interstate or international movement to be made mandatory. With this simple step, the movement of infected dogs and spread of disease would greatly decrease.

ACKNOWLEDGMENTS

The authors thank Dr Johanna Daily, Albert Einstein College of Medicine, New York, for her assistance in depicting the clinical picture of human B canis–associated disease.

REFERENCES

1. Alton GG. The occurrence of dissociated strains of Brucella melitensis in the milk of goats in Malta. J Comp Pathol 1960;70:10–7.
2. Olsen SC, Palmer MV. Advancement of knowledge of Brucella over the past 50 years. Vet Pathol 2014;51(6):1076–89.
3. Scholz HC, Hubalek Z, Sedlacek I, et al. Brucella microti sp. nov., isolated from the common vole Microtus arvalis. Int J Syst Evol Microbiol 2008;58(Pt 2):375–82.
4. Whatmore AM, Dawson CE, Groussaud P, et al. Marine mammal Brucella genotype associated with zoonotic infection. Emerg Infect Dis 2008;14(3):517–8.
5. De BK, Stauffer L, Koylass MS, et al. Novel Brucella strain (BO1) associated with a prosthetic breast implant infection. J Clin Microbiol 2008;46(1):43–9.
6. Hoyer BH, McCullough NB. Homologies of deoxyribonucleic acids from Brucella ovis, canine abortion organisms, and other Brucella species. J Bacteriol 1968; 96(5):1783–90.
7. Schoenemann J, Lutticken R, Scheibner E. [Brucella canis infection in man]. Dtsch Med Wochenschr 1986;111(1):20–2.
8. Rumley RL, Chapman SW. Brucella canis: an infectious cause of prolonged fever of undetermined origin. South Med J 1986;79(5):626–8.
9. Lum MK, Pien FD, Sasaki DM. Human Brucella canis infection in Hawaii. Hawaii Med J 1985;44(2):66, 68.
10. de Souza TD, de Carvalho TF, Mol J, et al. Tissue distribution and cell tropism of Brucella canis in naturally infected canine foetuses and neonates. Sci Rep 2018; 8(1):7203.
11. de Figueiredo P, Ficht TA, Rice-Ficht A, et al. Pathogenesis and immunobiology of brucellosis: review of Brucella-host interactions. Am J Pathol 2015;185(6): 1505–17.

12. Cosford KL. *Brucella canis*: an update on research and clinical management. Can Vet J 2018;59(1):74–81.

13. Carmichael LE, Zoha SJ, Flores-Castro R. Biological properties and dog response to a variant (M-) strain of *Brucella canis*. Dev Biol Stand 1984;56: 649–56.

14. Ke Y, Wang Y, Li W, et al. Type IV secretion system of *Brucella* spp. and its effectors. Front Cell Infect Microbiol 2015;5:72.

15. Bowden RA, Cloeckaert A, Zygmunt MS, et al. Surface exposure of outer membrane protein and lipopolysaccharide epitopes in *Brucella* species studied by enzyme-linked immunosorbent assay and flow cytometry. Infect Immun 1995; 63(10):3945–52.

16. Moreno E, Jones LM, Berman DT. Immunochemical characterization of rough *Brucella* lipopolysaccharides. Infect Immun 1984;43(3):779–82.

17. Hensel ME, Negron M, Arenas-Gamboa AM. Brucellosis in dogs and public health risk. Emerg Infect Dis 2018;24(8):1401–6.

18. Hollett RB. Canine brucellosis: outbreaks and compliance. Theriogenology 2006; 66(3):575–87.

19. Blankenship RM, Sanford JP. *Brucella canis*. A cause of undulant fever. Am J Med 1975;59(3):424–6.

20. Ronneau S, Moussa S, Barbier T, et al. *Brucella*, nitrogen and virulence. Crit Rev Microbiol 2016;42(4):507–25.

21. Chacon-Diaz C, Altamirano-Silva P, Gonzalez-Espinoza G, et al. *Brucella canis* is an intracellular pathogen that induces a lower proinflammatory response than smooth zoonotic counterparts. Infect Immun 2015;83(12):4861–70.

22. Zygmunt MS, Blasco JM, Letesson JJ, et al. DNA polymorphism analysis of *Brucella* lipopolysaccharide genes reveals marked differences in O-polysaccharide biosynthetic genes between smooth and rough *Brucella* species and novel species-specific markers. BMC Microbiol 2009;9:92.

23. Giambartolomei GH, Zwerdling A, Cassataro J, et al. Lipoproteins, not lipopolysaccharide, are the key mediators of the proinflammatory response elicited by heat-killed *Brucella abortus*. J Immunol 2004;173(7):4635–42.

24. Barrionuevo P, Cassataro J, Delpino MV, et al. *Brucella abortus* inhibits major histocompatibility complex class II expression and antigen processing through interleukin-6 secretion via Toll-like receptor 2. Infect Immun 2008;76(1):250–62.

25. Zhang H, Palma AS, Zhang Y, et al. Generation and characterization of beta1,2-gluco-oligosaccharide probes from *Brucella abortus* cyclic beta-glucan and their recognition by C-type lectins of the immune system. Glycobiology 2016;26(10): 1086–96.

26. Baldwin CL, Goenka R. Host immune responses to the intracellular bacteria *Brucella*: does the bacteria instruct the host to facilitate chronic infection? Crit Rev Immunol 2006;26(5):407–42.

27. Greene CE, Carmichael LE. Canine brucellosis. In: Greene CE, editor. Infectious diseases of the cat and dog. St. Louis (MO): Elsevier; 2006. p. 369–81.

28. Wang L, Cui J, Misner MB, et al. Sequencing and phylogenetic characterization of *Brucella canis* isolates, Ohio, 2016. Transbound Emerg Dis 2018;65(4):944–8.

29. Johnson CA, Carter TD, Dunn JR, et al. Investigation and characterization of *Brucella canis* infections in pet-quality dogs and associated human exposures during a 2007-2016 outbreak in Michigan. J Am Vet Med Assoc 2018;253(3):322–36.

30. Gyuranecz M, Szeredi L, Ronai Z, et al. Detection of *Brucella canis*-induced reproductive diseases in a kennel. J Vet Diagn Invest 2011;23(1):143–7.

31. Brower A, Okwumabua O, Massengill C, et al. Investigation of the spread of *Brucella canis* via the U.S. interstate dog trade. Int J Infect Dis 2007;11(5):454–8.
32. von Kruedener RB. Outbreak of a *Brucella canis* infection in a beagle colony in West Germany. Dev Biol Stand 1976;31:251–3.
33. Dillon AR, Henderson RA. *Brucella canis* in a uterine stump abscess in a bitch. J Am Vet Med Assoc 1981;178(9):987–8.
34. Carmichael LE, Shin SJ. Canine brucellosis: a diagnostician's dilemma. Semin Vet Med Surg (Small Anim) 1996;11(3):161–5.
35. Wanke MM. Canine brucellosis. Anim Reprod Sci 2004;82-83:195–207.
36. Myers DM, Varela-Diaz VM. Serological and bacteriological detection of *Brucella canis* infection of stray dogs in Moreno, Argentina. Cornell Vet 1980;70(3): 258–65.
37. Boebel FW, Ehrenford FA, Brown GM, et al. Agglutinins to *Brucella canis* in stray dogs from certain counties in Illinois and Wisconsin. J Am Vet Med Assoc 1979; 175(3):276–7.
38. Lovejoy GS, Carver HD, Moseley IK, et al. Serosurvey of dogs for *Brucella canis* infection in Memphis, Tennessee. Am J Public Health 1976;66(2):175–6.
39. Brown J, Blue JL, Wooley RE, et al. A serologic survey of a population of Georgia dogs for *Brucella canis* and an evaluation of the slide agglutination test. J Am Vet Med Assoc 1976;169(11):1214–6.
40. Brown J, Blue JL, Wooley RE, et al. *Brucella canis* infectivity rates in stray and pet dog populations. Am J Public Health 1976;66(9):889–91.
41. Rowan A, Kartal T. Dog population and dog sheltering trends in the United States of America. Animals (Basel) 2018;8(5) [pii:E68].
42. Flores-Castro R, Segura R. A serological and bacteriological survey of canine brucellosis in Mexico. Cornell Vet 1976;66(3):347–52.
43. Angel MO, Ristow P, Ko AI, et al. Serological trail of *Brucella* infection in an urban slum population in Brazil. J Infect Dev Ctries 2012;6(9):675–9.
44. Monroe PW, Silberg SL, Morgan PM, et al. Seroepidemiological investigation of *Brucella canis* antibodies in different human population groups. J Clin Microbiol 1975;2(5):382–6.
45. Lucero NE, Jacob NO, Ayala SM, et al. Unusual clinical presentation of brucellosis caused by Brucella canis. J Med Microbiol 2005;54(Pt 5):505–8.
46. CDC Centers for Disease Control and Prevention, Brucellosis. Available at: https://www.cdc.gov/brucellosis/veterinarians/dogs.html. Accessed December 5, 2018.
47. Dooley MP, Pineda MH, Hopper JG, et al. Retrograde flow of spermatozoa into the urinary bladder of dogs during ejaculation or after sedation with xylazine. Am J Vet Res 1990;51(10):1574–9.
48. Georgia Department of Agriculture, Canine Brucellosis (Brucella canis). Available at: http://agr.georgia.gov/Data/Sites/1/media/ag_animalindustry/animal_health/files/caninebrucellosis.pdf. Accessed December 5, 2018.
49. Kauffman LK, Bjork JK, Gallup JM, et al. Early detection of *Brucella canis* via quantitative polymerase chain reaction analysis. Zoonoses Public Health 2014; 61(1):48–54.
50. Keid LB, Soares RM, Vasconcellos SA, et al. A polymerase chain reaction for detection of *Brucella canis* in vaginal swabs of naturally infected bitches. Theriogenology 2007;68:1260–70.
51. Keid LB, Soares RM, Vasconcellos SA, et al. A polymerase chain reaction for the detection of *Brucella canis* in semen of naturally infected dogs. Theriogenology 2007;67(7):1203–10.

52. Phanse Y, Lueth P, Ramer-Tait AE, et al. Cellular internalization mechanisms of polyanhydride particles: implications for rational design of drug delivery vehicles. J Biomed Nanotechnol 2016;12(7):1544–52.
53. Dorneles EM, Sriranganathan N, Lage AP. Recent advances in *Brucella abortus* vaccines. Vet Res 2015;46:76.
54. USDA, Best Practices for Brucella canis Prevention and Control in Dog Breeding Facilities. Available at: https://www.aphis.usda.gov/animal_welfare/downloads/brucella_canis_prevention.pdf. Accessed December 5, 2018.
55. USDA, Brucellosis and Dog Kennels: What Breeders Need to Know. Available at: https://www.aphis.usda.gov/animal_welfare/downloads/CanineBrucellosisBro-finalfp.pdf. Accessed December 5, 2018.
56. Stull JW, Bjorvik E, Bub J, et al. 2018 AAHA infection control, prevention, and biosecurity guidelines. J Am Anim Hosp Assoc 2018;54(6):297–326.
57. Wanke MM, Delpino MV, Baldi PC. Use of enrofloxacin in the treatment of canine brucellosis in a dog kennel (clinical trial). Theriogenology 2006;66(6–7):1573–8.
58. Bodaghabadi N, Hajigholami S, Vaise Malekshahi Z, et al. Preparation and Evaluation of Rifampicin and Co-trimoxazole-loaded Nanocarrier against *Brucella melitensis* Infection. Iran Biomed J 2018;22(4):275–82.
59. Lecaroz C, Gamazo C, Blanco-Prieto MJ. Nanocarriers with gentamicin to treat intracellular pathogens. J Nanosci Nanotechnol 2006;6(9–10):3296–302.

Printed and bound by CPI Group (UK) Ltd, Croydon, CR0 4YY
03/10/2024
01040404-0019